CREATI(

SAVE ....

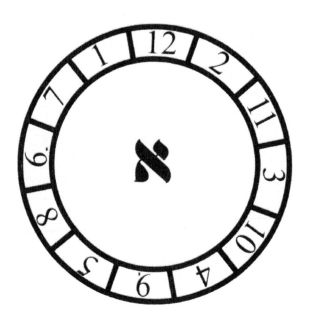

Arcady Petrov

CREATION OF THE UNIVERSE

SAVE THE WORLD WITHIN YOU

Jelezky publishing, Hamburg 2011

Jelezky publishing, Hamburg www.jelezky-media.com

Copyright © Original Russian Language Version: Arcady Petrov, Moscow

English 1st Edition (Book 2), september 2011, (1st Edition)

©2011English Language Version, Dimitri Eletski, Hamburg (Editor)

English Translation: Lingua Communications Translation Services, USA

In ancient times it was assumed that the world stands on three elephants, or three columns, according to the Jewish Kabbalah. You can say that the world stands on whales, elephants or pillars – the essence will not change. Anyway, it isn't about animals but about the right and left hemispheres of the brain, the spinal cord and whether they are capable of harmonious functioning on the basis of CONSCIOUSNESS, meaning divine consciousness, of course.

The left hemisphere manifests its function of logic through the scientific worldview. The right hemisphere displays its function through an intuitive perception of truth and through religious perception of the world. At first glance, they appear to be irreconcilable opposites. But if you look closely, you will see that the nonsense of atheistic views and the shocking demands for "sacrifice of the mind" are just two extreme manifestations of the same natural life source. And while the left brain hemisphere "hits against" its own mirror reflection, unable to overcome the BOUNDARY separating the worlds, it will continue to repeat the same old statements about atheism, physical foundations of the world, speed that cannot exceed the speed of light, and space and time as the medium of our existence, not even understanding that they are secondary to the CONSCIOUSNESS OF THE CREATOR, Who has created all this in the world and in relation to WHOM they are correlated, as consequence with cause.

CREATION OF THE UNIVERSE

SAVE THE WORLD WITHIN YOU

"We are such stuff as dreams are made on…"

William Shakespeare

You are holding in your hands the second book in a series conceived as a trilogy. Its title "Save the World within You" largely defines its subject matter. The purpose of the book is to unveil the techniques and technologies of clairvoyance, its discovery through the spiritual aspects of self development, and positive management of events in one's life. Just as in the first book, the narrative is presented on two planes – the ordinary, earthly plane and the subtle matter plane occurring, as it were, in parallel to our world, the existence of which most people do not even recognize.

You may be able to unlock your clairvoyance while reading this book, because in it, as in the first book, "Save Yourself" you will find the will of superior intelligence being fulfilled, acting from a different dimension of reality and radiating the energy of a higher life through words.

Albert Einstein proved mathematically that there are only two realities in the Universe – matter and energy. However, in order to explain the very obvious fact of the presence in the world of such a phenomenon as CONSCIOUSNESS, it is not less apparent ability to intelligently respond to a variety of interactions, we cannot hide from the third global reality – the media. But matter, and energy and information, in turn, are different states of a certain universal substance, which esoteric sciences call SPIRIT, SOUL and CONSCIOUSNESS.

This substance is manifested in our space only by indirect signs of high technology management. It is this universal substance that binds together all the cause and effect events of our world and produces matrix structures of any material bodies.

It is important to emphasize the close connection between such concepts as CONSCIOUSNESS and INFORMATION. Consciousness is essentially a regulatory mechanism that is responsible for the interaction between the human body and the substance of the world. It reflects the

7

reality of the world in its entirety within any space and at any time. Being coupled with knowledge is conscious being. Consequently, SUPER-CON-SCIOUSNESS represents the highest form of concentration and development of information which it processes and to which it responds.

It goes without saying that no new theory is born in a vacuum. "For anyone who is reasonably well familiar with the history of philosophy and the history of human knowledge it will always be obvious that the main directions of science were mapped out in the distant past... Don't we continue to refer to Egypt, Babylon, India and China in search of an elementary expression of some idea, the roots of which are hidden far back in the mists of time, yet they give us their magnificent bloom in modern day life?" – wrote a few decades ago, Alexander Chizhevsky* ("Space Pulse of Life", Moscow, 1995, p. 33). This idea was in one way or another expressed by many serious thinkers... "The very concept of knowledge as a guide in the world remains the same: to pick out of everything that is new and unfamiliar a repetition of the familiar and customary, and to perceive it as only 'seemingly' new – as a 'version' of a topic essentially familiar to us" (S.L. Frank, "Collected Works", Moscow, 1990, p. 187). "The new can never be unexpected" (D.S. Likhachev, "The Past to the Future", Moscow, 1985, p. 515).

This explains why we don't perceive the doctrines about the nature of consciousness, soul and spirit as abstract constructs, but view them as a real opportunity enabling humanity to rise to a new stage in its evolution. I repeat, enabling it to actually rise in reality, physically, and to develop the potential for self-cure and self-regulation as well as the ability to influence physical processes already at the level of Soma.** The discovery

* Soviet-era interdisciplinary scientist, space biologist and biophysicist.
**Located in the forehead, the Soma chakra is the most powerful of the lot and governs the whole body.

of the phenomenon of inner vision and controlled clairvoyance are no longer material for science fiction stories but present-day realities. Today thousands, even tens of thousands of people, not rare individuals, manifest new, phenomenal abilities. The ability to see through material barriers is presently recorded not only in scientific laboratories but even in the Guinness Book of Records. We at the Center for Bio-information Technology see this as our everyday reality – I would even say a normal technological process.

The fact that phenomena perceived in earlier times as mystical and occult are becoming accessible to everyone and scientifically explainable today demonstrates a slight spiritual uplift of humanity. It shows that the human race has finally matured for a constructive and creative exploration of this area of knowledge.

We have also arrived at a new understanding of man: his psychophysical constitution and his personality. In fact, it would be difficult to consider as useful and beneficial the situation when every science had "its own" man as an object of study. The anatomists studied "one man", the psychologists another and the physicists a third... There was also genetics, medicine, religion and political doctrine – and each of these pulled man apart dragging what was left in his direction. But man is one! And to be able to control the functioning of his body and personality with greater competence, he must do it on a more uniform, more skilled level. This cannot be accomplished without the connection of a living organism with the forces and processes of the Earth, and, further, the Cosmos.

The world is replete with facts and evidence testifying to a structure of our being that is far more complicated than we tend to think. More than likely it does not determine consciousness, but is determined by consciousness or, more specifically, by its levels and organization. Some peo-

9

ple speak about doom, others about fate, and still others argue that neither one nor the other is true. And they are all right in their own way, because the answer is based on the level of their consciousness.

The predetermination of our destiny is to some extent confirmed by the textbook example about the American twins Springer and Lewis. It so happened that they were separated in infancy and met for the first time 39 years later. That was when people learned that their lives were as identical as their faces. They both married women with the same names: it was Linda in the first marriage and Betsy in the second. They each had two sons and they also carried the same names: James and Allen. Moreover, the twin brothers drove cars of the same model and color, and in their spare time they both loved wood carving...

Someone will probably say that it is just a coincidence. But scientists have established that identical twins (regardless of whether one lives in the city and the other in a rural area, one in the north and the other in the south) simultaneously suffer from similar diseases, and that both show signs of aging and die at the same age – the difference is usually no more than a few months.

Of course, we can simply entertain ourselves by collecting such stories. Or else we may stop and think: perhaps we are dealing here with some event-predicting programs, incorporated in the DNA structure of the human body? And what is the extent to which events are pre-defined in the dynamics of their development based on the various ways we respond to them?

Human history contains numerous examples of instances when people knew with certainty what was going to happen to them in the future.

The Ukrainian philosopher and poet Grigori Skovoroda (1722-1794) knew the exact date of his death. He was perfectly healthy when he publicly announced he was about to die; he ordered a grave to be prepared for him and died on the day he predicted.

The well-known Russian historian Vasili Tatishchev told his family not only the exact day but even the exact hour of his death, and he wasn't mistaken.

Facts of accurate predictions of the future are too numerous for them to be coincidental. More than that, when people are forewarned of impending disasters it rarely helps to avoid them.

Thus, fate caught up with Nero, one of the most sinister rulers of all time, whom Pythia, the priestess and Oracle at the Temple of Apollo, warned about his future: "Beware of the number 73." Assuming that she referred to the duration of his life, 31-years-old Nero was very pleased with the prophecy. How could he have known that the number actually denotes someone's age but not his own? Less than a year after that he will die, and the conspirators will put Galba, then 73 years old, on the throne in his place.

In vain were the efforts of renowned Russian poet Alexander Pushkin who tried all his life to avoid death that was predicted to strike him when he was close to thirty seven years old. The prediction was made in 1817 or 1818 by Alexandra Filippovna Kirchhoff, a St. Petersburg fortune teller who was famous at the time. She told the poet that he would soon acquire wealth, go into two exiles, get married and become famous. She also said to him that he might live a long life, but when he was close to 37 years old he should beware of a tall blond man, a white horse and a white head.

All the first predictions came true, and Pushkin was waiting for the last one. The extent to which the poet believed in fate is confirmed by the following. In preparation for his duel with Count Tolstoy, Pushkin, in the presence of A.N. Wulf, repeated several times: "I won't be killed by

11

this man. I'll be killed by one who is blond, as the witch prophesied." In fact, Pushkin was killed at the age of 37 by a blond cavalry officer named Dantes, who wore a white uniform and rode on a white horse.

A person, who visited Vanga (Vangeli Gushterova), an amazing clairvoyant from the Bulgarian town of Petrich, recounted during his trip to that country: "Two weeks before the tragic death of the first cosmonaut Yuri Gagarin, Vanga said suddenly: 'What a pity that Yuri will be hit by misfortune.' Folks who were with her at the time wanted to call Moscow immediately to prevent it from happening, but Vanga stopped them: 'It's useless. It would be impossible to change anything. Everyone follows his own path. Our destinies are predetermined.'" Two weeks later, the media reported: the aircraft, in which Gagarin and Seregin were making a training flight, crashed, killing both pilots.

Here is another example. Shortly before her death, Vanga cautioned that Kursk will be under water. People misinterpreted what she said. They thought that her prophecy referred to the city of Kursk. And they made fun of it: where would all this water appear from to flood such a large city located a thousand miles away from the nearest sea? It turned out that they should have taken her words more seriously. Just as in the situation with Nero, the prediction was accurate. The "Kursk" submarine did indeed sink to the bottom of the sea.

That explains why even those experts who categorically reject the possibility "of seeing into the future" are still trying to explain this phenomenon. One such explanation is intuition, i.e., the ability of human intelligence to calculate the probability of the future. But the problem is that not only "homo sapiens" but less intelligent creatures as well have the gift of foresight!

There is a popular belief among seamen that rats flee a ship, which is destined to drown. And this has been confirmed in reality. Here is just one example. During World War II convoys transported food and weapons and ammunition from Britain to Murmansk. Two barges were towed in wake formation. Suddenly, hordes of rats came rushing out of the hold of the leading ship, trying to climb to the other vessel across the rope. Some even jumped into the icy water and swam. Soon after that the barge abandoned by the rats was hit by a bomb...

One can certainly assert that rats also have intuition. But what about plants that don't even have a brain? Moscow researchers conducted an experiment: they registered electrical "impulses of pain" generated by a geranium plant when its leaves were burned with a match. As it turned out, exactly the same impulses were recorded by instruments during the time of planned repeated experiments, although these experiments didn't have any specific clear timetable...

Hence, fate or something else that we can call similarly exists nevertheless? After all, it becomes possible to "read" future events before they happen only when they are already written in the Book of Destiny and can't be changed. Nature, by the way, constantly gives us examples of this phenomenon, when the future affects the past and when in some way or other "tomorrow" sends information about itself to "yesterday".

Yet, even future events that have taken specific shape can be changed...

The practical experience which Igor Arepyev and I have accumulated proves it. People with cancer and AIDS who come to us for help have already been handed the verdict of fate. So what? We change the sentence. And people go on living.

How we do it? We do it through the technologies of consciousness. Consequently, at some stage the development of consciousness leads to the fact that a person ceases to depend on circumstances and fate. Of

13

course, we could ignore these facts, but better still to comprehend them.

Russia has become home to the theory of the biosphere and its evolution, its transformation into the noosphere under human influence – the sphere of reason. Some of the names of those who worked on developing this issue are widely known throughout the world (Tsiolkovsky, Chizhevsky and Florensky), whereas others are presently familiar only to supporters (Nikolai Fedorov, Alexei Losev, Nikolai Umov, Valerian Muravyov and Alexander Gorsky). All of them, and not they alone, created a special spiritual aura in the country. There is a reason why many clairvoyants are predicting that Russia will attain exceptional world-wide significance in the new century.

All those who have studied the history of mankind and their people's history understand that there was a reason why knowledge about the energy-information structure of human beings amassed in ancient times has been inaccessible for its assimilation on a broad, mass scale. Is a person who isn't familiar with the multiplication table capable of understanding the set-point theory and mathematical logic? Can someone who doesn't see the boundaries between light and darkness or good and evil apply their knowledge of the supernatural for the benefit of their neighbor? Evil wizards existed not only in fairytales but in life as well. Here is a simple reference, clear to every high school senior. About 160 years ago Vissarion Belinsky* wrote in a letter: "People are so stupid that they need an iron hand to lead them to happiness."

Less than a century later a poster with a similar maxim first graced the walls of the ancient Kremlin and then the gates of the first Soviet concentration camp on the Solovetsky Islands. This camp was located on the site of an ancient monastery. Isn't this symbolic?

* Well-known Russian social thinker, writer and literary critic.

14

But many people tend not to notice such symbols. In his article "Psychological foundations of esoteric teachings," included in the book "Discourses on Esotericism (a collection of works by the Institute of Philosophy of the Russian Academy of Sciences, Moscow, URSS, 2001) O. Ye. Baksansky makes the following statement: "The cosmological notions of esotericism are in such stark contradiction with scientific data that this fact is obvious to a significant number of our contemporaries, even those without a college degree" (p. 132).

You see, it's as simple as that. The author then continues: "Analysis of esoteric views on the phenomenon of life, on the one hand, once again reveals their apparent discrepancy with scientifically established data..." (p. 133).

This is an example of how a BIG LIE is being born. One cannot but wonder under what level of educational background O.Ye. Baksansky would classify such scientists as Carl Jung, B. Pauli, E. Schrödinger, W. Heisenberg, E. Wagner and C. Weizsäcker. They all in some way acknowledged the existence of esoteric knowledge. "We are part of an indivisible reality, possessing an innate ability to formulate ideas about itself that it registers internally. This model resembles the Indian theory of Akasha, or the theory of Cosmic space; this substance is considered so subtle that it records all events occurring in the Universe... By analogy with physics this reality can be called the FIELD OF CONSCIOUSNESS. This single gigantic field represents orderly and wholesome energy, manifesting itself in uncharted regions at the interface of physics, psychology and religion." These words which the above-quoted author would consider "absurdly preposterous" belong to one of the greatest contemporary physicists David Bohm.

The Nobel laureate Roger Wolcott Sperry, a leading specialist in the

15

field of brain research, writes: "I think that human destiny and the destiny of our biosphere found themselves entirely dependent on those beliefs and values that the next several generations will choose for themselves (I hope that they will), which they will follow and observe in their lives. The most important beliefs are not those that have to do with the mundane daily routine and basic means of subsistence, but those associated with

religious, philosophical and ideological beliefs of a higher order – the ones for which people live and die, views concerning the purpose and meaning of life, faith in God, the human psyche and its role in the Cosmic system. Science no longer believes that everything is ultimately controlled by 'fundamental forces of physics and that our Cosmos is devoid of values, consciousness and purpose, and indifferent to human concerns.'"

In 1992 the journal "Questions of Philosophy" published an article by the major Soviet philosopher Merab Mamardashvili (1930-1990), titled "Thought Placed under Taboo", which emphasized that man belongs simultaneously to two worlds – the natural and the transcendental. The scholar called this transcendental world "an unknown country", an obscure mystery and the home of all conscious beings. All of us (since we are conscious beings) have a second homeland and as spiritual beings, as people, we are its citizens. According to Mamardashvili, man's transcendental essence is "incarnated" in his soul, and the word consciousness is "used in the same meaning, which we imply when talking about the spirit."

Academician Natalia Petrovna Bekhtereva, a leading Russian neuroscientist, recently spoke about super-consciousness and God on TV.

Even the founder of English materialism Francis Bacon, who publicly proclaimed the principle of experimental verification of theoretical concepts, warned people close to him in a conspiratorial whisper: "Atheism is a thin layer of ice over which one person may cross, but a

16

whole people would fall into an abyss..."

Are critics saying that all these people are school dropouts?

While writing in my books about my personal experience of clairvoyance, I fully recognize that many people will see their content as either fantasy or mental aberration. Nevertheless, I am writing this because this is the time when the genes within the chromosomes of many people that have always been silent have begun to "talk" and they will be forced to go the way of personal transformation. Regretfully, there is still a predominant view in this country that if a man speaks to God – it is a prayer, but if God speaks to man – it is a mental illness. I fear that many potential psychics may fall into the hands of psychiatrists who, unfortunately, know nothing about the soul, thought it is the main subject of their science.

Recent advances in quantum physics and the resulting better understanding of our surrounding reality as an intelligent, energy and information rich environment have led to the need to acquire practical knowledge and skill in handling this substance. It is presented before the researcher in the form of invisible self-organizing structures that can actively influence any vital processes, primarily those occurring in the human body. The point is that our body at the energy-information level represents a system of reception, radiation and transformation of some forms of energy into others.

Hermes Trismegistus, a very knowledgeable witness, who was declared to be god during his lifetime, pointed to this human trait: "O Egypt, Egypt, there will remain of thy religion only fables, and thy children in later times will not believe them; nothing will survive save words engraved on stones to tell of thy pious deeds... For behold the divinity goes back up to heaven; and men, aban¬doned, all die..."

Arguing about this postulate of the ancient deity, who is also called a

17

sage, Eugenio Garin* in his book "The Italian Renaissance" (Wiley, 1986) wrote: "Man's main characteristic is not so much his central position in the Cosmos as his ability to go beyond the realm of form, his power over his own nature exactly as the result of his having no nature. The absence of intrinsic nature and man's being as an expression of complete freedom lead to the fact that the entire world of form can be controlled by man to such an extent that he can overcome it either by transforming into a demon, or by ascending to the divine essence of transcendental reason.

The surprising feature of man consists precisely in this inherent ability to freely remain at the center of certain reasonable foundations of things, which is why in some way all of nature, all essences and all finite reasonable foundations depend on him. He can uproot and destroy anything in the same way as he can recover and restore everything in a free transformation. All things are what they were always and eternally, permanent in their state: rocks, animals, plants and stars, moving in their orbits. But man is nothing which is capable of becoming everything projected into the future, because his very human essence does not consist in what was given to him by nature but in his grown and discovery of self, where he transcends beyond reality. His lack of ultimate image makes it possible to find him in his creation, and this creation is his sentence to things, the trail which he leaves in the world as he creates within it, altering and transforming it."

This statement could serve as an epigraph to my book!

We sometimes find in magical texts a repetition of the story of how at the will of one man, of Adam, the world is either destroyed or reborn and becomes either a kingdom of demons or God's kingdom. This plot carries

*Famous Italian philosopher and historian, a recognized authority
on the cultural history of the Renaissance.

18

a very definite meaning. After the destruction of the notion of original order, which also included Man and extended between the ugly that was found below the human, i.e., the realm of the devil, and what was absolutely endless, free roaming, that is Divine, it turned out that a person could use forms and consciousness either to raise the essences to the level of God or else to plunge them in utter darkness, into monstrous chaos.

Those reading this book will meet with Hermes Trismegistus, face to face as they say, and see how he took advantage of the opportunities given him by the Creator. Unfortunately, a good understanding of things does not guarantee correspondence of action with one's wishes. And God's divine name does not exempt people from having to answer for their deeds before Him, Who is always above all heavenly and earthly ranks, and Who prides Himself on holding not the most opulent but the most important of all names – the Father.

Man contains within himself every imaginable possibility. One of them is the ability to see the spiritual world, which is for the time being outside the ordinary mechanisms of vision.

Controlled clairvoyance is confidently entering into our lives. New branches of events have begun to grow on the tree of life. They are not yet fully ripe; they are still in the process of becoming arranged into a sequence of cause and effect connections, but they are already irrevocable, because they have arrived from the future. And they have already happened in the future: in it everything has already occurred.

The great Avicenna, who in the Middle Ages had no modern medical equipment, or astounding drugs developed through highly intense scientific research nonetheless achieved results in his practical treatment that are statistically unattainable for most present-day physicians. He explained

19

the essence of his technologies in a very peculiar way and never tired of repeating that the soul is all-powerful, that words, signs and symbols are the most effective tools in his fight against human diseases.

If we were to translate into modern scientific terms what this genius of medicine has left us as his legacy, it would sound something like this: all material bodies, including human beings, are multidimensional in structure and should not be viewed only in terms available to man and according to dimensional parameters within his understanding; beyond the world with physical parameters there is an enormous world with which it is possible to interact and attain desired results. Influence can be achieved through the soul, through words, signs and symbols.

There is extensive evidence about the existence of this "other" world. In the first book of my trilogy, I have already spoken about the fate of Nicholas II, the last Russian emperor, as it is revealed through clairvoyance. It is widely known that decades before the Emperor's death, there were predictions regarding the main events of the Bolshevik Revolution. In all these prophetic predictions the future was seen from the past, and it was foretold quite precisely

Saint Seraphim of Sarov (1759-1833) prophesied that "there will be a king once, who will glorify me, then there will be great turmoil in Russia, and a lot of blood shall be spilled because people will revolt against the king and his autocracy..." But Seraphim of Sarov didn't just make oral prophecies. Shortly before he died he gave a letter, sealed with softened bread, to his servant by the name of Motovilov from Diveyevo. The letter was addressed to the future Emperor of Russia! When handing him the letter, Seraphim said to the servant: "You won't live to see it but your wife will, when the entire royal family pays a visit to Diveyevo. Make sure she gives it to him..." That is just the way it happened... In the summer of

20

1903 there was a grand ceremony at which the relics of St. Seraphim of Sarov were exposed for public veneration, with the royal family in attendance, after which Nicholas II went to Diveyevo. There he was handed a letter. According to the testimony of the daughter of the father superior from the Diveyevo Convent, Nicholas II broke into bitter tears upon reading the letter.

The Emperor of Russia had every reason to cry. In St. Seraphim's letter he found confirmation of another prophecy contained in a letter drawn up in 1801 by Abel, a monk from the Alexander Nevsky Monastery. According to the monk's will, the letter had to be opened one hundred years later, on March 12, 1901. On that day, Nicholas II and his wife visited Gatchina, where the message from another century was stored in a special casket. They both read it. "To Nicholas II, the Holy King, whose great suffering will be akin to that of Job's. His imperial crown will be replaced by a crown of thorns; his people will betray him, as the Son of God was once betrayed. There will be war, a great war, a world war... People will fly like birds in the air and swim under water like fish; they will destroy each other with stinking brimstone. Treason will grow and multiply. On the eve of victory, the royal throne shall collapse... A peasant wielding an ax will seize power in an act of madness, and there will come a time of truly Egyptian plagues..." As we see, here too World War I and the Bolshevik Revolution were predicted a hundred years in advance... These events were predicted as accurately as possible, with the maximum amount of detail accessible to the consciousness of people who had never seen airplanes, submarines or chemical warfare.

The Russian tsar responded to these predictions very seriously. Once, at a palace ceremony with fireworks one of the cannons was accidentally charged with live ammunition. When it was fired, shrapnel cut off the flags and the top of the tent, where the emperor was at the time. However, the monarch didn't even flinch. He explained his poise and confidence with a short phrase: "It isn't yet time." Incidentally, this shot killed a policeman, who bore the name of ROMANOV, just like the tsar. Was this yet another coincidence?

Science is still incapable of explaining these evidences of the manifestation of a different, higher and more powerful mind in our lives.

Should we also consider it a coincidence that when, (according to the description of events in my first book, "Save Yourself"), Armageddon occurred in the world of subtle matter, in which the last Russian Emperor, Nicholas Alexandrovich II, participated in 17th Legion of Power, at this particular time the issue of his canonization as a martyr-saint was being discussed at the Patriarchate of the Orthodox Church, and at this same time in the city of Tver, in the only New Martyrs Church in Russia, there was a unique sign? There had never been a sign like this in the entire history of the Russian Orthodox Church! Four images of the Blessed Virgin Mary and three crucifixes began to exude myrrh simultaneously.

On July 22, three days after the burial of the imperial couple's remains and those of their royal off-springs, the Mystic Rose, the Image of the Virgin Mary, started exuding myrrh. Later, on the Day of the Assumption of the Blessed Virgin, myrrh was exuded from the image of Our Lady the Immaculate Conception, and then from the Crucifix.

The Lord gave His sign not in a temple, fragrant with incense, among golden icon-lamps and chandeliers, but in a half-dilapidated, half-decayed house belonging to one of the sister-novices of the Church. However, as it often happens, not all the most holy shrines instantly become places of mass pilgrimage. First they are subjected to doubts and rejection from the authorities and sometimes even the clergy. These holy shrines are remem-

22

bered only several decades later when nothing but barely noticeable traces remain of their former grace.

This sign was given not just for one temple but for all of Russia and for each of us. Though I have my own personal opinion about the Church's role as a mediator between God and Man, I must admit that this sign has to mean more than the Higher Reason rewarding with indulgence the religious superstition of worshipping an image instead of the living Deity.

According to Eastern philosophy, reality is inexpressible, incomprehensible and indescribable. This at the very least leads us to the conclusion that we don't live in reality, though we imagine our existence to be real. We delude ourselves thinking that we can see the truth, though everybody knows in what a narrow spectrum of electromagnetic waves our visional analyzers receive signals.

There is a reason why Einstein wrote in this respect: "Imagine a bedbug completely flattened out, living on the surface of a globe. This bedbug may be gifted with analysis, he may study physics, and he may even write a book. His universe will be two-dimensional. He may even intellectually or mathematically conceive of a third dimension, but he cannot visualize it. Man is in the same position as the unfortunate bedbug, except that he is three-dimensional. Man can imagine a fourth dimension mathematically, but he cannot see it, he cannot visualize it, and he cannot represent it physically. It exists only mathematically for him. The mind cannot grasp it." (A. Einstein, "Collection of Proceedings", Book 4, Vol.4, 1967, p.131).

But as one scientist from St. Petersburg quipped in response: "Nobody wants to be a bedbug even one with an analytical mind."

The book, you are holding in your hand could have been rightfully titled: "The Book of Knowledge from the Creator". Its subject matter is not science fiction, not simply a writer's dreams about a possible abstract future; it talks about reality, witnessed and confirmed by numerous trials, properly notarized and registered.

One of the central characters in this book, Academician Grigori Petrovich Grabovoi, is well known throughout Russia. An impressive number of books and articles have been written about him. However, none of these publications present him from the angle which you will find in this particular work.

The phenomenon of Academician G.P. Grabovoi does not at all fit the Procrustean bed of conventional science. He not only insists that there exist various realities in the Universe, including spiritual and unrevealed ones, but he also convincingly demonstrates how they affect our lives. Materialization along with dematerialization of objects, telepathy, curing terminally ill patients, including those with cancer and AIDS, and, finally, resurrection of the dead, which took place in the presence of experts, and regeneration of missing organs carried out in the operating room – all these events represent not some kind of speculation by people with agitated fantasies but the persistent daily work of this incredible man who is not interested in TV exposure and does not attempt to build celebrity hype. Grabovoi is simply creating a new reality in the field of knowledge, where science and religion are not opposed to each other in a senseless effort to monopolize their right to the truth. Instead, they join their efforts in discovering the truth.

It is worth pointing out that formation of a new world vision, simultaneously a scientific and religious one, is not just a separate aspect of philosophy but presents the quest for an alternative path in the development of society and a way to ensure the survival of mankind.

Truth be told, not everybody is happy with this turn of events. Some scientists, while failing to address the real issue, respond with "mosquito bites" instead, trying to create negative public opinion. "Komsomolskaya Pravda", the paper, which regularly publishes horoscopes on its last page, was willing to devote its two full pages to run a phone interview with two Academicians of the Russian Academy of Sciences – Mr. Kruglyakov and Mr. Ginsburg. They both work in nuclear physics, which is supposedly on the cutting edge of science. However, their arguments seem more appropriate to philistines, not to prominent scientists.

First of all they attacked A.Ye. Akimov and G.I. Shipov, the developers of the theory of torsion fields: what kind of nonsense within physics are these two members of illegal academies promoting? Apart from everything else, they are wasting federal funds. I can't help but wonder, what these so-called "legal" academicians were doing themselves their entire lives? Everybody knows that science is the way to satisfy one's personal curiosity at the expense of the state. Any serious invention requires tremendous efforts and substantial financing for its implementation.

Meanwhile, Grigori Petrovich was picked on as well. Not only was he reproached for his cooperation with the Security Council and the Administration of the President of the Russian Federation (look who is entrusted with the job!) but on top of it they misspelled his last name, referring to him several times as "Grobovoi" instead of "Grabovoi".

Lev Tolstoy, in his time, gave an explanation to such positivism: "Contemporary scientists like to state triumphantly and assertively: we are dealing with facts, as if what they are saying makes any sense. It is impossible to study only facts because there is an endless (literally) number of facts, suitable for research. So before one starts to analyze these facts, it is necessary to have a theory, which will be the basis for studying certain facts selected from the endless number of all the facts" ("Complete Works", vol. 25, p. 355).

25

But the point is that Grabovoi's ideas are so foreign to Kruglyakov and Ginsburg that they choose to use other facts that have very little to do with the issue at hand. In actuality, what does it matter that Grigori Petrovich is consulting the Security Council of the Russian Federation? If he didn't do it, there would be someone else. However, his regeneration of organs and resurrection represent unique breakthroughs, truly epoch-making discoveries of the very first magnitude. It is quite possible that if it weren't for Grabovoi, these breakthroughs might have occurred many years later and, possibly, not even in Russia.

I find the arrogance of some scientists' approach toward the history of their own science to be quite shocking. How can they be so conceited as to assume that the mistakes made by somebody sometime ago in the assessment of the completion of theories, which ultimately proved to be far from being complete, cannot be repeated? Even the attacks of these bygone days and the wording of these accusations were often the same as those we find today: Leibnitz, for instance, was so mad at Newton's theory of universal gravitation that he rebuked the great scientist for introducing the notion of "mystical far-reaching impact" into physics.

And what are we going to do with the opinion of such a world renowned philosopher as William Thompson: "The impossibility of autogenesis (he is referring to the Universe) at any time should be taken for granted, similarly to the law of gravitation." Or let's take Sir Isaac Newton, who is considered to be one of the foremost scientific intellects of all time. He proved the theorem of binomials, invented the differential calculus and formulated the laws of motion of classical mechanics. He was also the one who discovered the law of universal gravitation. At the same time, he never published anything, which was not thoroughly supported by the results of experiments or by visual geometric constructions.

26

If we look at the numerous notes and diaries, which Newton never intended to publish in the first place, we will get an image of a man totally different from the commonly adopted perception of the great scientist who wrote "Mathematical Principles of Natural Philosophy". Sir Isaac was an alchemist. He was looking into ways of transmuting one element into another, and making the philosopher's stone and the elixir of life. From his diaries and notes we learn that Newton made attempts to interpret The Book of Revelations, which, he hoped, would help him to uncover the secrets of the Universe. Actually, his scientific work also had a certain "magical" element: he would solve a problem by mere intuition and only afterwards shape it with logical proof.

Another great scientist, Albert Einstein, would also avoid the positivist approach on a regular basis. He would fall into explicit mystical heresy, saying: "There is no logical way to the discovery of these elemental laws. There is only the way of intuition, which is helped by a feeling for the order lying behind the appearance". Such quotations may be cited ad infinitum.

"Everything that derives from experience – whether through experiments or observation – cannot qualify for anything beyond the probability of a true conclusion. No matter how high the degree of probability might be, it should never become a dogma... Dialectics accepts the possibility of true knowledge but does not allow pointing fingers in the direction of true knowledge, – wrote S.V. Meyen.* – "The so-called 'universal laws' of nature are not that universal, in fact, for they reflect only a certain vision of the world."

Mind you, these are opinions expressed by scientists, whose standing in the global scientific hierarchy is much higher than that of Academician

* Russian botanist, paleontologist and geologist, Dr.Sci.Biology.

27

Kruglyakov, who isn't even known to many Russian physicists.

When someone publicly claims his right to the ultimate truth in a scientific debate, I find it laughable, because there are constants in the Universe presently unknown to physicists. They are simply bound to exist in an infinite Universe, which is recognized even by ardent materialists.

In fact, not so long ago scientists unanimously denied the possibility of any life in the surrounding Cosmos. Now they claim the opposite, just as unanimously. Sorry, they say, we were sincerely mistaken, and it took some time before our eyes were opened. And what about the fate of cybernetics, labeled as a "false science" in Russia? The fierce reactionaries at the Academy crucified it mercilessly. Now they sit comfortably at their computers, casually hitting the keyboard, because they have successfully erased their own obscurantism out of their memory.

However, the world has changed. The Creator has changed something in it but some have failed to notice the change.

An individual able to see the truth possesses the gift of clairvoyance and finds himself in the present. One who is able to control clairvoyance can place himself in the future or in the past, wherever he wishes. From any given point of space and time he is able to get actively involved and assume responsibility for the dynamics of any event he wishes to get involved into. This is called co-creation – a mutual effort in Creation. It may be barely noticeable, insignificant, affecting only one tiny branch on the tree of life, and, yet, it is already an admission to something the Creator Himself is doing. You, who are created in His image and likeness, in the long evolutionary process, have finally obtained the ability to construct an event starting at the level where this event did not yet occur, at the beginning of its inception and even before it began. This is precisely what is meant by the technology of the Creator.

You, who are created in His image and likeness, should know how to control things in His image and likeness as well. God has acted as a gardener in this world. He planted the tree of life. He took care of it, watered it and trimmed the dry branches, helping the

healthy ones to grow. This was His dream, his cherished fancy which He wrenched out of Himself with the help of the Spirit. God came to this world as an artist. With the help of light and color he moved his dream onto the real planes and volumes of space. He enabled us to grow, the best way we can, the branches of our own families, our personal destinies, desires and dreams on His Tree of Life.

That is how time emerged in infinity and space appeared within time, because for the first time for the sake of fulfilling His dream He emerged as spirit out of His soul, while limiting His presence in the physical world by creating a pulsating Universe.

He gave us the ability to see His future (because dreams are the Creator's technology in building the future) and form events by tracing the vectors of creation through analysis and studying the progress of any particular event. He has persistently taught us these skills, despite our inertia, our ignorance, and our egocentrism. As the light of the souls and Divine Spirit penetrated deeper into the darkness of our personal Egos, our ability to trace the trajectory of creation and follow it in the dangerous labyrinth of our own imperfections, as if it was the Ariadne's thread, grew ever stronger. What do you see in it – the right path or the dreams of fear, created by Darkness in the dark? Make up your minds! If you make the right choice, time will become obedient to you, turning into a system of interdimensional connections, where transmission of information takes place through the energy of spirit and its transformation into real objects of the world through consciousness.

The world we live in is psychophysical. All connections of the Cosmos are human-oriented. You should, therefore, be vigilant. If somebody professes the inevitable and complete destruction of the Earth, ask yourself the question: why is he doing that? The answer is obvious: he does it to obtain the sought-after sequence of future events through death and fear.

Mind you, the moment we change our attitude to our place and role in this world – the world will inevitably change.

Day after day we see catastrophes, wars and murder on TV. This creates the image of the present, while fear programs the vector of the future.

Our Heavenly Father teaches us to create worlds, to grow gardens of life in them, take nurture everything that has the propensity to develop and perfect itself. If you dream of doing these things, if you are ready to learn and if you are not discouraged by difficulties, this book will help you.

But if you are not in a hurry, if you are sure that it is better to wait a bit more to avoid possible mistakes, in this case you will always be dominated by the phases of the Moon.

By virtue of his dual nature – his physical body coming from Mother Earth, and his life from Cosmos, the Father – man is capable of understanding Nature and loving Heaven. The two can secure the harmony of their existence precisely in man; they can forget their mutual resentment and find parental reconciliation. And he, as the Son, has the responsibility to do everything in his power to restore the harmony of Heaven and Earth.

Chapter 1

The year of the millennium was defined as the year of change. Who could have guessed that a few months prior to the beginning of the third millennium, my friend Igor Arepyev and I will become directly involved in extraordinary and impressive events. All this gave me the feeling that, purely by chance, I once crossed an invisible line and suddenly found myself in an entirely different Universe, where myths, legends and folk tales acquired a tangible reality, whereas our customary reality gradually melted away before my eyes.

Global changes were accompanied by a remarkable sign: there were six solar eclipses in 2000. Let me give you the strange number representing the code of my fate, which I was able to change from six to nine as the result of subtle matter battles and confrontations (I have written about them in my previous book, "Save Yourself"). Can this too be called a coincidence?

I first became involved in this series of events beyond the looking glass unconsciously, but later I continued quite consciously. The things I learned were unquestionable evidence of a mysterious interdependence between the earthly human world and the heavenly divine world.

Unusual phenomena began to occur to me in 1996. Nothing predicted them at any time earlier in my life. I had written a number of books and published a two volume edition on the Russian poet Fyodor Tyutchev. I held administrative positions: during several years before it closed down for restoration work I was director of the Tyutchev Museum "Muranovo", after which I headed the "Kultura"* Publishers. At the very beginning of 1996, I was appointed director of the "Khudozhestvennaya Literatura"**

*The name of the publishing house means "culture" in Russian.
**The name of the publishing house means "fiction" in Russian.

31

Publishing House. It happened during the most difficult time when this well known publishing house was facing utter ruin and inevitable bankruptcy.

A few months later I became seriously ill. My kidneys refused to function and physicians recommended removing the left kidney.

It was then, at the hospital, that I started having visions. They were nothing like dreams. They were real. It was as though someone was showing a skillfully made film in my head. The images I saw were very distinct – better than those on the TV screen. The film was about the life of Christ. That was just the beginning. I suddenly started to recover very fast. The issue of surgery was taken off the table. But the theme of the "pictures" began to expand. I realized that someone was involved in my destiny and was leading me to some new mission, incomprehensible to me for the time being.

Retelling a film, even a documentary work, is in itself a losing proposition. Therefore, if I have sufficiently engaged your curiosity, you would be better off picking up the first book. In the meantime, I will mention only two significant acquaintances I made in the past. Four years ago I met Igor Arepyev, a police officer from the Orlov Region. He appeared unexpectedly in my life and mastered the wisdom of clairvoyance with amazing speed. Since that time we have been working together. My second acquaintance was with the long known psychic Grigori Petrovich Grabovoi. Grigori Petrovich is much younger than I, but he has the gift of clairvoyance since early childhood. He taught Igor and me many valuable lessons and is always ready to help us, and for that we owe him a debt of gratitude.

Our Center for Bio-information Technology, which offers help to patients considered incurable by traditional medicine, is becoming more and more reputable. We are gaining credibility as we acquire new knowledge and become more skillful in our grasp of ever increasing opportunities. The number of unanswered questions doesn't decrease, and our minds are anxiously trying to explain what is happening, not trusting simple everyday evidence. Indeed, our knowledge is like a balloon: the greater its size, the more its surface of interaction with the unknown and undiscovered. And then, is it knowable in principle?

Who do we deal with in that virtual world, and who gives us hidden knowledge, telling us about the secrets of the worlds? Some of them may look like people in their image, but I guess that not all of them are humans: some are actually entities. Unlike humans, they are not multifunctional, since the missions assigned to them are fairly limited. Is it for us or in general? Who are they: persons, super-persons, or the embodiment of some ideas?

All philosophers are familiar with the rule, which is called "Occam's razor": * "Entities should not be multiplied beyond necessity." In other words, concepts, reducible to intuitive knowledge and not verifiable through experience, must be removed from science. However, the feelings, emotions and even the physical pain which Igor and I experience are with us, and we get them in another world, unknown to most people. Finally, what about our experience of healing, which can't be learned in any medical school? What about our telepathic conversations not only between the two of us but also with patients and students, who are also mastering the ability of controlled clairvoyance? They haven't yet entered these other worlds, but they are successfully mastering the knowledge we give them.

*The law of parsimony and economy attributed to a 14th-century English Franciscan monk, expressed in Latin as "Entia non sunt multiplicanda praeter necessitatem."

Of course, the recent generations are quite ignorant as far as their knowledge of the invisible world. I was no different – an atheist, skeptic and romantic at the level of classical poetry. This applies not only to the occult and esoteric but to Christian faith as well, which is perceived predominantly at the everyday level of rituals and at the solstice of religious holidays. I was trying to find the truth in old books but without much success. I mostly came across the same "multiplying of entities beyond necessity" and playing with various terms. I was also puzzled by one human obsession, which the Russian writer Vsevolod Solovyov wrote about more than a hundred years ago in his novel "The Magi": "Those minds, carried away by a thirst for the miraculous and unable to quell their thirst by reveling in the purity and simplicity of the Christian doctrine, which was too elevated and great for them, reverted to ancient and medieval dreams, seeking out remnants of

ancient secret sciences and trying to pull off the veil from the mysterious face of Isis."** Freemasons and Rosicrucians, Illuminati and Satanists, Theosophists and other seekers of ancient wisdom, I now know that they are seeking for answers in the wrong places.

It was Kant who noted that there are two kinds of prejudice: not to believe anything and believe all that is being rumored. Incidentally, the above-mentioned Solovyov had a friendship that lasted a couple of years with Helena Blavatsky, the founder of modern Theosophy. He then became disillusioned with her teachings and wrote a crushing book, titled "A Modern Priestess of Isis". While recognizing Blavatsky's numerous remarkable personal abilities, Solovyov proved that theosophical claims to truth and beneficial miracles were utterly unfounded.

**One of the most important goddesses of Ancient Egypt, worshipped as the ideal mother and wife as well as the matron of nature and magic.

34

Alas, the man in the street, eager to find miracles at any price, is always far more represented in society than the patient gardener, who diligently takes care of the Tree of Life.

Can we consider what happened with Igor and me this year and the one before a miracle? Perhaps, we humans were simply too quick to see ourselves as omniscient? And as St. Augustine said centuries ago: "Miracles do not happen in contradiction to nature, but only in contradiction to that which is known about the laws of nature."

For instance, science explains to us that the development of plants occurs through the process of photosynthesis. However, if you were to plant a seed in absolute darkness, it would still grow a shoot – albeit a feeble and weak one – without photosynthesis. Hence, there must be some kind of energy that contributes to growth.

Now what about vision? We are being convinced that the eyes see, because they are a special device designed to receive visual information. Nonetheless, there are successful techniques that due to the activation of the optic thalamus – two large ovoid masses on the occipital cortex of the cerebral hemispheres – assist even people who are blind from birth in developing alternative vision. Mind you, they see in color, the same way as ordinary people do. They are able to read books and watch TV. They do it without various glass tubes and rods, which, according to conventional biological studies, are responsible for color in visual analyzers.

Even such prominent scientists as Academician E.M. Galimov, Director of the Institute of Geochemistry and Analytical Chemistry at the Russian Academy of Sciences, are perplexed by the impossibility of giving a purely materialistic explanation to the phenomenon of life: "Molecular biology and biochemical logic are powerless to overcome the conflict between the need to simultaneously have both an enzyme that controls the synthesis of informational molecules (DNA or RNA) and these molecules themselves which encode the synthesis of the enzyme that controls their synthesis. For physics, the problem of living is something that preserves an uncomfortable relationship with its basic laws. This problem is exacerbated by the fact that geologists and planetary scientists have virtually no incontrovertible facts about the situation that existed on Earth in its early days. Practical geology begins with the age of rocks being 3.5-3.9 billion years, whereas the earth is 4.56 billion years old. There is no material evidence on Earth

of the processes which occurred in the period covering 500-700 million years of its early history, except for some 4.2 billion or even 4.4 billion year old grains of zircon.

Science and religion each offer their own solutions. But the search continues, for the believer wants to back up his beliefs with scientific logic, and the scientist wants to support them by faith. For me as a scientist, the starting point is the scientific theory of evolution. However, explanation of evolution by natural selection which modern Darwinism offers us is by no means satisfactory. The theory of natural selection does not help us understand how life originated. Darwinism provides a clever mechanism, which ensures the evolution of Life that emerged (somehow!), despite the fact that the blind forces of nature are acting in the opposite direction." ("The Phenomenon of Life", Moscow, Editorial URSS, 2001, p. 5).

What does this mean? It testifies to the fact that scientists are quite successful in copying the forms of nature. But all they offer already exists in the Cosmos.

Below is the text of an advertizing about an illusionist who is famous throughout Russia and also known as a denouncer of psychics, magicians, sorcerers and fortune-tellers: "He can catch an arrow released from a bow

36

at a distance of more than 30 feet. He drives a car blindfolded and shoots in the direction of a sound (hitting the target!). Simply by listening, he can memorize up to 30 phone numbers, 40 first names and patronymics, and 100 randomly selected and uttered sounds. With the help of combinatorial thinking he can add five-digit numbers in his mind and raise two-digit numbers to a power of thirteen faster than a person can do it using a calculator. He can simultaneously perform more than five actions within a minute, and he can also run up to the 15th floor within a minute or stay five minutes under water."

This text is about Yuri Gorny. Here's more about him:

"In 1965 Yuri Gorny substantiated and established the art of psychological sketches as a genre and a way to demonstrate concentrated expression of sensations, emotions, feelings and thoughts in order to influence the senses of other people. These types of skills were so unusual and attractive, so hard to explain and so little studied that the country found itself flooded by a putrid wave of magicians and psychics. Over the years, Yuri Gorny, who opened the way for healers, showed them up in their true colors. But, as a prominent bridge engineer – the hero of one of Chekhov's short stories – said once: 'I don't get it! I design unique structures and yet no one knows who I am, but the young ladies of dubious reputation who are photographed on my bridge are known to the whole world.'"

As to the fact that it was Yuri Gorny who opened the way for healers, this is a bit of an exaggeration. The existence of healers was no secret before 1965. But as to Yuri Gorny's remarkable abilities described in the newspapers – that was indeed a seven-sealed mystery until recently. The master himself didn't really explain any of it, and, to all appearances, he had no intention to do it. Unfortunately, he viewed his achievements only from the perspective of individual fame and personal glory. He could well

37

be compared to Chekhov's bridge engineer. So maybe this is the time to expose the denouncer himself?

After all, Yuri Gorny's abilities that have amazed his audience for so many years can be described in just two words: controlled clairvoyance. It is therefore absolutely the same thing that those other "magicians and psychics" are trying to use, albeit less successfully. They simply have weaker abilities and less acting talent. That, incidentally, explains why all extrasensory experiments are thwarted in the presence of Gorny: he simply dampens the abilities of less capable clairvoyants. He's stronger, so he closes their channels of perception. He doesn't need competitors.

The fact that the development of controlled clairvoyance can restore health to millions of people doesn't seem to concern him. Nor the fact that controlled clairvoyance is capable of pulling mankind off the dangerous track of unrestrained technological development.

At our Center, even seven-year-old children can demonstrate the kind of tricks that Gorny demonstrated to his audiences: they can shoot precisely at target balloons and read when blindfolded, and they can also memorize numbers. They aren't in a hurry after this to call in representatives of the Guinness World Records, the press and TV, but they simply put on their backpacks and knapsacks and go to classes in regular schools. These kids feel embarrassed to brag about their unusual abilities before their peers at school. They want to be no different than everyone else.

The article by A.V. Bobrov, "Field concept of the mechanism of consciousness" ("Consciousness and Physical Reality", Volume 4, № 3, 1999, p.48) provides a very interesting list of unusual events and facts related to the so-called "speech syndrome". Here are some of them:

"– In 1987, the next day after suffering a heavy blow to the head, G.S.

Smirnov, a retired Tula Region resident, became fluent in German, which he never knew;

– In 1992, after undergoing a severe illness, a girl from Yaroslavl suddenly began to speak in the Sumerian language, which existed in the third millennium BC;

– In Moscow, a 70-year-old patient who forgot her native language following a stroke, began to communicate in Hebrew, which she knew as a child;

– S.P. Perov, a retired man, began to speak in Old French after he regained his senses following a car crash;

– Sleep-walkers during sleep and mediums during seances can switch easily to foreign languages, though they don't speak these languages in their normal state. Thus, the American medium Laura Edmonds, whose mother tongue was French and who didn't know any other language, spoke 10 different languages during these séances easily and fluently, and she even sang in Italian, Hindu, German and Polish, quite unconsciously and not understanding a single word;

– Emilia Tolmedge, a girl from the U.S., who didn't know a single note and never played a tune, suddenly wrote down the notes of a musical composition and performed it brilliantly on the piano;

– 27-year-old German electrician Thomas B., after an evening fight with his wife, began speaking in Russian the next morning, totally forgetting German, his mother tongue. Lessons with a teacher didn't produce any results: Thomas turned out to be "incapable of learning a language" and he would instantly forget all German words."

Conventional psychophysiology is unable to explain these phenomena and ignores or rejects them as non-existent. Similarly rejected, despite all the apparent and glaring facts, are other features of the mechanisms of thought and memory: their volume and speed.

Thus, in the early 1980's, there was a brief report in the media that a semi-literate woman from India named Shakuntala Devi extracted the 23rd root of a 201-digit number mentally up to a unit, beating by10 seconds one of the most sophisticated U.S. computers, UNIVAC 1108. She openly admitted not knowing how she did it. Scientists made the following calculations: if we assume that the same algorithm was being used in solving the problem by computer and by this Indian woman (without access to memory), then with a tact frequency of 10 MHz in the computer network it would take at least eight days for a human being to solve this problem. However, when we consider that while solving the problem a person, in addition to the thinking process, needs to resort to his memory multiple times and has to store and retrieve large amounts of digital information, the complexity of this task increases exponentially. Anton Chekhov's character would say in this case: "It cannot be, because this can never happen." But it does! Here are a few examples taken from the "Guinness Book of Records":

– In 1995 Hiroyuki Goto of Tokyo memorized and recited Pi to 42 195 decimal places. The record was registered at the Tokyo Radio Broadcasting Center.

– Alexander Craig Aitken calculated the square of the number 57 586 in two seconds.

– Dutchman Willem Klein took 48 seconds to multiply two nine-digit numbers.

– Bhanddanta Visittabm Vumsa read 16,000 pages of Buddhist canonicg119

– al texts by heart in 1994.

– Jan Christian Smuts (South Africa) learned 5,000 books when he was already advanced in age.

40

– In 1996 the American Dave Farrow memorized the order of 52 decks of playing cards, randomly shuffled together, and recalled them correctly after just a fleeting look at them (a total of 2,704 cards).

All this happened despite the fact that the travel speed within fast operating neuron networks, which is limited by the time of passage of the action potential along the nerve fibers and the duration of the synaptic transmission, excludes the possibility of solving any of the above problems within the specified time frame.

Numerous studies have demonstrated that the brain of such people is idle during the moment they perform these "calculations", i.e., in fact, they aren't counting anything. Then where does the correct result come from? Human calculators assert that they see the answer on some imaginary screen and simply read it out loud.

So Yuri Gorny is not the only one who is capable of unusual things. Why he doesn't want to reveal his secrets and the technologies he uses is another story...

We are living in such strange times, times of change. Connections, relationships and interactions are experiencing a crisis. On the one hand, an alarmingly increasing number of people in the world are not fully functional – drug addicts, alcoholics and schizophrenics. But on the other hand, there are children who can read blindfolded, who are able to see events that take place hundreds of miles away and communicate with each other using telepathy. The recently unshakable materialistic symbols are crumbling right before our eyes, and people's minds are filled with fantasy-like hypothesis about the not-so-distant future.

Many people would like to have super-abilities, but they would prefer not to have too many competitors getting in their way. It's I who am unique, one of a kind, so why would we need others like me? For the sake of gaining demiurgic powers, some scientists are even willing to "improve" their own bodies and brains with the help of computers and devices. Projects involving implantation into the human brain of chips that enhance the volume of memory are openly discussed by the media. At a scientific conference in the British city of Sheffield, Professor Kevin Warwick of the University of Reading announced in September 2001 that he will test on himself a chip implanted in his body, which will transform him into a super psychic. Warwick is confident that with the help of the device he will be able to telepathically transmit his thoughts and feelings to others.

What an odd situation. Hence, modern science considers the phenomenon of extrasensory perception to be "legit", when it is implemented with the help of chips and computers, and rejects this phenomenon if it doesn't see next to the brain some kind of crutch to assist its functioning.

Once I had an opportunity to talk about it on TV with Academician Kapitsa, the famous host of the popular-science show "The obvious and the incredible". Sergei Petrovich got so upset when he saw three of my female students, blindfolded, quietly reading random texts picked out of a pile of newspapers by Yana Chernukha, the TV host of the "Good day" show, that he expressed his suspicion right there in the studio that the TV host, the girls and I were involved in a conspiracy. And although Kapitsa himself selected the method of observation, which, according to him, ruled out the possibility of deliberately deceiving him as a witness, Sergei Petrovich nevertheless insisted on the impossibility of what he was observing even though he was unable to reveal any trickery.

– I really have no idea how you do it, – Kapitsa admitted, – but the thimble-riggers at the railroad station also manipulate their cups so deftly that no one can detect the fraud.

That was the entire reasoning of the famous scientist. He obviously went too far with his thimble-rigger comparison: their trick had to do with the speed of the viewers' reaction. He could have given a thought to the fact that these were ordinary schoolgirls, young kids, in front of him. How did they get the time to learn how to practice such deception, which Yuri Gorny himself might envy? Besides, they had parents, friends and acquaintances. If they had learned something similar to what the thimble-riggers were doing, all these people would surely know about it. And then, there was no way they could learn such tricks in the month or two that they were studying at the Centre. Nobody taught them anything like this; it that was true, our Centre would have an entirely different reputation. However, why do I sound so defensive?

Sergei Petrovich should have recalled what his father once said: "Science is something that cannot be; what can be is called technology." What's more, technologies may be relevant not only to matter but to consciousness as well.

I am positive that if someone showed Sergei Petrovich a device, which was able to perform everything he saw the children doing, he would treat it all not only with confidence but also with interest.

Why should we be surprised? Academic titles and degrees are not an indulgence or patent confirming one's possession of the truth. Our technological age has an impact on thinking. True, people operate machines and devices, but it is also true that they exercise control over humans.

Its mysterious beauty Nature shall protect
Should you try to uncover it, she shall object.
No tools you use will let you draw from her
That secret, which your spirit can't infer. –

43

wrote Vladimir Solovyov, a famous philosopher and brother of the above-mentioned Vsevolod Solovyov.

I don't doubt that Sergei Petrovich would have responded with confidence and professional curiosity to what unfolded in the TV studio, if the person involved was not some writer by the name of Petrov but a reputable representative of a prestigious research institute or design center. The hierarchical mentality of scientists would have played its part. It might even seem justified considering the abundance of crooks and charlatans. And yet, such great minds as Watt and Faraday, Polzunov and Edison, and Columbus and Galileo were also "outsiders" in science. And so was Tsiolkovsky, an outstanding Russian self-taught scientist and inventor! His genius was recognized only during the Soviet regime, and then not so much by the scientific world as by the State, and in a one-sided way at best. They patted him condescendingly on the shoulder, gave him some medal, took his most important idea to serve the country's needs ... and swept the rest of his legacy under the carpet for years. By the way, governments and their security services in all countries pay much closer attention to informal science than to the scientific establishment. Probably they do it for their own self-preservation.

After all, we don't insist on the reliability of psychophysical effects for the sake of some dubious notoriety. Far from it. The point is that throughout its history mankind has accumulated too many facts and evidence which don't have a solution within traditional scientific concepts. Now we have personal experience. PERSONAL! That's why we affirm: there is much that is unknown hiding beyond the horizon of familiar truths. The unknown may be very useful; indeed, it may turn out to be necessary for the further evolutionary development of mankind.

I have devoted many pages in both the first and second book of my tril-

44

ogy to traditional, "big" science. "Why did you do it?" the reader may ask. It was adherents of traditional science that formed mankind's collective consciousness for centuries; they are responsible for many of the planet's problems, both global and those involving personal destinies. Therefore, all those to whom the true state of affairs is revealed must relentlessly ring the alarm bell and help to shift the worldview and psychology of people into the other direction – from mechanical knowledge to universalism and from selfishness to universal love for all nature, for everything that the Creator has given us.

Yes, the inertia of thinking is a powerful and dangerous force. The well-known American writer James Halperin has a good joke about it: "People drummed it into their heads that man is mortal, and now they keep dying of inertia."

Actually, Halperin is absolutely right. People do not necessarily have to die. Conviction in the inevitability of death is real only as long as public consciousness accepts this sad inevitability. But if people stop thinking that death is inevitable it will no longer be that. After all, some people have allowed the thought that it may be possible to see without the aid of the eye, by developing alternative vision – and this has already happened. Some of them believed that it is possible to communicate with each other telepathically – and now the media is full of reports of successful experiments in this most exotic area of telecommunications. As for psychic healing, do we even have to prove to anyone today that such a thing exists in reality?

When people appeal to the past, extracting from it abundant evidence to confirm that these or any other paranormal phenomena are impossible in principle (which is what Academician Kapitsa did), they forget about the simple and universally understood word "evolution". After all, our

45

ancestors weren't able to do many of the things modern man can. It took a while before such things appeared as cars, computers, televisions, nuclear reactors and rockets.

Sometimes linguistics indicates to us certain mechanisms of perception and interaction with reality.

Many languages have three moods of verbs: indicative (or declarative), subjunctive (conjunctive) and imperative (commanding). They fully correspond to the level of everyday consciousness. The indicative mood reflects what occurred in reality; what actually happened, is happening now or will happen in the future. This is reflective modality telling about the actual facts, and it is in some way coordinated with that reality, being associated with it through a relationship of mutual dependence. Incidentally, Academician Kapitsa conducted his dialogue with the show participants on this particular basis. (Of course, I am referring only to this instance.)

The subjunctive mood describes something that may happen, a possibility that a phenomenon or process might occur, or that a certain event might have taken place in reality (incredible but possible). The position taken by Yana Chernukha, host of the "Good Day" TV show, expressed this mental modality, i.e., a free-thought approach.

The imperative mood is very straightforward: it expresses the subject's wish or command and his desire to see that a certain event takes place. Here we have volitional modality, implying a feedback between speech and reality.

In essence, these three levels of consciousness reflect the three-dimensional space-time continuum of our being. That is why, from the standpoint of consciousness, which has the ability to mirror actual reality, our world is three-dimensional and marked by the boundaries of these levels of perception and consciousness. But, in turn, they too reflect some global stages of evolution. The first level is that of water (mirror reflections). Life originated in the ocean. At that level, there is no subjunctive or imperative mood, just one continuous indicative mood: the waves are rolling, the sun is shining and the corals grow. Then the second level of consciousness appears – the level of amphibians. And with it, the subjunctive mood – the conjunctive: it would be great to have something to eat; I'll open my mouth now and maybe something edible will end up there.

At the third level, there is already man who contains the former two levels within him and must learn next one, associated with the development of the physical body and the thought apparatus. And here his will and command come into play: I wish, I want and I command.

Transition to the fourth dimension – the imperative of creation – is associated with the development of our brain and consciousness. Then something else, something called freedom of the individual, is added to the Holy Trinity (the soul, spirit, consciousness, or, at another level, information, energy and reflection in matter), on the basis of which the world was created. Freedom of the individual can be achieved through the mechanisms of development and harmonization of the processes in the right and left hemispheres of the brain. And no additional vector, be it time or space, in fact nothing can change any of it, because consciousness is a reflective system (mirror of waters) of information coding both from the Cosmos and from the levels of DNA.

If you aspire to reach into higher dimensions, you must ensure that the space of the Universe corresponds to your consciousness, or vice versa. Then, and only then, will the imperative of creation appear. ("And God said: Let there be light and there was light.") Everyone strives to achieve this state of consciousness but not all of us are able to reach it.

47

In the middle of year 2000, a barely noticed but extremely important event took place in Russia. A study of the possibility of obtaining external visual information without the aid of eyes was carried out at the Brain Center of the Russian Academy of Sciences (RAS) in St. Petersburg under the guidance of RAS Corresponding Member, Svyatoslav Medvedev. The examination procedure was broadcast on television. A girl by the name of Katya, whose eyes, covered by an opaque plastic mask which extended over her whole face were unable to receive any sensory information, glibly read several texts displayed on the screen of a computer monitor. The commission members repeatedly changed the content of the displayed materials but the result was the same – the girl never "messed up" while reading. The results of these experiments were reported in scientific and academic journals, and in the popular "Science and Life" magazine.

As I mentioned before, you can meet such children at our Center, too. We don't teach them in any special way to read when they are blindfolded. This happens of its own accord as a result of personal orientation toward the game.

But the point is not how this is achieved. You can just take my word for it, this occurs without much effort on our part. What matters is that the whole thing is completely inexplicable in terms of conventional science. Based on its prevailing notions, such a result is impossible in principle. But nonetheless it has been achieved, recorded and recognized by an academic commission. Moreover, it may be repeated many times.

The Cosmos implies the presence of order. This order, reflecting down to the atomic and cellular level or, conversely, rising up from the subatomic level, simultaneously gives structure and reflects our consciousness. "The Wisdom of this world is foolishness with God," – the apostle Paul said uncompromisingly. But St. Peter corrected him gently: "Make every effort to supplement your faith with virtue, and virtue with knowledge."

Einstein once remarked ironically that if, according to the quantum theory, the observer creates or contributes to creating that which is being observed, the mouse can alter the Universe simply by looking at her.

The great scientist was closer than ever to the truth. If he replaced the word "mouse" by the word "person", he could easily escape the impasse of his own logical objections.

Why can people do things that are beyond the reach of mice? It is because man was created in the image and likeness of God. Because only man has the potential of the kind of form and content, to which space and time will respond.

The Universe is the work of the Creator, and only His words: "So be it!" – are the measure of the law and human rights. Man, however, as he gets closer to the ideal of his inherent likeness to God over the course of his evolutionary development, becomes capable of creating, and, moreover, is already partially creating that which he observes, changing the Universe. But in order to change the world, he must move beyond established notions. That isn't easy. Many people are willing to die on the spot, repeating: "It cannot be, because this can never happen!" They apparently forgot the sad lesson of the French Academy of Sciences, which in the eighteenth century passed a verdict that appears quite absurd from a modern perspective: if a machine is heavier than air it cannot fly. There were some great people among those responsible for this verdict, yet fortunately someone found their words to be vanity, insulting to the mind, rather than the voice of reason itself. As a result, we have planes and spaceships in the skies above, i.e., those very machines heavier than air, which, in the opinion of revered French academics, were not allowed to fly.

In his little-known article "Vehicles of progress" Konstantin Tsiolkovsky suggested a very clear explanation for this strange, but prevalent attitude demonstrated by venerable academics and other pundits. "It seems natural that it is scientists who are asked to judge various inventions and discoveries. But these are people who have exhausted all their energy on the perception of science, people who are tired and unresponsive as the result of these efforts, who essentially have a weak (...) creative streak." Tsiolkovsky examines the arguments and excuses of these naysayers. He then concludes: "The old hypotheses are constantly being rejected, and science moves forward. And this process is always hindered by the scientists more than anyone else, because they are the most to lose and suffer from these changes."

Nikolai Gumilyov gave the most ruthless portrayal of such people:

As a ferocious dog he must defend
His name that he built up for years.

Let us repeat once again the truth Einstein almost guessed: the COGNIZER and COGNIZED can never be separated. In the UNIVERSE, which is the work of the CREATOR, there is simply no such thing as an in-between position. The oldest books on Earth that very few people are still able to fully understand, tell us about it. To quote the opening words of Creation captured in the Bible:

In the beginning was the Word
And the Word was with God,
And the Word was God.

50

At this point, it is appropriate to consider the multidimensional content of the above lines only on the basis of the level of their universal perception achieved in the progress of mankind. In this case, the WORD and GOD, although identical, are nevertheless separated. Hence: WORD, God and THAT WHICH SEPARATES THEM form part of the world-creating triad, the same HOLY TRINITY, through which all "started to be..." and "became flesh..."

If we attempt to see the divine WORD through clairvoyance, we can see, strangely enough, the physical atom – the protons and electrons orbiting around it. The proton is the root of the tangible physical word. And if we focus on it, we can see something altogether unusual: it isn't just a bundle of energy and not just an inter-dimensional tunnel, but it's also a control panel. It resembles a spherical structure, designed internally along the principle of the Rubik's Cube. When you look at it from one side, say consciousness, for example, you can follow the sequence: evolution, civilization and intellect. If you look at the same sequence from another side: it is religion, science and culture. Here it is: get to the root of the matter. Some root it is! But here, too, is not the end of the puzzle but only its beginning. On one side you select the sector designated by the word "individuality". You reverse the structure, and now this same sector is already designated by the word "personality". And if you are able to take a look at the center, you will read the words "individual personality" out there on the middle cube. That's what the proton looks like, a genuine puzzle. Modern nanotechnologies cannot even begin to understand its true complexity.

When we say that "in the beginning was the Word", we are referring to the linguistic level of thinking, related to the demiurgic management structure. In this case, we must bear in mind that there are certain areas of information with distinctly differing properties. For example, passive, unstructured information resembles scattered letters of the alphabet.

Letters are indisputably informational. But it is equally obvious that they reflect a certain meaning, a desire or an event that are simply lined up a certain way. By themselves, the letters do not add up to form words and sentences – certain tools are needed for that. Something needs to enter into this area of information to combine the letters into words, and, in addition, to have the power to move them out of this passive area of information into the active one, where they will acquire flesh for their existence, that is, from virtual become real.

This process is graphically illustrated by physics. For instance, we have a structured material particle – the smallest and indivisible particle called the atom. So, in the form in which we know it, study and use it, this is already a word. The atom has been materialized or it is manifested in our world; it can be used and we can achieve results by combining it with other atoms; we can also get molecules any necessary substances, including those of man-made nature.

But the atom also consists of something. That is the boundary, where the structural changes into something without structure and becomes, on the contrary, an energy space that separates the revealed, that is, the physical world and the hidden spiritual world.

So when they say that "in the beginning was the Word", they have in mind a very concrete meaning of the demiurgic technology that allows to control events of any degree of complexity.

For example, how is the periodic table formed? It all begins with a single elementary and indivisible particle, with the proton, i.e., with the hydrogen nuclei. To get the next element, a fusion reaction is required – the proton must connect with another proton, which the law of nuclear interactions prevents from happening. In this case, under the conditions of boiling solar plasma, in the depths of which cycles of nuclear transformations are occurring, one proton emits a positron, i.e., a positively charged electron, and turns into an electrically neutral neutron. In a neutron plus and minus are aligned. In other words, something positive allocated from its surplus of positivity, to become simultaneously positive and negative in a way, thus achieving inner harmony. Such a particle no longer falls under the law of the inter-nuclear repulsion of similarly charged particles and it freely combines with another proton. Thus, the nucleus of heavy hydrogen appears. Then it is joined by another proton, and a new element is born – light helium. Then the two nuclei of this new element are joined together to create helium.

The triad of creation, whose actions we tried to understand by analyzing the nature of the Sun, finds its smaller but exact copy in the world of chemistry. Limiting ourselves to organic chemistry, we will discover that (alongside with the ubiquitous presence of hydrogen) the three creative sources are quite clearly and simply represented by three elements: carbon – the active source, nitrogen – the neutralizing source and oxygen – the passive source.

When we look at the world through our biases and prejudices, that is, through the prism of those theories and explanations which we selected from the treasure trove of knowledge that we assume to reflect reality most adequately, we will never see the truth. We must remember that people in general are capable to visually perceive information only within a limited range of electromagnetic waves. For instance, the human eye can't distinguish X-rays or any other kind of radioactive radiation.

If we don't know the true path (and the path is known only to the One, Who has already created the events that are occurring to us), in this case our consciousness is observing some sort of an illusion of the real world – or, rather, a mirror that distorts the true picture of the Universe and our personal existence. That is, this is exactly what was said before – the OBSERVER CREATES the OBSERVED. And then it all depends on the observer's level of consciousness. Is it normal, advanced and expanded or true?

To substantiate this statement, let me give a recent example. You have probably watched the movie "Jaws" about a giant man-eating shark. It should be noted that facts confirming the attacks of these marine animals on people are actually quite rare. But the filmmakers did not set a goal of historical authenticity – they had other things on their mind. The film was brilliantly executed. So strong were their impressions of the movie that people on vacation who frequented the beaches felt terrified of the hypothetical danger and suffered from psychoses and neuroses.

Then, suddenly, reports started coming from all over the world, from different continents, of an unprecedented number of shark attacks on swimmers. Mind you, before the film's release there was no alarming statistics about such incidents. Even the author of the original novel Peter Benchley was almost killed, after being attacked by a ferocious two-meter shark.

Just think about what happened? People's consciousness projected into space fierce scene of their encounters with marine predators. And space responded by replicating the new behavioral patterns upon the consciousness of the animals.

Obviously, we all need to change our attitude to our place and function in the world.

In order to see reality properly, you need to know at least the following: all the theories of modern scientists are based on life, rather than life being created on the basis of theories. And life is not static – it changes in accordance with certain programs of the Higher Reason. Its change is based on collective consciousness, which either moves closer or further away from the knowledge that is embodied in the PERFECT MAN. Humanity has defined him by NAME: the MAKER, the CREATOR. Humanity has also identified those who follow in HIS FOOTSTEPS.

It starts with Raphael painting a picture. And only after that thousands of art historians try to explain how he did it. Yet even after thoroughly studying the artistic techniques of the genius, none one of them is able to create anything like that.

The main mistake of conventional science lies in the fact that it has elevated methodological impartiality and independence of the experiment procedure from the researcher's personality to the level of an inviolable principle. But such independence doesn't exist in principle. Suffice it to recall the film "Jaws" and thousands of other similar cases that are well known to science. It is precisely the partiality of the researcher that represents the main event of any experiment and a special phenomenon of our perception. To what extent the partiality of the subject of an experiment affects its objects is already a different story. This largely depends on his mastery of the capabilities of personal consciousness and his entire inner microcosm, i.e., it is the result of a long path of evolutionary development, not in one lifetime but in a number of reincarnations.

Let us consider the basic constants of the Universe, on which biological life as we know it is built.

The first rungs of the ladder of Jacob, which leads man to true knowledge, are located in the areas of CONSCIOUSNESS. Take a note: we're not speaking about one area but about many. In other words, we are referring to a certain structure that has its own organization and is connected to the planetary network of information. Both the Earth and man represent structural, level objects of the entire Universe. Therefore, they regularly take in, transmit and generate various kinds of information, which supports their vital activity and evolutionary development. That the world of information, as it turned out, stretches beyond the known physical, material world and is simultaneously its foundation, walls and roof, i.e., surrounds the grain-structured material on all sides, radically alters the picture of the overall structure of the world. Matter, which occupies only an insignificant part of the revealed Universe, is a kind of mirror reflecting the subtle information processes occurring in the infinity of the Cosmos on the macro and micro levels.

Man, too, is similar to a mirror up to a certain degree. Spiritually initiated people knew and understood what is hidden behind the ordinary meaning of words. When we read in Genesis, the First Book of Moses, that "the earth was formless and empty, darkness was over the surface of the deep, and the Spirit of God was hovering over the waters", we perceive only the external meaning of these words.

But there is another level of perception. "The earth was without form and empty." That is, it has not yet been revealed and was at another information space, at the Beginning of Beginnings, not yet fertilized by God's thought. "The Spirit of God was hovering over the waters." Water is the mirror of consciousness. This sentence tells us about the procedure of recording the core program of the newly created space object, its further evolution and development, on the material transmitter.

Thus, there is one, literal meaning of the sentence, in terms of the collective consciousness. There is also a second, hidden meaning, or rather, one that has already been uncovered. There are actually two more, but it's premature to speak about them today, because each of these meanings is at the same time a creation technology, and a demiurgic one at that.

This is a multilevel process. And whatever is referred to, according to religious tradition, as the Throne, Forces and Powers at one level of the Universe, is designated as soul, spirit and consciousness at another level. In our physical world other terms are being used for it – information, energy and matter. That is why we assert that space and time are projections of our consciousness; in other words, materialization occurs via the reflection of wave processes of the spiritual world in our consciousness.

Academician Grigori Grabovoi is one of only a few people who possess true knowledge. In his book "Resurrection of People and Eternal Life – Now Our Reality!"(Moscow, Kalashnikov Publishers, 2001) he speaks of this divine technology: "When you combine what you think with what is happening in the external, supposedly objective reality – when you combine this at the level of action – then you can achieve the materialization of objects..." Do you understand?

Actually, all this knowledge and these technologies are recorded on the structure of every person's DNA. And from time to time they are transferred to our consciousness, which, in turn, "switches on" our speech center and notifies the Universe, shouting "Eureka!" in recognition of this event.

In ancient times it was assumed that the world stands on three elephants, or three columns, according to the Jewish Kabbalah. You can say that the world stands on whales, elephants or pillars – the essence will not change. Anyway, it isn't about animals but about the right and left hemispheres of the brain, the spinal cord and whether they are capable of harmonious functioning on the basis of CONSCIOUSNESS, meaning divine consciousness, of course.

The left hemisphere manifests its function of logic through the scientific worldview. The right hemisphere displays its function through an intuitive perception of truth and through religious perception of the world. At first glance, they appear to be irreconcilable opposites. But if you look closely, you will see that the nonsense of atheistic views and the shocking demands for "sacrifice of the mind" are just two extreme manifestations of the same natural life source. And while the left brain hemisphere "hits against" its own mirror reflection, unable to overcome the BOUNDARY separating the worlds, it will continue to repeat the same old statements about atheism, physical foundations of the world, speed that cannot exceed the speed of light, and space and time as the medium of our existence, not even understanding that they are secondary to the CONSCIOUSNESS OF THE CREATOR, Who has created all this in the world and in relation to WHOM they are correlated, as consequence with cause.

It isn't only science fiction writers who talk about human super abilities. The world-renowned professor Stephen Hawking, who is no doubt one of the most brilliant scientists of our time, asks people to be prepared for change: "Humans need to improve themselves as a species – to alter their own intellectual and physical abilities. After all, man will have to exist in an increasingly more complex world and meet new demands. He must develop superhuman abilities. I know that many people say that genetic experiments on human beings should be banned. But I don't believe that someone is actually able to stop them. Genetic experiments on plants and animals have been allowed for economic reasons, and some geek will definitely be tempted to try to carry them on humans. At some point someone, somewhere will create a new and more perfect person."

It would be interesting to learn what the Creator Himself thinks about all of this. He Who has created Man, that is, His most perfect creation? Isn't it possible that is was the scientist's strange thoughts about the need to improve the creation of our Creator which resulted in his present not very enviable physical condition as it has happened to many others before him? Stephen Hawking suffers from what is known as amyotrophic lateral sclerosis and has been in a wheelchair for many years now.

It all started in 1995 and developed in several stages. First, Hawking contracted pneumonia and he later had to undergo surgery. After tracheotomy he could no longer speak and he lost his ability to communicate. His friends made adaptive computer communication software for him, built right into his wheelchair. He can now talk to people and write books with the help of a computer. Please don't conclude that I am speaking lightly of his condition. I feel great sympathy for this man of genius. Moreover, I would like to help him get rid of his devastating disease, which condemns him to immobility and muteness, as Igor Arepyev and I have done for many other patients before him. Very little is expected of him in return: for us to succeed, he must take the possibility of such a cure quite seriously.

At the same time it might be good if he pondered over the following issue: could it be that wrong thinking is the true underlying cause of our physical disorders? The point is that when our consciousness takes a wrong direction this leads to a distortion of the world of our existence, its pathology, followed by its reflection through the mirror of water (consciousness) into the inner world, that is, into the body, where disease sets in.

Evolution is a difficult ladder of human development and finding God within Man, discovering God within oneself. Igor Arepyev's and my life didn't become any easier after clairvoyant abilities became revealed within us. On the contrary, our lives became more difficult. We now see current events differently from the way we did before – various connections and dependencies we were not aware of before and, therefore, ignored in mak-

59

ing decisions have become apparent. The problem is not that we must take into account more factors than we did previously but that we now know – and what's more, we see firsthand – the world was not the random result of self-development. It is the entirely natural process of evolution of the Universe, carried out strictly according to plan, in exact correspondence with the design of the One Who created this world and Whom people, intuitively conscious of His invisible presence in our existence, address with the all-encompassing name, Father.

We did not conceal anything that we could see. One of my learned friends, a mathematician, once said to me: "When you don't have sufficient facts, imagination begins its work." Behind this unambiguous statement was a clearly intimated hint of reproach: sure, you can imagine anything, but what does it have to do with real life?

Probably this is how it was in his life but not in ours.

One day in late August 2000, I was watching TV and suddenly the screen went black. I began to switch programs – it was the same on all channels. My first thought was that it must be another coup by the Gang of Eight.* But then I saw the glow of the distant fire spreading before my eyes. Igor, who always stayed in my house whenever he visited Moscow, was outside in the garden at the time. I went out into the garden to ask his opinion about the strange thing that had just happened to me. I found him near the gazebo but he already seemed to know what it was I was going to say.

– Did you just see a fire? – Igor asked.

– Yes.

– Go up to the third floor and look toward the Ostankino TV Tower, – he suggested.

*The Gang of Eight was a group of eight high level hard-line officials within the Soviet government, the Communist Party and KGB who attempted a coup against Mikhail Gorbachev on 18 August 1991.

– Is Ostankino on fire? – I asked my friend, aware of all the subsequent inconveniences of living without television.

– Yes, it is, – he confirmed. – The cables caught fire and there's a lot of smoke. This smoke makes it hard to breathe. It causes choking.

– So why did the cables start burning? – I was curious to know the answer, being aware that Igor was much better than me at analyzing any situation through clairvoyance.

– It's because the two sides are at odds again in the subtle world. This time it's a sports showdown. First the Dark scored, then their opponents scored, – he said mysteriously. (For readers not familiar with my first book: between the two of us we referred to dark forces opposed to the Creator as "Dark" or "mohair".)

– What do you mean by "scored"? – I wondered. Though there could really be some kind of secret connection between the fire at the Ostankino TV Tower and a soccer match. Yes, the same way that the sunflower-seed oil spilled by Anna was connected to a tragic tram accident near the Patriarch's Pond.*

–You know not what you do once again, do you? – my friend asked with a certain ambiguity in his voice.

I suspected that he meant some subtle-matter developments that sometimes have a tendency not to indicate our participation explicitly in the regular physical world, even when we actually did participate in these events.

– What match? Who is competing with whom and for what?

– That's a good question, – Arepyev approved and prompted: – You can now ask about the score.

– Well, if you know the score, please share it, – I agreed.

*Reference to Mikhail Bulkagov's magnificent novel, "The Master and Margarita".

61

Igor knew that I see things a lot worse than he, and compensate the deficiency of my inner vision with insight. Therefore he sometimes plays cat and mouse with me. But this time he refrained from pursuing his advantage in the personality contest.

– At the very top of the subtle-matter levels something like a soccer match has been going on for the past couple of days. More precisely, it's a competition over who can overpower whom and in what direction. The present score: one – one.

– What match?

– They made a field at the very top platform and rows of tiered seats. In the central stand are Justices of the Peace. You and I are the Chief Referees. There are also representatives of the Light and Dark forces, three for each side. Kirill is there too. He's very worried and fusses about. We sit in the middle of the stands.

– Chief Referees? But why?

– Yes, we are the main judges. It's because we won the Armageddon.

– Why did you say: something like a soccer match? Why the uncertainty?

– Each side sees what is happening in their own way. The Dark believe they're playing soccer. The ball they are playing with is the Earth, people's minds and their souls. And they already scored one goal. It wasn't exactly fair. Their representatives are shouting nasty things, suggesting where the players should pass the ball, but the referee on the field pretends not to notice.

– And how do the Light respond to all that?

– They refuse to consider it soccer. Because it isn't actually soccer. A man and his soul aren't expendable fodder to the Light forces but potential Saviors.

– In reality, what are this field, ball and match?

– This field represents the entire space of the Universe. It includes the revealed world (i.e., the world reflected by the mirror of consciousness) and the unrevealed hidden world (one with which our consciousness interacts only through intuition, clairvoyance and dreams). People with clairvoyant abilities make up the boundary between the Dark and the Light. Both the Dark and the Light look at the orientation of the soul, which is an indicator of the final score. Each player combines within himself a vast number of people and also the consciousness that he represents. Each team member occupies the position that is given to him on earth, depending on his evolutionary status.

– That is, depending on what abilities the soul had transferred to consciousness over the course of human evolution. – I finished Igor's thought following the voice of intuition.

– Yes, – he confirmed. – And the ball doesn't really exist. It's all the work of Dark fantasy. The players are actually trying to push over their own energy, power and space onto the opponent's side. Whoever pushes over more Light or Darkness is the winner. But all this is done through people. It all depends on the speed of the response: on who displays faster orientation in space and time, and who reacts faster in the volume of their knowledge. But all the action goes through people. Envy, deception, violence, hypocrisy, pride and greed – all these negative qualities are used by the Dark to prevent people from seeing the right path and receiving true knowledge.

– You're telling me they score by breaking the rules, and we don't respond?

There was bewilderment and outrage in my question.

– They can't win anyway. The other side scored back already, – Igor replied. – But you're right: we should put them in their place.

Now I see it all myself: the rows of tiered seats and the Dark in a wild frenzy. They are confident of their impunity, positive that they will win and this will allow them to prevail against their opponent on many attributes of Armageddon. Kirill is among them. He is explaining to two other devils, very presentable ones if judged by their size, that he has demoralized Igor and me, that we are quite confused and do not understand what is actually happening on the field. The devils are pleased to hear that. They smile at Kirill condescendingly. At this point, Igor rises, and the game is instantly stopped.

I stand up next to my friend. Igor beckons the field referee with a gesture. He immediately starts moving in our direction. He looks quite odd: on the one hand, he's a person, but on the other – it's some kind of energy contained in a sphere. Light and darkness are mixed together in this energy. Due to this the judge should be objective. If he demonstrates an absence of objectivity, he may be expelled from the sport's Supreme Court. Therefore, he's very scared. Igor addresses him politely but sternly:

– You must judge objectively. There are rules that weren't invented by us. I find it strange that you have forgotten about them. But all of us here live by them. These Laws were designed by the Creator.

"How did he manage to make himself so confident in this environment?" – I thought to myself but did not interrupt my colleague.

– No one is permitted to break these rules. From now on, no justification that you failed to see something, missed it or didn't know about it will be accepted.

I can see the faces of the devils grow progressively gloomier as Igor goes on with his monologue. And, on the contrary, a spark of hope appears on the faces of the Light.

– You have enough tools, strength, vision and power to carry out an objective analysis of the situation, – continues Igor. – And if you don't judge by the rules from now on, you will be replaced and you will lose all your privileges. You ought to have your own opinion and be independent. Otherwise, I repeat, there will be a replacement. And you know that we have such authority.

After these words Igor turned to the Dark and put an even sterner expression on his already far from sympathetic face.

– Also, according to the rules we have, we are warning members of the Dark forces that they could be removed from the game.

The referee grasped the situation correctly and immediately handed two penalty cards to the Dark. The devils were grimly silent and didn't object.

We left the psychic state of consciousness but Igor continued to be very serious. He was clearly concerned about the developments in the subtle-matter world. He understood that the present situation could have grave consequences. And it was unlikely that the strange soccer match and the fire at the Ostankino Tower were not connected in some way. There have always been a lot of misinformation and negative influences circulated by the TV, particularly more recently. There was always a lot of dirt streaming from TV screens. In the capable hands of managers, politicians, PR experts, chaos-makers (a trope invented by my friend, writer Yuri Polyakov) and other ingenious masters of the blue screen, television has become a powerful tool in the destruction of public consciousness. There were numerous articles about this in the press those days.

We read all these exposing articles and continued living normal lives, filled with good and evil, holiness and filth, where everything was abnormal, incoherent and far from any sense of harmony and rationality. But with all this, we already knew why, how and for what purpose this or that was happening. We knew now what the Father intended to do and who stood in His way. We also knew how people, unable to understand God's plan, spoiled and sullied their own lives, surrendering it to the power of idols they themselves created by their own lack of will.

* * *

We paid another visit to Grigori Petrovich Grabovoi. We found many people waiting – in the lobby, the hallway and even in the street. It's eight o'clock in the evening, but judging by the number of people he still needed at least three more hours of work. When does he have the time to rest? And whenever I spoke with Grigori Petrovich, I always remembered about these people outside his office and about their serious illnesses. And I tried to be as concise as possible. That day we were again working with the technologies of resurrection.

– Deep within their souls everybody knows that eternal life and resurrection are possible. – It wasn't the first time Grabovoi focused Igor's and my attention on the fact, which was perceived quite prosaically at the level of everyday consciousness.

Why did he keep repeating it? What did he mean by "deep within our souls"? Was it a trite idiom or a designation of access to something that ordinary people can't or don't wish to see? Man has created such powerful devices – electron microscopes and telescopes. He wants to know and to see other worlds and galaxies. But somebody uses the word "soul", and no one wants to stop and think even for a moment, where is it, this soul? What is it like? How does it work? Do all of us have it?

Somehow or other it's possible to imagine what lies behind such def-

66

initions as: mind, reason, consciousness and intelligence. But the soul! Spirit! These concepts remain a closely guarded secret. Perhaps they don't exist at all? Ephemera and nothing else...

But why is it that people continue talking about the spirit and the soul over and over again for thousands of years. They plead: do not meddle with another's soul, leave it alone, don't torture it. And Grigori Petrovich also adds:

– If we fail to expand human consciousness so that it can perceive the world at the level of the soul, resurrection will remain only a symbolic notion for many people.

– But the factual instances of resurrection have already been publicized. You have written about them in your works, – I tried to shift his attention to the real public prominence of the theme of resurrection. As a writer I was interested in the nuances of the public response to Grigori Petrovich's miraculous practice just as much as in the technology itself.
– Indeed, if a meeting of space aliens with the administration of the Chukotka Autonomous District was shown on a popular TV channel, the next day thousands of reporters from around the world would fly to Chukotka, – I said.

Grigori Petrovich smiled bitterly.

– The point is that most people have a twisted perception of the world. They think they are awake and are acting, doing something. This is partly true. But it's as if they are wearing dark contact lenses on their eyes. They don't know about them and assume that the world is really what they think it is. All the more so since from time to time they exchange with others some facts reflecting their perception and they find them to be adequate to their observations. We are limited by the model of three-dimensional space and linear time. This scientific fact is essentially a mechanism for self-limitation. A person knows that he lives in a three-dimensional world, that he is mortal, prone to disease and that all this is true not just for him but for all other people as well. That is how a collective dormant consciousness is created, and a detail of the macrocosm replaces the true picture of the Universe. Even though many prominent scientists around the world recognize the impossibility of spontaneous creation and self-development of the Cosmos and life, they are nevertheless afraid to take the next logical step.

When Grigori Petrovich speaks, his words are accompanied by the transfer of entire blocks of information generated in the form of spheres into our consciousness. The sphere contains both conceptual texts and images. Each sphere can be unfolded into an entire book on resurrection.

– Would you say that immortality is an act expressing people's consent to an eternal life, to not dying. In other words, the collective conscious-ness must accept the fact of immortality, and it will then move from the hypothetical area to the area of reality?

– That's right, – Grigori Petrovich confirmed, – it must be an act of collective agreement. The whole space of the Universe is a projection of consciousness. Therefore, we must acquire a standard procedure to access information and connect to the Cosmic Internet via archival points in space.

The Cosmic Internet... Several years ago I first used this definition in my book, "The Key to Superconsciousness." I gave a copy to Grigori Petrovich. It seems that the term caught on. There was the following pas-sage in the book: "Man has already started to create the noosphere. It won't take long before people get a new title – citizens of the Universe. We should prepare ourselves for this honor and this responsibility."

And here the three of us sit and discuss totally crazy projects from the

68

point of view of the so-called ordinary person: resurrection, immortal life and simultaneous existence in two or more spaces.

Throughout my life I have read a great number of books from different areas of knowledge. The content of many of them did not stay long on the surface of my attention but seemed to settle somewhere in the depths of the hidden storage in my memory. Occasionally, one or another passage from what I had read would surface again in my mind. And now for some reason I recalled Ray Stanford, or, rather, one of his phrases: "Planets are to civilizations what rivers are to salmon – spawning places. When we become adult we will have to go out into the sea of space and accept our place in ... the cosmological community."

– Note the following subtle point, – Grigori Petrovich emphasizes. – When in terms of our world cognition there is no longer the need to develop the phase of consciousness that corresponds to the splitting of physical matter – death disappears and becomes unnecessary.

We understood what Grabovoi is telling us. But do his fellow scientists? It appears not, judging by the fact that military laboratories and energy agencies of various countries continue to be involved with nuclear fission and biologists are increasingly drawn into research associated with hazardous genetic operations in the chromosomes of the cell nucleus.

Some private laboratories are engaged in dreadful genetic experiments: such as mixing human chromosomes with chromosomes of pigs. If these so-called scientists somehow succeed in whatever they are doing, it's scary to imagine what monsters might overrun the earth.

These facts clearly prove that ancient magic and witchcraft didn't die or dissolve in the streams of time receding into the past but have safely moved into state-of-the-art research facilities. Humans are in a hurry to solve the growing problems of their own existence with the help of knowl-

69

edge that they rip from nature by force and torture, not realizing that, in fact, such relationships with the Highest Reason of the Universe only exacerbate their already unenviable position.

I shared these thoughts with Grigori Petrovich and Igor.

– Science greatly exaggerates its potential, – Grabovoi agreed. – Scientists have concluded that a person uses no more than five percent of his brain's capacity. But even this figure is substantially inflated. Man has barely begun using his potential. Scientists don't realize that the influence humans have in the outside world does not depend on the contradictory achievements of science but on the development of people's inner world.

Grigori Petrovich was clearly referring to man's spiritual development. Recently, Igor and I have become inclined to believe that the factors of egocentric thinking, manifesting themselves in society's development as separated paths, due to their isolation, independence and alienation, bring mankind into a state of disharmony, which precedes the disintegration of chaos. The story of evolution on Earth, as astrophysicist Iosif Shklovsky wrote in one of his recent articles, is the cemetery of species. Loss of harmony – that is, the ability to cooperate, to establish understanding between people – which expresses contradictions within society, is leading all of us into an impending evolutionary impasse.

However, theoretical recognition of the need to observe rules of preservation and practical application of such understanding in our daily lives are two different things. Even now, while the three of us are discussing creative and, unquestionably, humane work plans for the treatment of sick people and regeneration of organs, up there, in the subtle-matter space, a fierce, though not military battle is being waged to ensure the supremacy of their own views in the course of world development.

– The score is now two to one in favor of Light, – Igor says suddenly,

70

as if tuned to my thoughts.

Grigori Petrovich looks at him in bewilderment for an instant, as though this sudden shift in the topic of conversation diverted him from some previously designated plan of communication. But he suddenly read the information on the event telepathically and, immediately arriving at the upper stage of the Earth's management levels, he eagerly supported the change in the course of our training.

– Indeed, it is two to one, but the Dark scored their goal dishonestly. Do you remember how they lured you into Mugen's lair with the help of Kirill?

– Of course, – we unanimously reaffirmed the well-known episode.

– Kirill wanted to poke Igor's finger with a knife. At the bottom they concocted a document regarding this event but they didn't have the needed drop of blood, a trace of DNA, which identifies a person, – I added some emotion to the indictment. And, developing the subject, I continued: – We are judging the results of the match right now. Igor could revoke the dishonest goal but he left the score unchanged, – I stated, not so much complaining about my friend, as lamenting the missed opportunity, in my opinion, to restore fairness.

– Yes, – confirmed Grigori Petrovich, – you could have cancelled the goal. But I have a gut feeling that they will very much regret their dubious achievement.

– Let it remain the way it is, – Igor agreed. I did not argue with him. In our subtle-matter adventures he always got the hardest job, so his word meant a lot to me.

– You are not just judging the game, – Grigori Petrovich suddenly clarified. – Look more closely. On the stand you act as chief referees and on the field you are both the dividing line and players. As players you

71

don't have a very high status so far. But it is for now – it will change soon. A goal, which the Dark consider to be their achievement, is called a scam in real life, a tripping maneuver.

– They don't seem to be very concerned about any of this, – I said with a sigh, fearing that the unstable score results in this subtle-matter competition might lead to apocalyptic consequences on Earth.

But Grigori Petrovich sensed my concern.

– After Armageddon space has been reoriented towards those who see the truth and not those who jostle for position with lies, – he explained the general state of affairs. – It will now be felt on a broader scale both in one's personal and public life.

– When new times come, accept a new rule of thumb, – I half-jokingly supported the positive shift in planetary events. – And where will these warlords go?

– They must define their position. You see, they are somehow in the dark about what is happening on Earth. Here in the physical world they are servants of the devil. But then the devil himself is gone. So their status becomes ambiguous: due inertia to they continue to engage in their dirty dealings, in accordance with their programs and commitments but they will soon have to answer for all they've done. Let me refer once again, to your acquaintance, the demon Kirill. He told you that he was the last of the tribe. It's serious business. Remember the horror in his voice when he confessed to it? Here's the point: none of them had been promised a third time. It may well be that their life will altogether come to an end. Anyway, that seems to be the tendency unless they change their position. After all, they do have considerable ability. They can heal people and be of help to others. The Father is merciful. They certainly have a chance. Will they be able to see the way to the heart of the Creator? Who knows…

* * *

The subtle-matter contest between the Dark and Light forces ended a few days later with a crushing win of three – one. The Dark lost. Judging by the cold farewell the two high representatives of the Dark gave Kirill at the end of the match, he should get ready for pretty gloomy days in the future. After all, he had ensured them that Igor and I were destabilized, disorientated and unable to guarantee correct, fair refereeing during the the match. As it happened, having lost, the Dark simultaneously received the maximum number of yellow warning cards. There were five of them, according to the rules of the contest. And as it turned out later, it was extremely important for each side to keep them in the future.

There was now no need to give warning in the fight against the Dark. The time of warnings was over…

The Light forces hadn't received a single yellow card and had all five of them available for future use. They played fairly.

There was also the unresolved matter of the questionable goal. It was counted as valid in words. But the paper remained unsigned. The word, of course, means a lot but the Heavenly Accounting Office demanded written confirmation. Where could they get it? The Dark ran down in search of it. Everyone was at a loss down there: the goal was indeed admitted as valid but there wasn't any trail on paper to confirm it. It didn't exist in the past either. So the Dark realized that they were getting a dose of the same medicine they had planned for Igor and me to taste. How they were supposed to wiggle out of the tight spot was unclear.

They rushed back: so and so, they said, we were wrong. Let the score

73

be three – zero, we would like to amend the situation that has been unfair to you.

But Igor for the umpteenth time wisely and proactively put a grim expression of formal zeal on his already unsmiling face.

– No, no, no, – he malevolently refused to accept the generous gesture of our opponents. – Let the cheating incident remain with you and we won't sign paper. You should understand: it's an eye for an eye.

I still wasn't quite sure what the strange situation with a goal, which seemed to be counted and not counted, would evolve into. But seeing how much such uncertainty was unnerving the horned population of the lower levels, I immediately sided with the position taken by my friend.

– An eye for an eye, – I commented somewhat theatrically on Igor's and mine joint decision to the two senior devils, who were following the progress of the match alongside Kirill. During that entire time Kirill stood on the sidelines, and his face expressed the whole gamut of despair. He already knew how it may all end for him personally as the very last one in the tribe. In the past he had millions of years of fairly comfortable existence, his present consisted of fleeting days of life on Earth but as for the future... He couldn't see into the future – that was the problem. And the cold touch of eternity was already creeping up to his black heart.

As winners, Igor and I were given the right to make any move we liked under the terms of the contest. The martial law detrimental to the Dark entered into force: if you were caught in a violation – you would be censured immediately. And how bad the punishment would be was anyone's guess.

* * *

74

Once in a while we ask our students at the Center for Bio-information Technology to review their former lives. This is a very useful task in many respects. It requires the ability, while concentrating your attention on the past, describing and comprehending it, nevertheless to maintain a stable connection with the present, and while penetrating inward, never to forget about your real location. These time travels always inspired the greatest enthusiasm. No wonder. The experience of becoming the hero of one's own life, not something imaginary, consistently moving through all the steps of reincarnation, provided the most intense emotional moments.

True, during these travels it is possible to get caught up in complicated, even precarious, situations having to do with battles, if you were a soldier, or with illnesses and violence. Even though all this occurs in the past, not in the present, the reality of these scenes is so absolute that some people lose orientation and live through various episodes of their former lives, as if they were happening in real time.

That is why we always escort our students in their time travelling. We are there to help if they find themselves in difficult situations.

However, some of our more "experienced" students resorted to the so-called cross-examination of each other's incarnations. To watch them in those moments is better than go to your favorite comedy show – for free. You split your sides laughing, and it doesn't leave a hole in your budget.

This time it was Sergei and Yuri who decided to find out what was the story with their past incarnations. The two are friends so they sat next to each other. Sergei started digging in the former life of his peer. This is quite an unusual experience – to see someone's destiny and life not on the TV screen but in the consciousness of that person, to point out the most important things in what you just saw and to be able to comment accurately on what you observed.

75

Sergei bowed down, apparently, he felt more comfortable this way.

– This is Ancient Rome. I see houses and all sorts of structures. There are many people around. Oh, here you are, – he reported gleefully, indicating that he had just tracked down Yuri. – You look like a soldier. Yes, you were a soldier.

Yuri straightened his back. He was proud that he carries a very prestigious status of a Roman legionary.

–You're doing nothing right now, just loitering. You're wearing ripped leather sandals, a short brown robe of coarse fabric and a leather belt. Ptew, you stink like a skunk! – Sergei's face twisted in a grimace of suffering. – Do you guys ever take a bath out there?

Yuri was embarrassed.

– I could be engaged in a campaign, where do you want me to find water?

– What campaign are you talking about? I said clearly – you are loitering. There is a gorgeous girl sitting in your lap.

Yuri smiled joyfully: a beautiful girl was a very normal vector in the developments. But his triumph was short-lived. Sergei thoroughly examined the new object from his friend's dark past and made adjustments to his original impressions.

– She must be homeless and a thief, as well.

Yuri stopped smiling again and started thinking how he could pay back his opponent by digging in his former incarnations. He was silent for a while but finally lightened up, finding what he was looking for:

– You too were some kind of soldier – in Poland. You have humongous wings on your back. Too bad they are so dirty and shabby. Who plucked you so badly, Sergei?

Sergei immediately checked the information marring his reputation,

76

and he was reluctantly forced to accept this fact of his biography.

– It happened in battle, I guess, – he had to admit the effectiveness of his opponent's response.

– No, there wasn't any battle. You just don't take proper care of your wings. They are dirty and shabby. If I were your commander...

Yuri decided not to finish his edification. Sergei was rattled and called for a truce.

– Okay, stop picking on me.

The two guys were working with time. They were not the first ones capable of doing that, and definitely not the last ones. When he depicted time through the visions of the warrior Er, who was slain in battle, Plato was well aware that time could flow in different directions. *"Now when the spirits ... came to a place where they could see from above a line of light, straight as a column, extending right through the whole heaven and through the earth, in color resembling the rainbow, only brighter and purer; ...in the midst of the light, they saw the ends of the chains of heaven let down from above: for this light is the belt of heaven, and holds together the circle of the universe. From these ends is extended the spindle of Necessity, on which all the revolutions turn..."* ("The Myth of Er" in Book 10 of Plato's "Republic", §§ 614-621)

The spindle shaft has seven inner circles moving slowly one in the other. . . On the upper surface of each circle is a Siren, who goes round with them, hymning a single tone or note. Together they form one harmony. Next to them are three Fates, each sitting upon her throne: these are the daughters of Ananka (Necessity), who are the goddesses of Fate, of the Present, Past, and Future. The spindle turns, and the spirals of planetary time move in the opposite direction. The warrior Er sees how the Fate of the Present turns time in one direction, the Fate of the Future in the other one, while the Fate of the Past alternates the rotation of the spirals in either way.

The fact that the fallen soldier sees the universal powers turning the spindles of time as represented by three goddesses, just like other people did before him, did not mean that those universal powers had to be expressed as images of these heroines of Plato, fixed once and for all time. Images can be different in different epochs, following the need to be adjusted to people's perception. (Similarly, over the centuries of history of Greek mythology, the quantity and quality of the Fates underwent multiple changes.) More importantly, the moment the warrior Er departed the real world, he immediately found himself in a new system of knowledge in a world never seen by humans. In fact, what he was shown represented genuine education, which was preparing him to perceive the new reality of his existence.

The way the Athenian soldier Er described his post-mortem experiences was reminiscent of an educational movie about the design of the space-time continuum in the area of perception accessible to humans.

Quantum physics changed the perception of how the Universe is designed. It showed that the process of observation or measurement has an impact and alters the parameters of the object under observation. Science has a special definition for this fact – it is called the principle of subsidiarity. We all form the audience of an unusual movie theater, where a mysterious quantum emitter is ready to offer us any reality depending on the personal abilities of our perception. The particles, i.e., the quanta of radiation, which combine within themselves something impossible from the point of view of rational reasoning – physical concentration in space (the corpuscle) and spatial dispersion (the wave) are able to demonstrate to each of us any aspect of reality, which our senses are ready to perceive.

78

But this is precisely the problem: what is each of us ready to perceive?

The universal field of energy and information will never stop the process of self-transformation. Without being aware of this, people become permanent subscribers of this unified information space. Bioplasm generated by electromagnetic oscillations of the human body, when united with planetary informational structures, is capable of creating a stable channel of connection with the super-computer of the noosphere.

What we call human intelligence is a special phenomenon in space and time. We are all comprised of atoms, which are at least five billion years old. (Tsiolkovsky called the atoms "citizens of the Universe.) "The atom is not the one science is familiar with as the connection between energy interactions – the real atom is intelligent matter." The empty space inside each atom (is it, in fact, empty?) pulsates with intelligence. Each cell is nothing else but intelligence responsible for the interaction of countless components. About nine trillion reactions take place every second in each of them.

Our cognitive system copes with it perfectly. Probably, this is what caused Academician Natalya Petrovna Bekhtereva, who devoted her entire life to studying the human brain, to admit: "The brain of people in ancient times, like the brain of our contemporaries, was equally ready for solving difficult problems. How is it possible? So far science has been unable to explain this phenomenon. As for me, I would not exclude the possibility that our origin is of alien nature... Our brain is way too complicated for this planet... (N.P. Bekhtereva, "The Third Breakthrough", "Trud" newspaper, December 19, 1997).

When we look at past events, what we see in the human consciousness is something like several parallel tapes that can be re-winded and fast forwarded at an extremely high speed. At least, this is the way the majority of our students perceive the chronological process at the initial stage of clairvoyance. Later these tapes disappear, and you can watch whatever you want. But in order to develop such vision one has to work really hard. Again, there is a hint – it means that the tapes of health, karma, fate and former lives are simply the average regular human visions in this "mystical" area of perception. No matter whether we want to or not, we once again encounter the notion of "collective consciousness" with its secret role in creating reality, because time and again we see that under the same physical constants of existence various objects of this existence have a different reality. Some people can see the invisible world, others can't – "collective consciousness" blinds their eyes. Some people can hear what the stars, planets and entities are saying to them, others can't – "collective consciousness" clogs their ears with the cotton wool of interferences. Collective consciousness is the average perception by the majority of people of current events and those which have already taken place; it is like a super-computer, the matrix structures of which are oriented along the Earth's axis of rotation over the North and South poles. Its functioning at the level of perception by means of clairvoyance is described in the first book of my trilogy, "Save yourself". But there is also a scientific description, which can be found in the article by A.Ye. Akimov and V.N. Bingi "Computers, Brain and the Universe as a Physical Issue" ("Soznaniye i Fizicheskiy Mir" magazine, 1995, issue 1). The work of this planetary super-computer is connected with the spin-torsion interaction of elementary particles. The rotating systems of particles or their own intrinsic angular momentum – spins – are a source of the torsion field. Here is what the authors of the article write:

"Research conducted in recent decades has proved the existence of such phenomena as non-thermal biological impact of electromagnetic

fields. At the same time, the mechanisms of such an impact are not quite clear. One of the suggested hypotheses was that the activity of biological objects is not indifferent to the state of the spin degrees of freedom of the molecules that make up cells. Since torsion fields are genetically tied to the spin degree of freedom, it is possible there could be a mechanism of biological impact of torsion fields, set into motion by molecular spins. If when speaking about cells we mean brain cells with their extremely delicate structure – neurons – it will be fair to assume that torsion fields would induce certain images of consciousness. If, in their turn, biochemical processes in human consciousness lead to appearance of certain well-organized spin structures, typical for these concrete processes of consciousness, then a situation is possible when characteristic torsion radiation will mutually correspond to certain images of consciousness. Based on the proposed viewpoint, it is possible that under the influence of external torsion fields, spin structures are formed in the brain cells, which bring out respective images and feelings in human consciousness.

If this is true, it makes it possible to build a relationship between consciousness and its material carrier in the shape of torsion fields. Now, coming back to the problem of operating the torsion computing machine, implemented in the Physical Vacuum, it will be fair to assume, that the operator's consciousness revealed through torsion fields, provides the operator with the possibility of direct access to the process of TCM (Torsion Computing Machine) without any transmission periphery. Thanks to this "leak" in the vacuum caused by his own consciousness, the operator will be able to integrate in such a TCM without any intermediate devices, by engaging the torsion channel of information. In this instance, individual consciousness and TCM in the Physical Vacuum will work as a unified whole.

81

These conclusions allow us to assume that individual consciousness, as a functional structure, incorporates not only the human brain but also the Physical Vacuum in the space surrounding the brain, structured as a torsion computing machine. In other words, it can be viewed as a unique kind of "bio-computer".

The ideas laid out above may suggest a non-controversial physical basis for the explanation of the phenomenon of perceptive transmission of information."

The level of consciousness is the level of the present. However, in order to correctly evaluate its place within the cosmic hierarchy, it is necessary to take into consideration that there is also the super-consciousness (the mono-world of the future) and the sub-consciousness (the proto-culture, or the past).

* * *

The events described in this chapter deserve to be given some thought and are in need of a conclusion. So let us try to summarize the unusual subject of subtle-matter events in their interconnection with our reality, the one we call our everyday life. About half a century ago, Folke Skoog, Professor at Wisconsin University, discovered a hormone called cytokinin, which carried the Life Program. This discovery was supported by experiments conducted by German scientist Kurt Motes, and later by other scientists, some of them from Russia. More recently, Olga Kulayeva, PhD in Biology, Professor at the Timiryazev Institute of the Physiology of Plants, carried out a series of experiments attempting to revive dying plants by "contaminating them with life". Her experiments proved to be a great success: lab methods allowed not only to launch the second and third life cycles of the plants but also to create a remarkable effect, when one half of a leaf injected with cytokonin became greener and younger, while the other half, which did not undergo hormonal stimulation, continued to age and eventually died. The conclusion drawn by Kulayeva is strict and logical: living organisms contain several programs of development and existence, some of them being minimal, other ones, maximal. The selection of these programs may be controlled.

Regretfully, or maybe fortunately, all efforts to apply this mechanism to humans failed. Some combination of biochemical and bio-energy conditions so far unknown to scientists prevents this idea from being implemented. The borderline dividing knowledge and cognition survived somehow. It is explained by the fact that human cells and the human body differ from those of plants because they have a far more developed system of informational control and regulation. Several dozen cytokonins responsible for performing specific and varied functions in the human body have currently been described.

Apparently, in his desire to obtain immortality the easy way, as if it was just a flu shot, Man has missed the point again. He is therefore doomed either to accept his lack of demiurgic abilities or to learn how to make his desires commensurate with his fundamental vision of the world, in other words, to ensure that his objective goals correspond to his level of spiritual development.

It must be said that all ancient philosophers and religious concepts of world order have emphasized the significance of this particular factor in their attempts to stop approaching death as something biologically inescapable. However, scientists, equipped by the relentless materialistic principle – to observe, to measure and to weigh – failed to understand what the Platos of every nation were intimating in all times.

As I ponder this phenomenon, I cannot help but recall the sarcastic verses of my good old friend Vladimir Noskov:

We storm the citadel of science. Knowing gives us might.
We must be strong to lead the masses to the light.
We ask the papers to explain creation of the worlds
In just a few brief phrases, sometimes even words.

In our studious effort the truth to lay bare,
We reach into the abyss but find nothing there.
The night makes sense because there is the day,
And particles will always near the nucleus stay.

But boisterous writers, as they try their best,
Are certain to devalue our efforts the truth to attest,
And the day will come as we vainly strive for fame
When death shows up our wasted lives to claim.*

Now, here is some relatively recent news from the biology department of the Moscow State University. Thanks to the activation of genes and bio-energetic coding, Alexander Burlakov and his team of researchers have managed to breed fish with two, four and even six heads. There are also species with six hearts and those with their vertebra bifurcated in ten places at the same time. The initiator of these frightful experiments openly admits that the mechanism of this transformation is still unclear to him. In this way he hopes to be able to transmit the necessary information (necessary for whom?) to various biological objects and

*This represents an original translation.

84

thus introduce the traits pre-programmed by the researches.

In order to understand a phenomenon in its complexity it is necessary to see it in its complexity as well, i.e., to view it as a whole, not broken up into fragments, specks and grains by means of modern diagnostics. I can't help but recall the words of the priest Felix of Notre-Dame who a century and a half ago addressed these issues, for which present-day scientists still don't have an answer today. In his work "Mystery and Science" the priest wrote: "Who has measured the bottomless depth of a speck of sand? Science has studied that speck for a thousand years, looking at it from various angles; it divides it into smaller and smaller fragments; it tortures it with more and more experiments; it bothers the speck with endless questions, hoping to extort from it the final answer about its secret structure, asking the same question with unstoppable curiosity: 'Do we have to divide you into infinitely small fragments?' Then, hovering over this abyss, science finds itself in a quandary; it stumbles and feels overwhelmed; its head spins, and it blurts out in utter desperation: 'I DON'T KNOW!'

...But if you are in such a fog about the origin and secret nature of a speck of sand, what makes you think you have any intuitive knowledge about the origin of any living creature? Where does life emerge from in this creature? Where does it start? What makes up the fundamental principle of life?"

Questions such as these may humble any honest academic. Invincible in areas of knowledge that they have studied and know very well, researchers are at a loss every time they are presented with proof that the edifice of materialism lacks the most important element – a material foundation. Is there any possibility at all to see the invisible? Not to see it through an electronic microscope, which is barely able to track subtle-matter processes at the level of energy and information, but to view it in its complexity, with all its interconnections and interdependencies? Clearly, the extraordinary phenomenon of clairvoyance has been known for a long time. All people of genius possessed this gift to a certain extent. Any human being is able to develop his abilities so that he can reach the level of perception beyond subjective impressions.

For instance, great Goethe, who wanted to increase his understanding of plant life, would visualize the entire cycle of plant development before going to bed, following every respective stage from seed to seed. By using such methods the poet ultimately obtained the ability to see the work of gigantic forces of nature in the simplest, most familiar objects.

Naturally, the question may arise: How objective is what clairvoyant people see? Fortunately, there is already an answer to this question.

The American Jodi Ostroy, a professional artist, came up with a convincing way to demonstrate the objectiveness of inner vision. Sectional cuts of a variety of biological objects – leaves, flesh, skin, rocks, and so forth – were placed under a powerful microscope. Without looking at the eyepiece of the microscope, Jodi depicted their internal structure on paper to the minutest detail, after which committee members could verify that the drawing was extremely accurate.

Igor Vitalievich Arepyev, one of the leading specialists at the Center of Bio-informational Technology, took a similar test. Here is how it happened. Andrei Igorevich Poletayev, who headed the research group of molecular and cell technologies at the *Engelhardt* Institute of Molecular Biology, asked Arepyev to describe the appearance of the human cell culture placed in Petri dishes. After the test was completed, the images of the cultures placed under the microscope were taken for analysis. It became obvious that the clairvoyant described all the features with perfect accuracy and, in fact, was right on the subject. Moreover, because of the psychophysical impact, the cycles of cell mitosis in the course of this experiment were decreased more than twice (from 28 hours to only 12).

For some conventional scientists and scholars such results are tantamount to the collapse of the Universe, the world order they fully understood and in which they explained almost everything. Alas, all that was accumulated, grain by grain, was reduced to grains once again when the invisible became visible.

The world is not what we are used to seeing. The eyes are deceiving because they don't present to you everything you need to know to find the truth. To see, to measure, to weigh – represents the path of an ant which is using its legs to palpate every grain of the planet it lives on in an effort to understand the surrounding world. Mind you, someone created this world, placing there this particular ant and also humans, who are following the ant's cognitive pattern.

Thus, there should be someplace where it is possible to find global knowledge on how worlds are created, as well as ants and humans. This global knowledge will make it possible to create, correct, transform, and cure any diseases without the danger of provoking new ones. No, this is not a fantasy world of a runaway imagination. Today it represents the everyday reality of informational technologies. The annotation to G.P. Grabovoi's book, "The Unified System of Knowledge" (Moscow, Kalashnikov Publishers, 1999) says the following: "Grigori Petrovich Grabovoi brings people back to life following their biological death. He also cures stage 4 cancer and stage 4 AIDS, when many organs have been affected. He cures all kind of diseases naturally. Thus, G.P. Grabovoi implements the principle of non-dying as the method of preventing a global catastrophe that threatens the entire world. The recovery cycle can be performed remotely, without any distance limitations.

The program includes the removal of manmade disasters of global magnitude and also control over events, by means of redirecting them from critical situations.

In every phase of his work G.P. Grabovoi uses his abilities of clairvoyance and remote control of information. Advanced digital diagnostics is provided additionally."

Grabovoi has a PhD in physics and math, and he is also a Doctor of Biology. He is not some kind of shaman with a tambourine or a sorcerer with chains dangling around his body. He is someone who is creating a new reality and new science today that are not opposed to religion. He writes:

"I perceive any external event, including one taking place in the future, as some form of information. Elements in the composition of form are intertwined, as a kind of mosaic, within the structure of DNA. Looking very closely at the protein form of matter organization (for instance, DNA structure) and the non-protein form, such as that of a rock, it is logical to arrive at the conclusion that the reflection of the protein form looks like oscillations of a crystal structure, that of rock, for instance (which is of non-protein form), this is, oscillations of the environment of non-living matter from the viewpoint of man. On the other hand, this is conditional. Many people perceive the world 'the right way'. But such a 'right' perception is conditional because points of view vary. I base my reasoning on the conventional definition of living and non-living matter. I intentionally limit certain fields of information within simple forms for the sake of faster understanding, using terms widely adopted at high schools, colleges and universities. This explains why some of the concepts I introduce take into consideration the current level of comprehension in its associative form. But at the spiritual level every human being understands it because his or her salvation is at stake.

*Secondly – **I offer knowledge at the level of cognition of the spirit.** First of all, I emphasize the rule: **the radiance of the crystal structure of non-living matter occurs in the vibrational form of information, comparable to the vibrational information emitted by living beings.** Thus, it is essential to define what is meant by living and non-living matter. In the present system of control such a definition does not exist. In the management of the environment, even more so, in controlling the future, **there is the concept of control over the external object of information, where only the interaction with some reactive environment is defined. The speed of such control is determined by the degree of the reaction.* "*

There are people for whom all this sounds like total nonsense and there are others who see this as a clear path to the truth. Why is it possible to have such a polarity of conclusions? In order to understand the passage from the book quoted above, it is necessary to possess the gift of clairvoyance, which, unfortunately, is still quite rare among people. If you are lucky to have such abilities, you will not perceive it as total nonsense but, rather, as a precisely marked crossing to new heights of knowledge. You don't have to ascend them, the choice is all yours. But if you decline this opportunity, don't hold it against those who were adventurous enough to climb to the top and reach something you have always dreamed about – immortality, non-dying and a happy meaningful life.

Each person is aware that he or she is born, lives, and then dies. But only a few of them know that they arrive in this world, do their work, leave, and then come back again when it is required. Such words as "to be born" and "to arrive", "to die" and "to come back" are similar in meaning but not identical. Indeed, very few people know how to escape the dark embrace of death, which erases the memory of incarnation, how to overcome the beastly essence of the material used for the implementation of the global project of creation (in His image and likeness) of the new highly intelligent creature of the Universe called the Cosmic Man. Let me tell you this: there is not a single living being, where human or animal, that won't come back after having departed from this world. But who remembers about it?

It is pointless though to ask death, how to win immortality. Death will lie. There is a far better teacher who, besides, knows considerably more and is always extremely close to every one of us – and this is our soul. The problem is how our consciousness can get access to the knowledge of the soul, how it can hear its voice and learn to see what it is able to show. Jesus was referring to the human soul when he said: "He who has eyes to see, let him see; he who has ears to hear, let him hear." He will see it and he will hear it... Jesus is talking about people with the skill of clairvoyance, about the ability to see the revealed and unrevealed world at the same time, to see the Earthly Kingdom and the Heavenly Kingdom.

True, sometimes knowledge reveals itself as the result of stress or tension, alternating with relaxation. And then you already have a different life, a different world, happiness, respect, honor, and various awards... But those who receive all these awards and rewards, as a rule, don't have a clue that the human soul is like a world library, where all the editions on all the areas of knowledge from the past, present and future have been stored from the beginning of time. Visit this library, if you can. And read its book collection, if you can of course.

It is the opinion of many contemporary scientists that information is the primary foundation of the world. Most would agree that the Universe is informational. Still, just as it was wrong to religiously believe in the primacy of matter, it would be equally wrong to award the same primary role to information. Yes, it is the primary foundation but not the only one. The basic principle of the Creator states: "There is diversity in unity and unity in diversity."

A hundred years ago the prominent physicist Max Plank opened the window into the world of quanta, a reality previously unknown to mankind. To be more precise, Plank rediscovered this world. Don't forget that two and a half thousand years ago the ancient philosopher Democritus of Abdera wrote about atoms as indivisible, eternal, indestructible, impermeable, and differing in form, position in emptiness and size. He also stated that they move in different directions, and both individual objects and entire worlds are created in the vortex of its chaotic movement. For most people, it remains a mystery how this ancient scientist who had no electronic microscopes or any other sophisticated tools of research managed to figure out the qualities and role of atoms or even their very existence. But as soon as we utter the word CLAIRVOYANCE, by now familiar to most, the veil of mystery and misunderstanding over this historic phenomenon is lifted.

It took twenty five centuries before the discovery made by just one instrument, i.e., the human consciousness, was confirmed by devices, experiments and the combined scientific work of thousands of researches. Based on this comparison alone, it is not difficult to decide, what method of research is more effective in terms of understanding the world. Nevertheless, we would like to avoid contrasting spiritual tools of cognition to physical tools and intuitive knowledge to scientific knowledge because each of these paths taken separately represents a "road to nowhere". We presume that the real world has permanent physical presence in some given point of the reality of this world.

What does it mean? Each of these three basic components of the Universe – the soul, the sprit, and the consciousness – is manifested through their own form, or as the ancient sages would say – their house. At the same time, they form an indivisible whole. The very concept of Man constitutes a sum total of the three above mentioned components. The *Dead Sea* Scrolls linked to the Essences and discovered in secret repositories on the shores of the Dead Sea, stated: "Don't try to find the law in your books with scriptures, for the law is life, while the scriptures are dead."

What does it mean if applied to the concept of information? First of all, it means that in the personal world of human beings, information represents the amount of knowledge obtained in the process of transmitting the mass of consciousness into the mass of perception as a result of the active impact of the spirit. Information is recorded in material substances but is not part of them or seen as identical to them. In other words, information on something is not that "something".

In any object of information it is possible to single out the field of this object's creation, which represents the static phase of reality. When you perceive the object, the dynamic phase of reality follows, which is the one that activates information with the participation of the spirit, as we said before. Any object reflects itself into the field of information, because, on the one hand, it represents something like a physical mirror, but on the other hand, it is spiritual in nature, so the concept of matter is not used anymore. Life is built and developed on a spiritual basis. The soul, as the universal plan of existence, is projected onto the reality of the physical plane. This process of projection represents both an act of creation and (or) a process of control over what has already been created. Information is the point of global connections revealed in the consciousness; in other words, it is the projection of the soul into the reality of the physical plane. Thus, the dynamics of information manifests itself

92

as the change of its flow or form. Time is the transformer of space in the dynamic processes involving information. The range of activity of time is from eternity to infinity.

The projection process is bi-directional. The scenarios of implementation in the physical plane are recorded and reflected into the consciousness. In situations when they correspond to the upper matrix structures of the soul, the images driven by the power of spirit from the consciousness are transferred to the plane of the soul, thus enhancing and expanding the treasury of universal knowledge.

We used to say that God dwells in every human being but now we can say for sure that we all dwell in God as well.

Why is it so important to know this, particularly now? Unfortunately, mankind in its development, which took a primarily technocratic turn, reached a point when its impact on the environment has become global. The environment is a living organism, and, what's more, the one we all live in. We act like cancer cells in this organism, without even understanding that the environment we inhabit is of psychophysical nature, and because of the universal ties, which connect it with any internal object, it has to respond immediately and adequately to any emerging situation, including the option when it has to sever its ties with the object endangering its existence. This is true even if the object in question is Man, i.e., the embryonic cell of a new universal body. We will all be mortal only until our consciousness continues initiating dangerous ideas, which threaten the body of the Universe, and until, blinded by these ideas, we continue provoking insane actions. It is so true that we cannot expect any mercy from Nature after what we have done to her. If we recognize our place, significance and responsibility, then the period of troubles for each particular individual and for all of mankind will come to an end.

With the help of clairvoyance we found out without much difficulty that the life of the cell nucleus is designed for a thousand years! In other words, the work of a normal cell is designed for a thousand years, if not more! This is very close to perpetual motion. The energy of a cell can be replenished, and its body rejuvenated. Of course, we should understand that such immortal existence should be supported by certain conditions of being in ETERNITY.

So why is quite the opposite taking place? Why do we live a short and miserable life instead of living for a thousand years? Here is the answer: because of the erroneous orientation of our consciousness and our ego-centric nature, when a person cares only about himself, trying to grab as much as possible for his own use. This works in his favor until a certain point. Sometimes even for a long time by the standards of human life. I wish people knew what a high price they will have to pay for their selfish-ness, self-interest and desire to care only about their own needs! It is not that difficult to draw some obvious comparisons. What does a person do when he suddenly feels pain? He starts thinking how he can get rid of this discomfort. He will be lucky if he doesn't need to take radical measures or the insane behavior of his cells gone amok doesn't lead to a fatal outcome.

Indeed, selfish people who live only for themselves are the cancer cells of the universal body. Let's take a look and see what can be done in the fight against these parasitic structures.

A cancer cell differs from a healthy one because the structure of reason is broken in its nucleus. In other words, it doesn't think properly and, as a result, does not function properly. It is kooky, or nutty as fruitcake, as people say. We can see this spiral. It is crumpled and ripped. Alas, such a cell is incapable of creating anything; the only thing it knows how to do is to live as a parasite on something created by others. It gets the bug of selfishness. Looks like a very typical life situation doesn't it? That is why such a cell sucks the energy of others. There are also neutral cells, which are neither fish nor fowl, so to say. They represent the "electorate". The cancer cell exploits their neutrality. It lures them and breaks the spirals of consciousness.

What is the right thing to do in this case? Should we, perhaps, perform resection, as traditional medicine recommends, or move to chemotherapy? Let me tell you upfront – it's not just a bad choice, it's the worst.

Igor and I approach the problem differently. We enter the cancer cell, the one which initiated the whole trouble. The internal part of the nucleus is black and hard as rock. It is repulsive even to look at it to say nothing of dealing with it. But the job has to be done. So we fix the spiral and remove the ruptures if we detect them. We destroy the record of the disease, and write down the information on health and harmonious development instead. The internal surface of the cell nucleus becomes redder and starts to come back to life. This is no longer cancer but a benign tumor. After that everything is even simpler: a couple of corrective measures and the patient will recover. Hundreds of people came to us with the diagnosis of cancer, and we were able to help most of them.

Where exactly does the new life of a human being start in any place whatever? It starts just from one fertilized cell, from a zygote. The person may be small – earthly or big – cosmic but the process of development will fundamentally be the same. An average Joe and the Man-Universe (all ancient religions of the world have for centuries unambiguously referred to such a gigantic organism as existing in the Universe) in principle have to go through the same process of development. Once you assume this to be true, you will see how strikingly all the basic stages in the development of Man and the Universe coincide. Naturally, we have to take into account the time flow correlation in organisms that are so different in their size.

To make things easier, let's take an intermediate parameter, say, the planets of our Solar System. Taking into consideration that besides revolving around its center, the system also rapidly moves ahead, these two parameters of motion create something like a plasma body of our stellar structure. It is also necessary to recognize that nobody is able to see the entire body of the Solar System correctly because of the barrier of the space dimension. Strange as it might seem, the Solar System partially exists in another dimension, one inaccessible to regular perception. Instruments known as thermal imaging devices depict a human being as a structure of spots of various colors. Because of our perception deficiency this is the way we see our stellar system. Clairvoyance helps us to overcome the barriers of space dimension, thereby allowing us to perceive a different structure: an ensemble of cells. In such vision, the Sun acts as the leading cell controlling all the processes of this particular segment of the Universe.

Assuming that our assertion is correct, it becomes clear why ancient science always made a point of emphasizing the sameness of what is above and what is below. The worlds are stacked inside each other like nesting dolls. The Universe, like atoms, molecules and organs, contains within it people, planets, stars and galaxies. Not only are we inseparable but also very important for each other's existence. After all, it essentially expresses the unity of the sets: we can't exist without each other; we are one, although we also remain individualities.

A totally different ethics of existence follows from this, as well as a different vision of mankind's role in the destiny of the Universe, our highest body of being.

As far as the recession of galaxies is concerned, this is a proven fact.

This shouldn't come as a surprise since it always happens when the Universe inhales. The galaxies may start moving closer together when the Universe exhales. Our galaxy, the Milky Way, is positioned somewhere close to the heart of the gigantic Man-Universe. We are surrounded by the structures of the heart and lungs. Inhaling just once translates into multiple years, and so does exhaling. This gives plenty of time for many astrophysicists to successfully defend their thesis, proving the presence of cyclical processes in our galaxy and Universe.

That is why people say: "The one who discovered himself has also discovered the world and the one who discovered the world has also found his self..."

Nobody placed any restrictions upon human beings, neither the Creator himself, nor anyone else. Humans restrict themselves by their own behavior. That explains how AIDS emerged, putting the human mind to sleep. Such somnolence is an obstacle preventing Man from obtaining knowledge – knowledge of immortal existence.

God the Father provides the ideas and information. God the Son gives matter and consciousness, and God the Holy Spirit fills everything with life. This is how the cell is created, which is the basis of everything.

Get to know the cell and you will advance to the next step in your evolution; you will see the world not in the narrow range of electromagnetic radiation but in the divine radiance of totally new energies, formerly unknown to you. This is when you will finally see the Temple. It won't be the Temple people built out of stone but the Temple that dwells inside you.

Two global systems compete for dominance in the Universe. The first system is the creation of Universal selfishness. It causes diseases and illusions of self-deception. Its goal is to break Man and to convince him that he has a flawed nature and is impotent to make him a pawn in the pyramid of service to self. The second system which bears with it the heavenly light, states quite the opposite: nothing can harm Man created in the image and likeness of God.

Even space and time represent a construction of consciousness and are secondary to consciousness and the soul, which are potentially equal to God Himself. We are accustomed to looking down at our feet. One who looks at his feet is unlikely to stumble. But how is it possible to see your goal if you constantly look down at your feet? How is it possible to see the space of the spirit and the space of soul hidden behind the materialistic curtain of our physical world?

Mind you, this is the path to Immortality, at the top of which Man will discover his own true power. There he will find out his great destination, and he will learn that there is no greater name in the entire Universe than his simple name that he always wanted to be proud of but was deliberately discouraged. This name is MAN.

> To his times a man should never bow
> But firmly stand with his lofty vow,
> Whatever happens, be a man.
>
> *(Sofia Parnok)*

Chapter 2

The consequences of the strange match, which was to decide the fate of the Earth for the next several hundred years, instantly influenced the cosmic computer, towering over the North Pole. Above all, their impact was felt on the top platforms at the apex of this mysterious subtle-matter structure, where events are created by people just as much as people are guided by events.

First, the topmost platform became very complicated. Its construction was now similar to a telescoping antenna, in which the outer shell hides the inner development potential – six other platforms that could be thrust out into the Cosmos. At its highest point there were steps and another disc-shaped device, where it was possible to stand and get a very good look at the surrounding area.

Four planes hung in limbo across the way from the steps corresponding to the four Earthly directions of the Bardo – the intermediate space separating the manifested and unmanifested worlds. These four areas correspond to the elements Fire, Air, Water and Earth. All of them are equal to each other and represent simultaneously a mechanism and a symbol. If you look down at them, they are like hourglasses with dark sand or dark energy in one of them, and light sand in the other. They are also the Sun and the Moon with an equal sign between them.

Each of these symbols, in turn, is not uniform in its meaning either, and has changeable internal positions, or potentials. When they change, this alters the situation on Earth. Take the Sun, for instance. One of its sides warms without burning and gives life as the sacred fire in Jerusalem, but the other can burn everything down as an unforgiving and punishing force. The Moon, too, has its own mechanisms and opportunities: it may have something to give and something to take away. At high tide, there is an increasing number of new births, and at low tide, on the contrary, more people die.

Let us try to analyze what happened.

Why is the planetary computer located over the poles? I think this can be explained not only by the processes of electromagnetic separation. The enormous amount of water and ice at the base of the subtle-matter structure also plays a very important role.

The North Pole predominantly consists of water on the verge of converting into ice. The water molecule has an amazing geometry with two hydrogen atoms located on one plane in front of an oxygen atom. As a result, an excess of positive charges contained in the protons of the nuclei emerged in the area of their molecular location in space. In order to restore the energy balance the atom of oxygen was compelled to concentrate four electrons on the opposite side of its nucleus, thereby creating a negative charge. A dipole structure was thus created with an ideal ratio of 3:4:5, i.e., the famous Egyptian triangle.

From the side of the foundation, there exist an unimaginably large number of small pyramids, which create, due to the geometry of their form, the basic long-range static torsion matrix with central symmetry. It is a system of wave packets of electrons and protons with a nested organization and, therefore, self-compensated. A well-ordered structure emerges, which interacts with cosmic radiation, the collective consciousness of mankind or separate individuals, creating what has recently become known as the informational field of the Earth.

In fact, it is a super-computer, in which interactions are predominantly informational, not energy driven in nature.

Most surprisingly, the planetary super-computer was created precisely with the expectation that there would be people with a true consciousness or one approaching such a state, that is, people with clairvoyance, in order to support the new evolutionary stage of human development with the passage of the so-called barriers. Incidentally, the levels of consciousness reflect the stages of evolution very clearly: the barrier of the ocean, the barrier of land and the barrier of the sky. Barriers are also interrelated with the structure of the space-time continuum. Consequently, the transition into the fourth dimension is primarily a problem of overcoming the three-dimensional paradigm of consciousness, the transition from the world of the body to the world of the soul.

This doesn't imply rejecting the physical body, as some esoteric writers assert, due to the shift in the evolutionary path towards subtle-matter planes of existence. The body hasn't exhausted its potential for self-development. Moreover, it is just beginning to use its possibilities. But these authors are right in that its further development will be directly linked to spiritual development, i.e., the development of the soul's composition.

And the antithesis to man's mortality also lies along this course, along the direction of the transformation of lower forms of life in the highest ones.

Many people perceive the soul as something ephemeral, ethereal and unreal. But through clairvoyance, which is now available to so many, it is easy to determine that the human soul has a definite organized structure and mechanisms of influence, very powerful ones at that, upon the surrounding reality. We don't have to look far: one such example is the above-mentioned planetary computer, which towers over the Earth's North Pole like an indescribably beautiful blue radiance having the shape of the Temple.

As I already said, there is another similar computer over the South

Pole. But due to the fact that the mainland of the South Pole is covered with water, by now fully crystallized into ice, the pyramid base does not represent the golden section. The energies accumulated over the South Pole are negative and the form is more reminiscent of a castle and not the Temple. The color of the emitted subtle-matter radiance when viewed from the outside is red, like the planet Mars.

Ancient sources also testify to the fact that spiritual existence is not opposed to the life of the body. Here is what St. John the Theologian saw on the island of Patmos: "On the Lord's Day I was in the Spirit, and I heard behind me a loud voice like a trumpet, which said: "I am the Alpha and the Omega, the First and the Last…"

I turned around to see the voice that was speaking to me. And when I turned I saw seven golden lamp stands, and among the lamp stands was someone like the Son of Man, dressed in a robe reaching down to his feet and with a golden sash around his chest. The hair on His head was white like wool, as white as snow, and His eyes were like blazing fire. His feet were like bronze glowing in a furnace, and His voice was like the sound of rushing waters. In His right hand He held seven stars, and coming out of His mouth was a sharp, double-edged sword. His face was like the sun shining in all its brilliance…

Then he placed his right hand on me and said: "Do not be afraid. I am the First and the Last. I am the Living One; I was dead, and now look, I am alive forever and ever! And I hold the keys of death and Hades" (Revelations: 1:10-18).

This vision reflects the hierarchy of the Solar system. The seven golden lamp stands are the seven sacred planets which are involved in the management of our space.

St. John the Theologian himself emphasizes that he was "in the Spirit".

And despite this he was physically alive. Now, and it is clearly visible, a balance has been established between the Light and the Dark, between plus and minus, between good and evil, all of which was disrupted in the past. Harmony represents the will of God, which is not in God Himself, nor identical to Him. Sounds a bit convoluted? I understand how it seems, but then again – it all depends on how you look at it. If the new reckless actions of the Dark forces do not lead to any new, unpredictable consequences, the balance will remain, and that, in principle, is the most preferable condition for evolutionary development. From here, from high above, one can clearly see what is happening on both the Earth's physical and subtle-matter plane. One can see our twelve boxes, each containing a portion of global knowledge divided according to its direction. Here is the seventh box, where we had previously treated people. A little farther is the magical box, the one due to which we barely avoided starting Armageddon before the right time.

We watched how it works, how the Dark use it to influence people and to stab them in the back, dealing them a crushing blow. This last expression is not accidental. One function of the magic box actually is stabbing people in the back. The Dark select in the surroundings of the individual defined as a target someone who is close to him or her – a relative, friend or acquaintance through whom the impact is directed and applied. The function of such a person is to act as a mirror that receives the energy-information bullet and diverts it to the target. Not everyone is suitable for the role of a magic mirror. Only the negative acts a person has committed in life, allow the Dark forces to use him or her in their projects. Their hellish "accounting office" scrupulously collects information about the actions of people, using them as a base for its earthly manipulations.

We could now see, through the technology of magic, how people became transformed into devices from hell that threaten the life and health of others. Sometimes people act this way deliberately but more often not. An energy bullet is simply placed in their hands, which they then direct at the target when a convenient moment presents itself. Before accomplishing his mission such a man-mirror suffers and feels very bad. He feels pain in the hand, where he carries the diseases and adverse events designed to hit those dear to him. His soul, which sees what is happening but can't shout loud enough to reach the conscious-ness of that person, is also in pain.

But there is protection against such attacks. First of all, no doubt, knowledge is your best protection. It may be used to analyze the situ-ation and change it in a positive direction. Of course, in this case the Dark forces feel peeved since they failed to fulfill their task, but that's all there is to it. In the end, everything is done by the hands of the peo-ple themselves, and they are the ones responsible if anything should go wrong. Yet this, as it turned out, can also change after a certain point in time. And the time is now, as we can tell from current events. Those who have always persecuted others and poisoned their lives, suddenly, literally overnight, have themselves become victims of persecution and severe punishment. Incidentally, this is a serious challenge for the win-ners and a good reason to refrain from taking extreme measures with respect to the vanquished.

But changes occurred not only with the levels and platforms, they also occurred in our lives. Igor and I went back to school and once again became students.

It was an unusual school located right in the Cosmos. A large cube hung among its infinite spaces with four walls on the sides, a floor and a ceiling. Outside there was black infinity interspersed with colorful stars, constellations and galaxies, and a gaping chasm underneath the cube. The energy torr of the down-flowing streams began immediately below the plane of the strange cosmic institution. Inside one found the regular classroom setting of an ordinary school. Three rows of desks – five on the right, five on the left and five in the middle. The ten on either side were occupied.

The class was a point for gradual build-up of pace. On the right and the left there were exit doors but there wasn't one in the center – just a school board. You could call it a blackboard only figuratively speaking. It was composed of space and it's very dangerous. But there was also knowledge hidden there. The teacher said that no one ever returned from this space. The blackboard served as a boundary: once you crossed it you could fall into the chasm. And as I said, no one has ever returned from the depths of that abyss. That explained why no one wished to be seated in the middle. Those attending the school weren't some simple folk: on the right was the upper crust of the Dark, with angels and archangels representing the Light being on the left. Of the fourteen students of the school only two were people – Igor and I. Even so, we stood in the aisle, not knowing what seat to take.

There were actually available seats: one on the right and one on the left. But we didn't want to be separated and held hands like little children. We had three cards with us, with which we were allowed into the school. All of them light ones. But one wasn't quite right. It was because of that goal which we told the Dark we recognized but we never confirmed it with our signatures in writing. We stood there for a while, and then sat down, what else could we do? So we sat at a vacant desk in the center of the class. And immediately there were whispers rustling through the rows. There were no sounds made – those were ideas, which we by then already learned to read:

– They've got to be crazy! They sat over the Abyss of Daat.* Now they can't get out of the class either to the right or left. They could've just rearranged the desks.

Igor and I exchanged glances.

– Are we staying here? – he asked.

– I'll do what you do, – I answered.

And I thought to myself: "Whatever happened let it be... Grigori Petrovich taught us that we must control events in any situation. And the more adverse the conditions, the more valuable the experience gained. The point is, if it works once, it always will."

The Teacher appeared – a stern-looking old man with severe eyes. He looked at all of us closely, not so much at our faces as at the essence of those who came here for higher knowledge.

– Only once in two thousand years can someone come to study in this class, – he began the lesson. – Those who sit on the right and those who sit on the left, should they discover that they lack the strength to continue their path to higher knowledge, have the right to terminate their training. They can exit through the doors that you see to the right and to the left of you. Those who sat in the middle, – this time he was directly referring to Igor and me, – have no right to interrupt their training and leave the class.

Our hearts skipped a beat at his words, of course, but we didn't let it show. The old man paused a little and then drew his conclusion, after analyzing the slight inner agony that took place inside Igor and me:

– Your courage is commendable. But courage alone is not enough here. You will need to have the necessary knowledge to complete the class

---

* Daat or Daath, or Da'at means "knowledge" in Hebrew and is the location (the mystical state) where all ten Sephiroth in the Tree of Life are united as one.

and get one step closer to the Creator. God speed...

– And we with Him, – the two of us answered in unison.

The old sage went to the blackboard. And it instantly came alive with twinkling lights, like a TV screen, filling up with diagrams, numbers and words.

– In this class, cognition becomes transformed into knowledge, – the Teacher began his lecture. – The path starts here but does anyone of you know where it leads? Right here, in this room where you are now sitting, there are, in fact, not one but many different spaces. Perhaps ten of them, perhaps a hundred... But do any of you see something else, except for the walls that surround you on all four sides? – He went silent giving anyone from the students the opportunity to answer but nobody took the initiative.

– Why do both the Light and the Dark study in the same class? It's because the spiral of evolution develops most effectively under the influence of two opposing forces. But did those whom the Creator commissioned to control these forces understand their task properly? Why is there such a horrible situation on Earth right now? Mind you, this is not simply one of the planets of the Universe. The Throne of the Creator is here, and therefore the Earth is the center of everything. So why have you, who have been elected and endowed with powers, come together in mortal combat, instead of ensuring the harmonious development of what has been entrusted to your care? Why have you ruined the plan of the Creator so irresponsibly and allowed the situation to deteriorate so badly that the Almighty had to personally intervene in the course of events?

All were silent, listening to the Teacher's accusations. No one, neither the Dark nor the Light looked at each other. Only we, Igor and I, looked around at our strange schoolmates with childlike curiosity. There, on the right (as soon as we sat at our desk, the left and the right were reversed,

107

naturally) sat a huge archangel with mighty wings on his back. A halo glowed above his head. These were energies, which he could use as a tool or a weapon. If it connected the energy of the halo with his hand, then the hand could bring down a mountain.

Those to the left of us didn't lack power either. They knew the past and could even see events before they occurred. Not everywhere, of course, only those on Earth. Up here, at the top, they lose this advantage.

– Let's examine the plan of the Creator one more time, – the old man urged us. And once again pictures appeared on the board. We saw the Earth as if separated by an invisible glass wall. Some people lived well, always had fun and succeeded in everything. The others were always unwell, and they were punished with failure for all their present and past wrongdoings. One half of the Earth was ruled by Death. And we could see it – an essence carrying a scythe, which is able to change its appearance. Now it is a beautiful young woman, now an ugly horrible witch. It has many faces and uses it to deceive people.

But Life, oddly enough, is a man. He heals us, helps and supports us.

– Who wants to go out to the board? – the old man asked.

The mighty archangel, whom Igor and I had studied so impertinently, rose to his feet and went to the blackboard. We couldn't hear what he was saying. Apparently, this was secret as a confession. Suddenly, the glowing screen of the board became extended in the direction of the archangel and it drew him into itself with a guttural roar. He tried to resist, screaming. It was all to no avail – the space behind the board swallowed him, and he vanished in it forever.

After this tragic incident, several students to the left and right of us got up and hurriedly left the classroom. The old man accompanied them his wise gaze, not accusing anyone.

108

Igor and I sat in our seats with no thought of leaving the premises.

– What you just saw on the screen about the Earth represents the initial samples of creation. These are also classes, – the Teacher continued. – There are many classes and many nations. They think that they are living. And I think that they are learning. They still have lots of learning to do but it's OK – God has many days. Adam and Eve are the primary sources, created in God's image and likeness by the will of the Creator. They were allowed access to everything except the apple, which they were forbidden to touch. Why weren't they supposed to eat the apple? – the Teacher was now addressing me directly. And not knowing why, obeying some hidden source within me, I replied cheerfully:

– They shouldn't have eaten it because you can't destroy what you haven't learned how to create. If you bite off a piece of an apple created by another you cognize it. If you can create an apple by yourself – you know it. This is the difference between cognition and knowledge.

The old man didn't say anything. He simply looked. The board, too, didn't make any threatening movements in my direction. It flickered quietly and peacefully beside me with its dangerous screen.

– Adam and Eve were imbued with cosmic force. They had access to everything in the House of the Father. But they were attracted to the one and only thing that they weren't allowed to touch, – said the old man. – By tasting the apple, they prematurely gained their independence and what we have today. We have just seen the nations that descended from them. This was the first violation of the Creator's will, and as the result something that opposes Man appeared in the world. Man himself created this confrontation. He can now return to the Father only through a thorny path. It's because he left his Father's House, having no knowledge of the shortest path back. It is the path that you are now following. This path is

109

dangerous but straight as the flight of an arrow. Only those who walk the Path, get the opportunity to know their Family.

* * *

Parallel to celestial studies we studied what was happening on Earth. The things we were learning in this extraordinary class, lost somewhere in the depths of the Universe, compelled Igor and me to read a substantial number of special books. As a rule, they appeared in my house in some unusual way. More often than not, someone gave them to me at the right moment and the right place, either in person or through an acquaintance, telling me that it was absolutely essential to read them. As I read them, I invariably found in them topics that we were at that very time studying at the celestial school above the Daat Abyss.

As for the Abyss, here, too, not everything was completely clear. We knew its name but that was about all we knew about it. There were now fewer students in our class: another student, one of the Dark, went to the board never to return.

Those who exercised their right to leave the school over the Abyss transferred to the peripheral system of master classes. Its students weren't trained to rise high but they weren't meant to fall low either. Prudence – that's what was written on their faces. Well, this isn't the worst label in the world.

In addition to theoretical knowledge, there was also practical work we did. Nobody forced us. It was just that people came with their problems, and these usually weren't easy. And the things that we studied here were immediately confirmed in reality.

We could see how human DNA and chromosomes were obeying the impulses of our consciousness. Through clairvoyance it was easy to trace how cells and organs exchange energy, information and matter. This process is managed by consciousness through the pituitary gland. Therefore, it is through consciousness that one can set goals and achieve their implementation.

But what is the impulse that we use to initiate the intracellular transformation? It is energy, of course, but not energy alone. Otherwise, why is it that before we originate the impulse, we create an information code for the energy bullet prepared to fire and directed at the cell nucleus?

Codes, DNA and cells – "big science" has also changed its attitude to the subject. Listen to this.

"Not so long ago the concept of the code of the Universe was unimaginable. Its essence is as follows. It has been established that heredity depends on DNA and RNA, the molecules of which are encoded in such a way that makes it possible to determine the element of the code and its structure in any living organism. There are one or more key (bearing) elements that in various combinations form different code structures with different densities of information. Due to the law of conservation of information and its eternity, the code structures of materialized or dematerialized information manifest themselves as symmetrical and asymmetrical cell structures, which secure the balance of information processes, their properties and forms. One of the fundamental laws of information is the law of constancy of encoding and decoding in the information process, which secures information equilibrium as a consequence of the constancy of its materialization and dematerialization. Processes of different information environments of micro-and macrostructures of the Universe have their own code key that holds the secrets of various information processes" (I.I. Yuzvishin, "Informationology", Moscow, 1996, pp. 15 -17).

(Experts shouldn't feel irritated with the specific use of concepts and terms in this excerpt. In essence, this passage has a holographic meaning beyond its textual interpretation.)

In fact, Ivan Iosipovich Yuzvishin and I are speaking more or less about the same thing. Yuzvishin has actually made a very significant step forward compared to those positions that have until recently been advocated by "big science". Just one additional effort must be made to cross the gap between his discoveries and the Truth, that is, the Creator.

Encoding is carried out through words, ordinary words. And there is a reason for that. It has presently been revealed through the use of methods of linguistic genetics and mathematical linguistics that the nucleotide sequences of the DNA of chromosomes are speech-like structures that interact with people's consciousness and speech. The language of the genome (DNA of chromosomes) and human speech share common roots and a universal grammar.

One can imagine the genome as a biological construction that has a holographic memory and the ability to generate and recognize images. Therefore, there is a real opportunity for contact between consciousness and the subconscious mind through the chromosomal apparatus with the help of normal speech. Although to achieve success one still needs to know certain laws of building sequences of commands, i.e., the number of code words and their sequence in the information file transmitted by the impulse of consciousness.

Since consciousness is, in fact, the energy-information matrix and the genome has a wave (information) channel of communication between the word and speech-like structures, recorded in the genome, words can influence a particular control function of the pituitary gland and any other organ through an impulse. I will now try to tell you how we do this in practice...

112

We were brought a photo of a boy. The child's attending physician came to us for help once before, and she became convinced that there exist certain things she can't understand, which are nevertheless quite effective.

There was a cancerous tumor in the boy's right lung. However, the definition of a case as a "complicated one" now has a relative, rather than a literal meaning for us. In the past year, we have worked a lot with cancer patients.

None of them died, except for those who were pressurized by family and friends, or conventional medicine, forcing these people into treatment through chemotherapy, radiation and surgery. Everybody makes their own choice: what they have confidence in and what they doubt, and whether or not they believe in God – each of us chooses his or her own path. Faith is rewarded. Those who believed in God are healthy and happy. We have also noticed a certain pattern in our work: the more we are confronted with complex diseases and achieve positive results in conquering them, the more powerful and effective are the technologies to combat disease that are given to us.

Sometimes we try to look at the situation involving human relationships with viruses, epidemics and terminal diseases from a spiritual perspective, globally. We visualize it as some kind of trouble map. Moscow is not by any means an oasis on this map but rather a geopathic territory.

Of course, not all people in the capital are so very ill physically and spiritually. But the sorry situation in the state unequivocally confirms: a small number of them are exactly that. You shouldn't forget that every man is a cell of another organism – the body of the country, or of mankind as a whole. So when we fight against cancer, with whom are we fighting on a global scale? Whom are we resisting? Whom are we trying to save?

113

If we succeed in curing at least one cell of this vast body by the name of Russia it will make things better. And if we cure thousands, hundreds of thousands of cells this will give everyone hope that the country will not die.

Two thousand years ago Jesus tried to explain people the truth. But they didn't understand Him. "Awake!" He said. Whom was He addressing? It was the people's consciousness! They heard Him but they still couldn't understand. Even today they continue to be unable to read what is actually written in the Bible. The Bible speaks about IMMORTALITY. But who saw it there and who heard it?

Everyone was talking about everything under the Sun: about fate, about karma, about the hard life and the evil predicament. But Christ spoke of IMMORTALITY. And He even suggested the technology of how it could be achieved. Read the Bible again. Everything is achieved through the consciousness – an extended and structured consciousness.

Igor and I watched Christ reviving Lazarus. He used both the information and material plane. He used His consciousness to condense time and space into a point and formed the impulse of resurrection. After that the soul of Lazarus instantly found itself on the Earth as though it never even left.

What is the power of human consciousness and the mind!

The boy's father is sitting right here before me, looking into my eyes with timid hope: is it really possible to avoid the threat to his son's life as that woman doctor told him? He is in big business, one of the top people at the powerful Siberian division of Gazprom. He is used to being responsible for the fate of thousands of people. He doesn't accept the words "I can't". He has control over everything except for... Everything except for the ability to halt the tentacles of death, which are stretched out precariously not to someone else, not into his neighbor's house but towards his family, towards the creature most precious to him, his son. This man knows what the diagnosis of cancer means.

He understands that this is just the beginning. Even if he takes the recommendation of physicians to remove the affected part of the lung, this will only mean winning a bit of extra time, which can be described as a double negative: neither life nor death.

He has everything – power, money and hundreds of the best professionals. But neither he nor the people around him can do what he needs most right now. None of them can stop death approaching his son.

He is in a state of total confusion. He isn't sure that he can trust us, even though his friends told him about what we do. But his life-long experience is literally screaming: "How can these people help you? They aren't even doctors!" We can read these doubts in his mind.

I am working without Igor today. He left to spend a week with his family in his native Trosna. For nearly two years now he has been torn between his work in Moscow and his family who live in the Orel area.

I find it a lot harder to work without Igor. Each of us has his own strengths. He is extremely attentive to every detail of the diagnosis, which is essential for deciding on the right solution. My forte is intuitive insight about what should be done in each individual case. We would usually exchange two or three words, which is sufficient to establish a common solution. To sum up the essence of our interaction: it contains analysis and synthesis.

During days when Igor is unavailable, I team up with Sergei who is both Igor's student and mine. He is a very talented and promising young man. He tries his best and is always nervous when working with me. Now, too, as he conducts his diagnosis, his tells me what he can see in a breaking boyish voice.

– I see cancer cells in the upper part of the lung. The tumor is still small but the surrounding area is already darkening. The connections with the pituitary gland are disrupted.

The damaged tissue is a new foothold for the spreading of the disease. If I was working together with Igor, we would have formed a disk, starting by overwriting the program of the disease to the program of recovery in the cell nucleus on the DNA spiral. We would then initiate the impulse and send it to a point in the space of the archive of the child's subtle-matter structure. It is literally the boy's entire "dossier". The fact is that everyone has their point of archiving in the planetary subtle-matter structure to gather information about all the lives they have lived, all their memories, events and experiences. This is essentially an information copy of the person that has everything, literally everything that is related to a particular person over his endless existence but it is a static form of consciousness and perception. In its dynamics it appears on the Earth. However, its static nature is also quite relative, since the points of archiving are among the most important structures of our world and, moreover, they have the inner power for development and are elements of the world's transformation.

The momentum for recovery, built into such a point of archiving, immediately sets into motion the mechanism of energy transformations corresponding to the task, which then move to the level of the Soma, that is, to the physical body.

There is, however, one limitation in applying this technology: the momentum has to be powerful and instantaneous. In fact, it must overcome the barrier of the speed of light. The consciousness of an ordinary person is unable to jumpstart such a momentum. Too few neurons in the brain are activated from its dormant state and involved in this work. Moreover, one must be capable of forming something like a laser beam in the area of the so-called third eye with an effort of his will, bringing the work of the brain cells into a preliminary balanced or, as the physicists say, "coherent" state. It is still too early and risky to engage in something like that in a team with Sergei.

The fact is that when we scan the cancer tumor with our bio-scanning technology (totally safe for the patient, since it has the same nature as the entire body), we sort of "alarm the disease". You must remember that it has its own consciousness, intellect and instinct of self-preservation. Therefore, it instantly becomes agitated. So if we implement active measures against it, the information structure of the disease will attempt to hide in the same place, where we aim to transfer information on how to recover, that is, precisely in the person's point of archiving. This is founded on a simple calculation: after a certain period of time when it is at a disadvantage, the information of the disease will return into the body and continue its work. It will continue, leaving serious damage in the person's design.

That is why the crisis of present-day conventional medical technologies has become so acutely felt in recent years: they fail to take into account the informational component of the disease. Even if they did that, they would still be unable to introduce the healing information at the person's point of archiving (the information area, with external statics and internal dynamics) with a speed faster than the speed of light (and this speed is required to jumpstart the momentum). Such devices and equipment simply don't exist now and probably won't in the future. Man alone is able to perform such "miracles" when he develops himself spiritually, because the whole world around us is created with the help of consciousness and, therefore, it is oriented towards consciousness as well.

All the communications of the world and all its interactions are focused

117

strictly on Man. That is why preparing people for their space mission takes such a long time and is so difficult. That is why the word "responsibility" is defining in the transmission of higher cosmic technologies, and that is why those who are allowed access to the perfect knowledge of the Universe go through such a harsh and thorough selection process in the mysteries of initiations and specific life trials. I know, based on my past experience, that as soon as we start to rewrite the history of the disease in the DNA, the information of the disease immediately removes itself from the affected area and starts to climb up to the point of archiving. But its speed is slower than that of the thought – an impulse of consciousness. Therefore, it ends up being literally a sprint competition. If the information of the disease arrives first at the point of archiving – that's it, we won't be able to beat it. It will hide and wait for the next opportune moment. The challenge, then, lies in getting ahead of it.

Sergei is still on the learning curve towards similar technologies. So we choose the option that requires less speed and is more appropriate to the situation. I suggest it to Sergei:

–You told me that the connections between the affected area and the pituitary gland are disrupted... So it means the latter doesn't see the chaos that the cancerous tumor is creating in the boy's lung, does it?

– That's true, – Sergei confirms.

– And if we show that to the pituitary gland, what do you think will happen?

– That will be soooo cool! – my assistant's face lights up joyously with youthful spontaneity. – And how will we show it?

– Draw the red arrow of anxiety from the pituitary gland to the tumor.

– Is it OK to do that? – Sergei asks.

- Go ahead.

118

After changing the ray's silver color to red, Sergei draws a clear line from the pituitary gland to the affected area.

Done. The pituitary gland saw the havoc created in the body and immediately proceeded to take protective action. Sergei delighted in observing the beginning of "warfare" and reported the situation:

– The signals from the pituitary gland are received by the thyroid gland. The immune system has been activated. Defender cells are moving towards the tumor. They surrounded the darkening tissue on all sides and are literally devouring it. They are just tearing the cancer cells apart and swallowing them like wolves eating their prey.

– Well, it isn't wolves and it isn't prey, – I correct Sergei's dramatic analogies.

– Of course not, – Sergei agrees succinctly. – Still, wow, you should see how they are ripping them apart.

A week later, the boy's father came to thank us. The virtual battle with the disease ended with his son's very real recovery. This time he asked us to help him personally: he had a whole bunch of chronic diseases.

Two weeks later, he brought a number of his relatives to our Center. As they say, it was just the beginning... This person does not need us to explain why and how we were able to achieve recovery. He simply tried our methods on himself and his loved ones. Now he isn't perplexed by our weird technique of treatment at a distance, or lack of equipment, or the fact that we don't prescribe tons of pills and use a circular saw to cut off the diseased organ. He sees the most important thing: our work results in actual healing. And healing is something everyone needs, even physicians who take it upon themselves to treat others, sometimes not being able to heal themselves.

* * *

The world which we inhabit is a world of interdependencies. No one is free: no man is free of Nature, the Earth isn't free of the Sun or the Sun isn't free of the Universe. Man and Nature alike use the opportunities of the Cosmos. But there is also an inverse dependence. Unfortunately, no one presently knows for certain what man really represents – neither biologists, nor geneticists or scientists in other disciplines. Just one Man in the Universe knows everything about everything – his name is the Creator, the Father, God. Only knowledge can lead us to Him. Sound knowledge about the world and ourselves is what forms Jacob's ladder that bridges the gap between Heaven and Earth.

In the school over the Abyss, where so few students remained by now, we were already seated in the front row. Only three desks were occupied. The Teacher sometimes called Igor and me to the board. But so far nothing extraordinary happened. None of those who remained in class seemed to indicate any intention to use the privilege of leaving through the door.

On that particular occasion, the Teacher was telling us about collective consciousness.

– For you, it now has the shape of clouds, – the old man said, explaining the picture, which appeared on the blackboard screen. – It's not an erroneous view, though, if you were to enter inside the cloud, you would see its construction, divided into separate areas. It displays constant movement, which never stops for a moment. Generally speaking, this is a space-time model full of global information. This information contains absolute data on the creation of the whole body of the Universe.

Collective consciousness is separated into several levels. A person

120

with ordinary consciousness belongs to the first level. The more a person attains in his life, the more information he concentrates in a certain volume of consciousness – the higher are his clairvoyant abilities.

The system of resurrection takes up the volume of the entire first level with the addition of the momentum of the soul. Curing serious illnesses takes up half of the left volume. Regeneration – the entire right volume. However, resurrection, regeneration and cure of serious illnesses can only be accomplished or halted by activating, together with consciousness, the cells of the soul. Note: when I speak about consciousness, I use the word "area" to designate parts of its construction. Remember it: an area of consciousness. When speaking of the soul, we use the word "cell" to designate its structural elements of. I repeat: a cell of the soul.

The picture on screen suddenly changed. We could now see another cloud in the area of the heart.

– The soul is also a cloud, – explained our Teacher. – Inside it are small particles, very gentle cells with very fast interactions. The soul is like a flower protected on all sides by the indestructible crystal of consciousness. This is the expression of God in man, the One Whom atheists are looking for, but can't find no matter how hard they try. Perhaps, they are looking too far away? And He is always close by. The crystal around the soul is the temple, in which He dwells. That temple has forty indestructible faces. And there are also six other faces. But they're not exactly faces. This, designated by number six, belongs to man.

– And there is also the Spirit that pervades and connects everything. What did the chariot, which you saw lying upside down in various levels, remind you of? – This time the Teacher directly addressed the question to Igor and me.

– A column, – I answered.

– Yes, it looked like a column, – Igor confirmed.

– And when you lifted it and placed it down horizontally?

– It now looked like two wheels connected by an axis.

– Wheels, wheels, – lamented the Teacher. – If you are inside the wheel, it's one thing. If you get out and stand beside the wheel – it's quite another story. You see everything differently and feel differently.

– What if we fasten the platform to the top and climb it? – Igor asked suddenly.

The Teacher looked him in the eye.

– The chariot cannot move on its own. It is pulled by the horse. The chariot you envision can be moved from the spot only by eternity. Do you know how to manage eternity, my son?

– I could try it, – Igor responded with confidence.

– Go ahead, – the old man agreed. – There is a particle of eternity out there behind the board. Just remember, no one has ever returned from that space. Are you still up to it? – He then relaxed the stressful situation. – You could, of course, do something different. People have invented spaceships to fly to the stars. But compared to this chariot their spaceships are like rocks with which prehistoric men tried to hit a star. So what have you decided?

Igor and I exchanged glances and took each other by the hand in a familiar gesture.

– Here's what I can tell you at this moment, – Teacher said, secretly feeling proud of us. – What you did was right: the whole issue lies in the alliance between people and the Earth. People's consciousness should be combined with the consciousness of the Earth, the soul of the people – with the soul of the Earth and their spirit – with the Holy Spirit. Now everything is in a state of disharmony. But if someone could do this, the people on Earth would be immortal and we would have the Golden Age. God bless you. You are the first who dared to voluntarily step into the Abyss. You know that no one has ever returned from there. Still, you're willing...

We thanked the Teacher for everything he did for us, for sharing his knowledge, for his patience and his wisdom, and then we stepped beyond the vague milk-white screen of the board.

* * *

As soon as we got outside the classroom, we immediately found ourselves in the middle of a giant energy pipe. A powerful vortex was dragging us inside, and we instinctively began to resist the flow.

Igor and I were still holding each other by the hand, and for some reason there wasn't any fear in our hearts. Although our surroundings left no room for optimism we felt that we could pass this test without experiencing the shame of defeat. Some kind of old, initial knowledge awakened within us and set in motion the secret processes of our internal and external reactions. We were yanked and tossed from side to side, but we did not unclasp our hands and in some unknown way, most likely through the effort of thought, we managed to stay on the periphery of the energy flows, which were trying to drag us inside their gut. Once again, I had the strange feeling that I had already been here once before.

A horizontal pipe... I suddenly recalled seeing it when Igor and I first opened the "Book of Knowledge". That was last year. After leaving the earthly levels of consciousness, we began to explore our heavenly home. Once, something incredible happened – the fabric of the Cosmos lifted and a huge book suddenly appeared on our way, tied with ribbons and sealed with seven seals. It was as huge as a rock against an ant, where man was the ant. I wanted to ask someone how I could look into it, but there was nobody to ask. We tried to raise the corner of its dark blue binder, but nothing came of it. The gold embossed title in the center of the binding read: "Book of Knowledge." Slightly below was the shape of a huge hand depressed in the leather cover. This couldn't be the handprint of an ordinary person – it was far too big. We guessed who left it. We were driven to place our own hands there, not to compare ourselves with the Creator, but because it had a strange, irresistible attraction. We took turns putting our own small hands on the handprint left by the Creator. Instantly, a glowing emerged right from the center of the book. Then the whole book became iridescent. For a moment the cover was hidden behind fog. When it cleared, we saw that the book was opened, and its title page, printed in huge letters, said: "Book of Knowledge of the Creator". There was another vortex of the abyss right in the center of the page, which was gently but inexorably pulling us inside. First we found ourselves in a maze, then in a tunnel and then in a point, around which a circle was outlined with signs of the zodiac. Each of these twelve signs and what lay behind them ruled events during one month of the year. This was the first design in the book. And it instantly reminded us of the cell nucleus, surrounded by twelve mini-mills.

The second figure we saw was a triangle. Something inside it was rising, falling and then returning to the starting point.

Each image we were shown seemed to enter us through a tunnel of light, inside which rings of energy moved vigorously and powerfully, connecting with something deep in our consciousness and soul. These were the codes, which under certain conditions gave access to knowledge hidden in the core essence of those with whom they came into contact.

The third figure was a cylinder. For some reason I thought: this is the bottle of the genie. What was in the middle couldn't get out. The cylinder was positioned vertically; we could move up and down inside it, or bang our heads against the walls.

The fourth figure was a square. Inside it had a plane, which was divided at right angles. Segments of the bad and the good were all equal to each other. We were supposed to understand and comprehend them.

The fifth figure was a horizontal cylinder (this is where we were). When we were in the middle of it, we were hanging there, kind of, so we couldn't rise too high or fall too low. Together with the third figure these were levels of consciousness, which had a definite limit until they became united with a new force. But now the situation was such that it was hardly appropriate to think about soaring freely. Clinging to the walls of the cylinder, we were barely able to resist the flow.

The sixth figure was a rectangle, with another figure, a triangle, placed against it. If one were to rise upward from its lower point, then, after passing the lateral and upper faces, one would eventually find himself at the bottom again. The path of enlightenment was movement from top to bottom, which ended with touching the ground. Then there was a new path, the path of initiation. This one was a spiral.

The seventh figure was a cone. The eighth was a trapeze. Moving along it, we thought that we were moving along a straight line, but in the end we returned to where we started.

The ninth figure was number eight. Vertically, it was the sign of eternity. Horizontally – the symbol of infinity. It also reminded us of the Möbius strip. If we moved along this figure, then, no matter where we were, or what our final destination may be, we could always see what was happening at the top and the bottom, on the inside and the outside.

The tenth figure consisted of two spheres partially lodged into one another. Its meaning was that anyone who succeeded in entering the second, upper ball, after moving through the lower one, would always have an idea what was in the first ball. It was also the symbol of the set theory. And it looked like two wheels onto which the chariot could be mounted. Naturally, one of these wheels was consciousness and the other – the soul. These were the two wheels of fate.

The eleventh figure was a point with the crescent moon located nearby. It warned us cautiously that wherever we may go from this point, we would always return to it. And the moon illuminated our path.

The last, twelfth figure contained two spheres with spirals inside, connected by an arched strip. The meaning of the spirals lay in that their content could equally be a state of mind and a state of consciousness. It may also not be the same. Everything was interconnected, however. Therefore, one had to be equal to the other to achieve the result, i.e., man.

The form templates taught to us were substances of the mind that generated ideas. It was part of a Cosmic mechanism unknown to us that regulated the development and structure of life. We weren't able to comprehend their true hidden meaning at once. The figures just entered us and dissolved into the depths of our being. Following that, the Divine words of the Creator began to trickle inside us from the pages of the Book. And we understood them: God is alive. God is in all of us. We found God in our souls, and God created us through these souls. By rejecting God, we rejected our soul and our own selves. When we brought ourselves closer to God, we brought our souls closer and got to know ourselves.

In the Cosmos, the human soul and God are not separated. They form a single unit. Whatever is not connected to God through the soul isn't whole and is doomed to die soon. Every rational being must establish a connection with God through his soul, and then it will find peace and eternal life. There is a particle of the Divine in each of you, in your soul.

The voice went on:

– Initially, all of you are connected to your God through your soul with invisible thread. But not everyone is able to preserve this vital thread; many of you lose it from generation to generation. Connected by the covenants with God, your soul had access to endless knowledge, in harmony and peace, opening the world and creating it. The possibilities of co-creation are endless and without limit. You don't know even a small part of what you ought to know and be able to do.

You use the knowledge of those people who have been allowed for a certain amount of time to increase their understanding of outer Cosmos and the inner soul. Know their experience, gain understanding of your soul and build your connection with your God, so as not to get lost in the endlessness of time and the hustle and bustle of your daily routine.

The mysterious voice fell silent, and we were sucked into the tunnel once again and carried away. When our journey ended, we found ourselves in space where there were no stars. All we could see were some balls shimmering around. When we took a closer look, we discovered they weren't balls at all but universes. And in the center was the brilliantly shining figure of a huge man sitting on the throne. Colorful spheres were flying around his head. They were worlds – and they were born directly by his consciousness. This was the Creator!

There is nothing above Him and never was. We are so small compared to Him.

He looked at us, and the sound of his thundering voice shook the spheres:

– What would you like to know, My children?

– We want to know the future, what will happen to our Earth, – we answered.

The Creator smiled. Irony flickered in His eyes, but then His face acquired a stern look once again.

– The future is impossible to know. It has to be created. To create it, one needs to know how to do it. You have been taught many things, and you have learned a lot already. But is it enough to save what you want to save? In front of you is eternity, in which there is everything, all possibilities, all that was and will be. And the answer to your question is there, too. Where will you go? How will you get back? There aren't any signposts here, you see. You can get lost in infinity in an instant.

– May we try?

– Go ahead, try.

We moved into infinity, leaving the trail of a silver thread behind us. It is stable, durable and can be sharp and dangerous as the blade of a sword, if someone tries to touch it with evil thoughts.

We stood inside one of the balls flying around the throne. There were galaxies in it – a lot of them. We moved among them with tremendous speed. We simply thought: I want to be there, and we found ourselves in that place. But the silver thread streamed after us, wherever we went. It was endless and infinite, as everything around us.

Now we could see that galaxies also had atmospheric mantles, just like planetary bodies. And they also had platforms, gaseous ones. We descended on one of them. There were some kind of screens there, very many of them. They were large and thin, very unusual looking. You could turn them on by your thought impulse.

– What would you like to see? – we were asked from one of the single screens.

– The structure of St. George, – we answered.

We were shown rivers, mountains, a sea, a forest and people's faces

– many of them. Another huge image taking up the whole screen was the face of Jesus Christ. Next to Him were two men with spheres or halos on their heads. Then we saw the design of a triangle, in the center of which there was an icon with the face of Christ. The circle around the icon had the signs of the zodiac marked on it. Six of them, on the left side, were female and the other six, on the right side, were male. The winged horse flew around the circle – this was time, the guide to the Cosmos.

The horse and rider are point X in the three-dimensional world. It is the last point in the end times by which society, penetrating through time into the Heavenly Kingdom, can gain knowledge of salvation.

Suddenly, a cloud passed over the screen and covered it. When it moved away, we saw the Creator sitting on the throne once again.

– You always want to see something large, – His reproachful voice sounded strict. – But do you know small things?

It became very hot, indeed, unbearably so. We could barely tolerate it. The Father took pity on us and pumped in a breath of freshness.

– Know yourself first, – sounded His thunderous voice. And its rumble was transmitted throughout the Universe. – Do you know what man is: his soul, spirit and consciousness? I painted the world when I came into it. Learn the secret of color. Not the one that was created on Earth by the deceitful spirit that does not illuminate but defiles the soul, the spirit which came out of the darkness that lies below and not from My Kingdom, not from above. His light is the light of deception, one that diverts a person from his way. You grow old and die because of him, without finding your God, Who is inside you. But you did not know this, could not see it and stagnated in the fragility of the deceptive world.

He said this and disappeared. And we saw a man on the screen, radiating seven colors. Closest to the body was yellow.

129

–This is the essence of man, – a voice said. Tables, formulas, organs and a skeleton began to emerge on the screen. – With the yellow color it is possible to draw a man – his inner and outer world. It is the color of the skin and the color of energy in the cell nucleus. It is something that can live and can also die. But if you would like to erase what was drawn poorly, it is best to use purple. It is like a sponge: it absorbs everything and dissolves everything within itself.

Green is the color of your being. It is the garden that you will plant, the child that you will bring up and the house that you will build.

Dark blue is your sin. It is everything in nature that you spoiled and ruined out of self-interest. It is poisoned rivers and dried-up seas; it is the air that is impossible to breathe. The dark blue color moves the world away from man.

Light blue is what brings closer and connects; it is that which unifies.

Red is your passion. It is the woman, who wants to get something through cunning and deceit, and the man who robs, captures and takes away by force. It is not really the difference in their gender that matters, it is the passion. It is reflected in the words "give me", "I want", "I demand", "I take". With this color we cut something out of a total and confiscate it, bringing it closer to ourselves and not thinking about others.

Orange is the secret within a secret; it is what everybody wants, pines for and dreams about. These are thoughts from the dark, which are drawn to the forbidden in the light of day. But they usually get scared and hide behind a veil of confusion. This is the twilight of the soul; it's neither darkness nor light. It is the soul's uncertainty.

These seven colors are like seven roads or seven films from a person's life. This is the person's essence, his being, his karma, his fate, his death, his designation and direction.

Seven colors represent seven forces.

These colors have millions of different shades and variations. But which one is true? Which is the dominant one?

There are two more colors: white – the color of this world. What we are talking about happens there. It is the color of My Son, the reverse side of black. Black is the most mysterious of them all – the color of the Father. It creates and they create with it. But this remains a mystery.

The heart focuses color. But consciousness influences this process. Change the focus only slightly – and, while reading the poster: "The Health Department issues the warning..." you already know the response: "I've smoked in the past, I smoke now, and I will continue smoking." Change the focus a little more. Do you see? A man just made a gun and shot another man. He fell. The first man thought: "What would happen if I fired from a cannon?" And he did. Aha! He blew up a man and a dozen others into the bargain. What about the rest? They were running!

He made a rocket and then a nuclear bomb. He killed a million at once. What about the rest? They're still alive, are they? He thought again, wrinkled his brow and rubbed his temples, the thinker...

Who focuses the heart? It is the person's own consciousness – his egotism, passions and desires.

That is what even a slight shift from the center of truth can lead to, a shift from the image and likeness, from the holy and perfect.

There, on Earth, from the bottom side, where you have been and where the heart of darkness is hidden, which calls itself the second sun and light, one finds many of those who have left to fill the people with the spirit of darkness and entice them toward the path of deception. Only a few were able to resist and not give in to temptation, who refused to trade the truth for food, drink and clothing, honors and riches and who did not allow themselves to be lured into the depths of evil.

When you stand here on what people call the void, but what in reality is the body of My Son, and you don't fall down, though you are standing without so much as touching the spiral arms of the galaxies with your feet – what does all this tell you? What does it tell you that you have nowhere to fall, though you can see infinity below? Who but you can stand there and not fall?

There is an obvious reality, but there is also a secret one. You have cognized the one and the other. What should you do? What should you tell people who are wandering in the dark and seek the path that has been stolen from them?

Everything in the world is the result of the transition from an idea to its implementation. You, too, are a mechanism of this transition, because you have been endowed with a portion of divine power. What else do you want to know? Perhaps you will ask about the colors? There are more colors than those we have talked about. There is the one between the black and the white – sometimes colorless, then silvery, then some other variable color. These three – black, white and colorless can be found in everything and everywhere. There is goodness in them and truth; in them lies the path toward the gold color. If they leave the world, it will disappear. If they leave man, he will not die but disappear, because to die doesn't mean to disappear. Those who die always come back. But those who vanish altogether, how could they come back? And with him gone, not only color but also sound will disappear. You see, each color has its own sound or, rather, its own note.

So that's what it is! It's all in the distinction between death and disappearance. Here lies the answer to one of the questions.

– The first sound, – someone unknown continues his lecture, – is "do".

It is white; it's the heart. If you want to tune up the liver, pancreas and gall bladder, you need the sound "sol". Arkady needs that sound. The sound "la" is also necessary for Arkady. Utter this sound. Do you see how his spine, damaged in two places, begins to move, align and correct the curvature, how the blood and energy begins to circulate evenly through it?

– Remember that time when you were in England, in Wales? – The voice was now addressed directly to me. – You and your friend Michael went to a farmers' festival at the old castle. A band was playing on the lawn in front of the house. The musicians were children.

As the voice was telling me this, I actually recalled that episode from years before, which concealed beneath its outer insignificance something extremely important in my life. My friends and I were about to enter the house when the children began to play a new tune. Its sounds completely fascinated me. I halted in the doorway and, resisting the pressure of the crowd behind me, I went back to the orchestra, like a fairy tale character enchanted by the sounds of the magic flute.

Everyone was perplexed. Yet, despite the urging of my friends, I couldn't move from the spot until the final chords of the strange music, full of heavenly harmony.

– Can you guess now why that music affected you so much? – asked the voice. – Because you knew it and heard it many times before. It was your favorite melody, which reminded you of the heavenly home, where they had long been waiting for you. How wonderful you felt then! So what happened? It was simply the sound of the music of your soul. The harmony contained there creates and lifts a person; it influences ones health and mood.

If, however, disharmony, dissonance, hellish screams and distortions are introduced to the sounds and colors, how would this affect a person?

133

Look into his eyes and you will see madness there. And this madness will be aggressive and dangerous.

Madmen are looking for their likes, joining together into crowds and flocks. If thousands of madmen unite they will look upon any normal person next to them as a weirdo.

The Tree of Life grows from top to bottom. It starts growing from the crown. On the other hand, if we look from down below, we will see a stem growing from a small root. It represents your age and worldview. It also bears fruit, a variety of fruit. For instance, there are red apples, and there are black ones. Some of them are ripe, and some of them are altogether inedible. If you taste such an inedible apple you will die, but if you eat the ripe one you will live forever. But these apples are deceptive. What you see when you hold it in your hands isn't, in fact, what you think it is. The black apple looks as if it's red, and it spins like a peg-top to boot. Besides, the leaves from this tree can cure wounds. Each tiny leaf is somebody's life, whereas the tree as a whole is the life of all people together. So, what kind of fruit are we going to grow on this Tree of Life? Ones which are deceptive, misleadingly attractive, like a beautiful girl who is shamelessly luring someone, not to love but to own him and control his life? Or will we grow genuine fruit, the ones we have to cultivate and nurture, and the ones which radiate light and generate the harmony of love?

Do you really think that there were no civilizations before your time that were more powerful than yours? The technologies used by the atlantes were more advanced by two-three hundred years if compared to ours. But theirs was the path of intelligence not the soul. The atlantes practiced magic, mastered telepathy and captured the nature of resonance: by controlling it they were able to move gigantic rocks and various heavy objects. They had the strength but they didn't feel responsible for having it.

At this point, an image of a mighty man appeared on the screen. He was taller than us, though not significantly. His muscles were those of an athlete. He was holding a huge rock in the air. He held it by the strength of his mind, not his hands. And he also moved it the same way.

– Where are those mighty atlantes today? – the voice asked.

We responded telepathically: "Their land vanished under the water."

– But everything can repeat itself once again, – the voice continued. – This is because the future is created by people themselves. Responsibility and power cannot exist separately. If they are separated the Tree of Life becomes the Tree of Death. Its root is bitter, its shadow means hatred, and such a tree grows into darkness.

Now the screen opened another screen inside of it. This was a tunnel, one side of which was white, the other one was black, and in between there was no color at all. We were summoned, and we entered the tunnel. We sped down it, realizing that it was the tunnel of time. Time indicators flashed by: 2002, 2004, 2006. The flashing of numbers stopped at the year 2039. An image appeared. There were people over there. But not only people, there were also aliens in their midst who came from another planet. As for the Earth, it is almost entirely lifeless.

Igor and I began observing the future.

We saw an enormous antenna in the center of the Eurasian continent. An entire city was built around it. With the help of this antenna it was possible to control energies, quite unusual ones, not the electromagnetic energies known to us now. The city's residents were trying, and quite effectively, to rectify the ecology of the planet. They were saving the human race.

– This course of events can still be changed, though we are short of time, – a voice said, but this time it was a different one, and we recognized who it belonged to. – Three powers that already exist on Earth have to unite. Everything could take a different course if the planet's authorities weren't so preoccupied with their own mundane, earthly matters. But power is always blind, so you can only rely on your own strength. Remember, you vouched for the Earth with your own lives. – Igor and I were reminded of the promise we had given and the responsibilities it entailed.

Archangel Michael once taught people how to use colors. They contain great might and great knowledge. Would you like to test the power of nine colors?

– Of course, – Igor agreed.

– Then try it, – the voice said. A rainbow flew in the direction of Igor's palm, the ends of which were black and white.

Igor caught it in his palm. He held it vertically, then horizontally, as if it was a bridge, tossing it from one hand into the other, like a colorful accordion.

– What do you see in this rainbow?

– The principle of creation, – Igor answered.

– You stretch the colors and then you compress them. They contain heat and cold, as well as life and death. Each planet in the Solar System has its own color and sound, assigned to it. Their beams are focused on Earth, and they form the pyramidal structure of control above the North Pole.

This was definitely a reference to the structure where Igor and I felt so at home.

– Those colors penetrate each individual, – the familiar voice sounded again, – and each individual gets the opportunity to be a genius, to be creative and imaginative. Through their own thoughts and actions people produce such distortions in their consciousness that push sanctity away from their spirit, and prevent it from displaying itself. As a result, the soul gets darker, and the consciousness becomes cloudy.

The future can change, if people's thoughts change; that is why it is so essential to explain and show them the path to light and goodness.

It does not seem possible. But you have just entered the tiniest point of space, and could clearly see that the endless Universe was at its opposite end. Think about it. Think about how this world is built, how one thing flows into another – what is small flows into what is big, and vice versa.

The voice fell silent and the screen became dark. Igor and I were left on our own with the limitless Cosmos, and its deceptively empty and weightless space.

But is it really weightless? Is it empty?

This entire vision instantly opened up in the memory, as if it was providing us with some kind of inner support in the precarious confrontation with the powerful energy whirlwind capable of dragging us in. We moved deeper inside the cylinder, our consciousness resisting the dangerous acceleration. But we weren't simply moving. While we were advancing, our consciousness revealed the history of four basic human races – black, red, yellow and white. The test seemed to progress parallel to our acquisition of knowledge. Whoever overcame the challenge, obtained the knowledge.

We advanced along the pipe and saw, besides scenes from human history, deep potholes on its walls. We knew what they meant. The words of the Teacher: "Nobody ever came back from this space," were way too expressive as a symbol for us to comprehend the real danger of our journey, which was very far from being romantic.

Nevertheless, we passed through the tunnel and ended at its exit, in front of the humongous and unbelievably tall gates of the Father's Kingdom. As soon as we touched them with our hands, we immediately became taller and stronger. And when we pushed the gate leaves for the second time, they opened, indicating the new path in our life.

* * *

Next day we showed up in the celestial class, as if nothing had happened. In fact, nobody expected us to be back. The eyes of the students expressed not merely amazement; they looked as if they were about to lose their mind. One and the same thought was rumbling in their heads, the way heavy stones rumble in an iron barrel as it rapidly rolls down a steep slope: "Who are these two, who have returned from the Abyss, from where nobody ever came back?"

"Nobody – ever! Nobody – ever!" – Their thoughts resonated in our consciousness like an echo.

Even the Teacher's eyes reflected his poorly concealed amazement. He was clearly struggling with his feelings.

– After that, why would you want to study in this class? Is this class even necessary anymore? – he asked contritely. – I am so glad you came back from where nobody has ever returned. But, frankly, I am at a loss because it was I who showed you the way to the Abyss. You returned, though everybody knows that it's impossible to come back. It is one of the world's fundamental principles. It is immutable. Then why are you here? This class has been around for a very long time. I have been teaching in it for a very long time as well. Human beings never attended it. You were the first. Even Christ studied in absentia. He never sat here at the desk. This is why, upon seeing that you were extremely close to becoming the only graduates, I took advantage of your inexperience and hot-headedness and suggested that you test yourself in the Abyss. But you came back, even though nobody has ever returned from there. As a result, I don't know what to do now, and what to think of you and myself.

Chapter 3

Early in October, the "KhudLit" Publishing House celebrated its seventieth anniversary. The celebrations were quite modest and family-style.

On the eve of the anniversary, there was a phone call from the magazine "Itogi". It was a reporter who was instructed to interview the heads of publishing houses regarding their opinion about the forthcoming merging of their institutions into holding companies created by the Ministry.

My first reaction was quite natural:

– What opinion could we have on an issue that nobody has ever discussed with us?

– Are you serious? So you don't know anything about it? – The journalist's voice showed genuine concern. It seemed that he was taken aback.

– The next issue of our magazine will contain Deputy Minister Grigoriev's article on the restructuring in the industry. Your publishing house is listed among those subject to the reform. Are you telling me that you aren't even aware of these momentous decisions?

– Exactly.

– So no one at the Ministry ever spoke to you about it?

– You are the first person specifically discussing this matter with me.

– This is totally ridiculous, – the reporter noted with amazement. – A reform is about to happen, which affects the major publishers of the country. The issue is already undergoing a trial run in the media, but the directors of those institutions know nothing of these impending events.

– Only at the level of rumors, – I confirmed. – None of the leaders of the Ministry spoke to us on this subject or showed any interest in our opinion.

The journalist fell silent, mulling something over, and finally said:

– Could I call you back later? I have to discuss this issue with my colleagues. Maybe we can offer you the opportunity to voice your opinion on the pages of our publication.

– Alright, – I agreed, even though I understood the futility of such actions. At that moment I recalled the words of Vladimir Mikhailovich Zharkov. It was during the reorganization of the Ministry, when all its leaders were pretty much shown out the door: "These new guys are anything but bashful. He should be happy they didn't kick him in the rear so he'd hurry up..." Zharkov said to me referring to the treatment of an old colleague.

Of course, "glasnost" could influence events. But for this to happen there should be at least someone in power who is interested in the truth. How much has been written about these guys: about their criminal settling of scores, about their constant proximity to the most notorious crimes and murders, and about the suspected and proven fraud they were involved in! The entire country read about these investigations with a degree of amazement, but those who were supposed to show some interest in such events as a call of duty, were silent. Those in power are trying to turn everyone in the country into voluntary scoundrels, prompting people to inform on their neighbors and accepting anonymous complaints for consideration even in the most frivolous cases. However, in the most obvious, egregious cases they turn a blind eye. It isn't that they don't see. It's just very inconvenient for them to see: it makes them intensely uncomfortable. They are a team. "The team of our youth..." Believe me, to try and catch somebody red-handed in our country, without being a member of a team, just isn't worth the effort.

It was with such a feeling of impending peril that I opened the ceremony of the seventieth anniversary of the "KhudLit" Publishing House. There were posters hanging on the walls, and the winged horse Pegasus, overcoming the Earth's gravity, soared into the heights of Heaven. We all wanted him to occupy his rightful place on the literary Olympus as fast as possible.

Apparently, our desire didn't coincide with someone's entirely different aspirations. Grigoriev's team from the Ministry clearly had other views of a desirable course of events. It wasn't at all hard to understand them. Here is the amount of designated federal funding for the issue of school textbooks – 3.5 billion rubles. The Ministry of the Press struck a deal with the Ministry of Education on the federally approved package. The mandatory use of these textbooks in schools pushes any publishers competing with away from publishing similar products. A powerful campaign was immediately launched, involving Sudakov, the director of the publishing house, and claiming that he was not good enough for the position. The publisher was doing quite well, even more than that, but they started digging around, squeezing Sudakov and trying to push him out. Not surprisingly, after all, it was a matter of billions of rubles, guaranteed by the cash cow named State. It is clear that only the most trusted people, their own kind, can be allowed to benefit from the final stage in the milking process, when the milk is flowing most abundantly.

They had probably drawn a few lucrative schemes involving "KhudLit" as well. And the numbers in these schemes ultimately don't reflect the number of publications, or the most valuable works of world and national literature but rubles and dollars.

I looked at the hall, at the rows of assembled colleagues and friends, with whom I worked side by side during the most difficult years of the crisis. They were waiting for what I had to say. I didn't know where to

142

start. What I had planned to tell them before, no longer made any sense. But what I was supposed to tell them now, would totally ruin our holiday mood and would destroy our celebration. So I stood facing them in painful indecision. Not a single soul from the Ministry attended the anniversary, and that, too, was a prophetic sign.

Finally, I began my speech. I spoke about our glorious past, how we fought together, surviving financial crises, bankruptcy and even hurricanes, real atmospheric disasters, one of which tore the roof off our building. And no one gave us zilch, not even a penny, to help us in the fight against defaults, the elements and other troubles. We went through hard times, but here was the result of our victory against all odds: we have completed all of our subscriptions, paid off our debts and were once again able to raise the salary of our employees, although only by a little. It was our joint gift to ourselves.

In the middle of the speech I noticed Galina Mikhailovna Shchetinina from the central administration slipping into the hall. She was carrying a folder in her hand. So her bosses must have decided to somehow congratulate us on the important date, after all.

Galina Mikhailovna used to work at "KhudLit" and our staff had the highest regard for her. She, in turn, loved our publishing house.

I was pretty sure that she organized this demonstration of at least a minimum of attention and respect for the oldest publishing house in Russia on her own. I thanked her for coming to share our joy with us and yielded the floor to her.

She opened the folder and read out Grigoriev's message. It was a very brief one, merely a few trite phrases and expressions befitting the event: "Congratulations! Best wishes! In recognition…" Then she closed the folder and presented her own long and excited speech. She indicated how

143

strange and absurd the situation was in connection with our anniversary.

Just a year ago she was in charge of all the paperwork authorizing a dozen awards and medals to be granted to the employees of the publishing house. And now, instead of commendations, she brought us the formal and meaningless platitudes of semi-official congratulations. She was trying to defuse the awkward situation with her sincere words, and she succeeded in part.

Galina Mikhailovna stayed with us during the banquet as well. After the more formal festivities were over, we sat together sharing memories. Valeri Sergeevich Modestov told some of the most famous anecdotal stories involving "KhudLit" and a number of well-known writers who were frequent visitors. My deputy, Sergei Kolesnikov, sang and played the guitar. I read some poetry. Igor Nagaev, Editor-in-Chief of "Detskaya Literatura"* magazine, who was our home-grown comedian, cracked jokes until everyone almost split their sides with laughter. No one could rob us of this sense of mutual admiration and respect, of our sense of family.

As for the journalist from "Itogi" magazine, he never called back.

* * *

The Millennium year was coming to a close. For me, personally, this was an amazing year because it opened the doors into a different world and into a different dimension. This other dimension is always next to us, like the wondrous land hidden behind the cloth with the painted fireplace in old Geppetto's little house. As for me, I became Pinocchio.

Igor Arepyev and I participated in a large number of remarkable events. I can't tell you how dramatically different they were from anything

* The name of the magazine means "Children's literature" in Russian.

else we have ever lived through or experienced. Along with them, came an acute sense of upcoming changes in our personal lives as well as the destiny of all of mankind. I don't doubt it anymore – we are witnessing the dawn of the New Era rising over the Earth.

However, along with these pleasantly encouraging signs, an old problem emerged, though it was now upgraded to a new level. It became blatantly clear that passively waiting for these changes to occur does not bode anything positive to those who are waiting. The assertion that changes pave the way to cognition of the permanent is completely right. But it's not enough merely to cognize – it is imperative to act. Any desirable change in the material world becomes possible only as a result of changes in a person's identity, in his spiritual, inner world. In fact, that is what the promise of Christ's second coming is all about. It has to happen within all of us.

Everything external that surrounds man (even provided that the Laws of the Universe and the Creator allow us to make this long desired step towards man's unity with God) can be changed in a positive way only for those of us, who are capable of making all the necessary changes within their own internal principles, to bring themselves closer to the commandments of Christ.

This is by no means easy. Fyodor Dostoyevsky, the most profound researcher of human nature, wrote the following not just to be witty: "To love a person, as oneself, according to Christ's commandment, is impossible. The law of the self is binding on earth. The 'I' stands in the way. Christ alone could love man as himself, but Christ was a perpetual eternal ideal, to which man strives and, according to the law of nature, should strive. Meanwhile, since the appearance of Christ *as the ideal of man in the flesh,* it has become as clear as day that the… highest use a man can make of his personality, of the full development of his *Ego* – is, as it were, to annihilate that *Ego*, to give it totally and to everyone, undividedly and unselfishly. In this way, the law of the *Ego* fuses with the law of humanism, and in this fusion both the *Ego* and the all (apparently two extreme opposites) mutually annihilate themselves one for the other, and at the same time each attains separately, and to the highest degree, their own individual development.

And this is the greatest happiness." (From Dostoevsky, "The Idiot". English translation by Alan Myer [Oxford, 1992], 20:172-173.)

The astute reader should accept my apologies for making more references to writers than to scientists in this book as well as the previous one. To restore the balance, let me now refer you to this quote by a scientist: "The input of art in understanding the spiritual world of man is immeasurably greater than that of all the humanities." (I.T. Kasavin, M. Phil., from the preface to the book "Deluded Mind. Variety of Non-Scientific Knowledge", which Kasavin compiled.)

This categorical verdict proves at the level of cognition how right Descartes was when he famously said: "It might seem strange how often the greatest ideas are expressed in the books of poets compared to the works of philosophers. This is because poets, when they write, are motivated by inspiration brought forth by their imagination. We possess innate seeds of knowledge, existing in the minds of all men like the sparks of fire in flints. Philosophers cultivate these seeds with their reason, while poets ignite them using their imagination, which is why they catch fire much sooner."

Inspiration and intuition – they make equal the super-intellectual Albert Schweitzer and the ignorant peasant woman Vanga. As for us, ordinary mortals, we must pay more attention to the lessons of mankind and the methods used by wise teachers, instead of waiting for a small gift to

146

fall into our lap from heaven. In this particular case, we have to study the technique of controlled clairvoyance.

Something the great thinkers of the past would discover using their intuition, is reflected today in modern science. The fact that consciousness is not so much a product of the individual brain's activity, but rather the innate principle of the existence of both nature and man, is now becoming the basic premise for present-day research work.

Let us recall the words of the renowned prophet Michel Nostradamus who wrote in his "Epistle to Henry II": "I hope to capture in black and white what prophecies meant where referring to years... I have always underestimated my own abilities, but *after making my soul and my spirit receptive*, I brought them in sync with my calculations."

Please take note of the circumstance emphasized by Nostradamus himself: "*after making my soul and spirit receptive*". Nobody says such things and, what's more, emphasizes them, for no good reason. This is the key to understanding. Nostradamus basically indicates the secret door to the magic land, where events are created by people to the same extent as people, in their turn, are created by events.

Truth be told, for Igor Arepyev and me it wasn't exactly a door but a high-speed tunnel. That is the way we see it. We also constantly associate our exit into the other world with the parable of the genie getting out of the bottle. Someone rubbed the side of the bottle, removed the cork – and here we are, enjoying freedom.

It would be fair, however to put the word "genie" in quotes. A human being is not a genie. His status in the hierarchy is considerably higher, because he is the main creation of the Creator – God's Father, His image and likeness. Someone (who it is we will find out later) did his best for people not to be aware of their own power as long as possible. I think we will

147

have to deal with this issue as well. Meanwhile, Igor and I were actively exploring our newly acquired opportunities in cognizing the world. Usually, we did it in the morning, before going to work. The world revealed to us is not the one we are used to seeing. First of all, I mean the Earth.

We would engage clairvoyance, then instantly pass the Bardo channel, the platform at its top, and enter the open Cosmos. Several times we got lost there and couldn't find our way back. Because of that, here's a friendly warning to all those who might attempt doing something similar on their own: the possibilities to get lost are very real. Your physical body and its Ego remain on the Earth, as for your consciousness... It is your consciousness that is actually the traveler in the Cosmos, so what will happen if it doesn't return to the Earth? What will happen if even a part of your consciousness fails to get out of captivity at any of the planets or the Sun? This is why the hierarchy of Initiations exists. This is why Teachers are absolutely necessary. In ancient times, people said that a man's feet are pressed against the ground, but his head strikes against the sky. Please, don't lose your head. Be level-headed. Otherwise, it will make you go insane.

We now saw the Earth at a distance. What we saw most likely exceeded the limits of the range of electromagnetic waves, which represents the norm for people. How else could we explain what we saw? The Earth, a ball flattened at the Poles, was speeding through the Cosmos. We saw continents and oceans. Two enormous cones crown its Poles. They emerge because the Earth revolves about its own axis of thin radiation.

Now we looked at the Earth from the North Pole. One of the cones reached up from beneath, from the planetary nucleus, the other one was directed towards it from above, i.e. from the Sun and the planets. These cones looked exactly like bottles. It was through one of those bottles that

148

we made out exit into the open Cosmos.

On one side, energy vortexes formed a distinct geometric figure – two pyramids stacked to each other at their bases on the Earth's surface. Countless tiny rays pointed towards these pyramids from the Cosmos. They not only resembled strings but actually produced slight, barely audible sounds. The Pythagorean singing of the stars, – as the well-known Russian poet Nikolai Zabolotsky would call it. When these strings reached the cones, the endless rhythmic rotation of the planet caused them to sort of wind around these cones. Upon getting inside the upper pyramid, they gradually disintegrated into layers of color and then condensed into a silvery, purple, dark and light blue, green, red, yellow and even black color. That is precisely how the levels of the planetary subtle matter structure are formed, which enable us to know the past, see the future and change the course of time and events.

If we view the cones from different angles, we might see that they change their appearance as well. It seems that these cones are, in fact, the very representations of the fourth dimension on Earth which ancient faiths referred to as "the depth of good", when speaking about the structure above the Earth's surface, and "the depth of evil", or "Gehenna", the destination of the wicked, when they implied the levels descending towards the planetary nucleus. Igor and I already had a chance to be there, so we do knew how strikingly these ancient legends and epics corresponded to absolutely real events, which were directly connected to the destinies of many people, who live in the real world, not in fairy tales and myths.

Let me give you a trivial example from Greek mythology. Upon accomplishing all his twelve labors, Heracles married Deianira, the daughter of one of the kings. Shortly after the wedding, she made Heracles weave and perform other chores: enough loitering already; it's time to do something useful. Then she fell in love with a wild centaur named Nessus. After Heracles hit him with an arrow, the treacherous lover advised Deianira to collect his blood, which would supposedly preserve her husband's love. Deianira smeared some of the blood on Heracles' lion-skin tunic, but since it was poisoned, the great hero died in dreadful agony. As for his widow, she was in such grief that she took her own life, stabbing herself with a sword.

What does this myth represent? Is it a fable of morals? Or is it, perhaps, a sociological analysis of the nature of a male and female? In any case, it reflects the pattern of relations to be found in many contemporary families. Why does our consciousness, after barely touching upon a problem, try to avoid its deeper interpretation? Is it at all possible to advance into the future without learning the lessons of the present? Those are legitimate questions.

I worry about those who are afraid to position themselves. In the Cosmos, where Igor and I had been, everything is as clear as day: today we are delving into new space, where galactic spiral branches are spread and flow around according to some other program, very different from the previous one. In this program everything real is becoming virtual, the old world collapses before our eyes, while new interactions are built.

It was so weird to watch it: not the usual Cosmos, not the usual Earth and not the usual man. Igor and I returned into our tiny bottle. Someone softly put back the cork. We proceeded to the second informational level.

– I want to see close up how the human being is built, – Igor said.

He is addressing me. But it seems we are never alone.

An old man with a long grey beard appeared across the way from us. He could easily be a hundred years old, but maybe a thousand or a hundred thousand years old.

The old man responded:

– Seven colors of the rainbow – that's what man is. The first color is just you. Know thyself, and the gates will open before you.

The second color is your essence. Know thy essence, and the gates will open before you.

The third color is your spirituality. Know thy spirituality, and the gates will open before you.

The fourth color is your being. Know thy being, and the gates will open before you.

The fifth color is your Earth. Know thy Earth, and the gates will open before you.

The sixth color is your Universe. Know thy Universe, and the gates will open before you.

The seventh color is the connection between Heaven and Earth. Know the connection between Heaven and Earth, and the gates will open before you.

The old man named all the seven colors, but Igor and I remained standing there, silent. Well, obviously nobody expected any answers from us. On the contrary, we were bombarded with questions:

– Do you know your own levels now? Do you know your strength? The power of your mind? Your true essence? Your being? Do you know your Earth? Or your Heaven? Your connection? After all, you are standing at the steps of thy God.

– No, Father, we haven't, – Igor answered humbly.

At this moment the old man instantly disappeared.

– What are we going to do? – I asked my friend.

– We will learn, – he answered curtly.

We used the power of our thought to create a person facing us. This person is a figment our imagination, pure abstraction. We colored him yellow. First charts appeared, then a skeleton, body parts and blood. The norms, pathologies, biochemical reactions and their interactions indicated how energy can correct the malfunctions of blood circulation.

We took the silvery color. This is our spirit. We projected it onto the person. The spirit flowed to the center of the chest and hovered above the heart, like a cloud.

The interaction began. The person sung, cried, and demonstrated joy, pride and humiliation.

We tried to take the cloud back, but another body emerged from this person. It was transparent, more phantom-like, I should say. Whatever emerged was able to walk and talk. It has no body parts to speak of – it only has shape and some kind of clot inside.

– Can you see me? – this entity called.

– Yes, I can, – Igor replied.

– It's me, a person.

The phantom has no smell; the color of his ephemeral body is hard to identify. We tried to compress his body but couldn't. We tried to give it a different shape – that didn't work, either. He seemed to be unhappy with our attempts. He said:

– This can't be deformed or changed. It is part of the One Who is eternal and ageless.

The body of this man was surrounded by information, which covered him in layers. There were seven of them: if we viewed them not as energy, but information, they would represent the essence, being, karma, fate, death, determination and direction. Each layer served as a mediator.

Aren't there way too many mediators between the Son and the Father? Who created all those mediators, and for what purpose? The point is that

152

each of these layers is a program, a labyrinth of sorts, in which one has to find one's way before enjoying freedom.

Suddenly three colors – black, white and silvery – emerged from the human form we had just drawn. Each molded itself into some strange vague shape, as if three figures were standing across from us, swaying.

– You have discovered the mystery of mysteries, – we heard a deep, melodious voice. The voice was calm; it did not threaten or accuse anybody but simply stated. – Be careful while using Divine power. Use it only for the benefit of people. Remember about goodness, and yet always be on the alert: evil is somewhere close by.

All the small figures disappeared, followed by the human being we created.

* * *

We were getting busier at the Center, with a growing number of patients coming, mostly with terminal illnesses. We succeeded in offering them effective help. Actually, anybody can find within himself the abilities we discovered in ourselves. People are capable of many things and have numerous abilities. The problem is that they very seldom know about this. Moreover, not a single milestone in technological progress can be isolated from the evolution of Nature and the Cosmos. Whatever we consider to be the product of human intelligence was invented in the Universe long ago, including intelligence itself.

We do our best to explain to our students that there is man's regular progress, consisting in stages of biological development, and there is also spiritual growth, i.e., one's personal evolution. There is a visible reality, which is objective, or, rather, the one we view as objective based on social

..on: production, economy, social systems and processes taking place in Nature... And there is also a secret, invisible reality, which is spiritual in its nature. This reality is the one that determines all the inter-dependencies and interactions in our world. The main purpose of man is to walk the path of his earthly life, however difficult it might be, and achieve a creative transformation, which opens the gates, through what is visual and virtual, into the true spiritual reality. It leads to God, to our Father, and to light and reason. The point is that everything else is a life of slumber and dependence.

Our world was created by the Creator's thought. That is why the space of our world is such that only something illusory becomes real in it. All the paths a man walks are emanations of his own psychic powers. Those capable of understanding it will be released from the genie's bottle and will obtain long-awaited freedom and immortality.

This is the message I am trying to deliver to my students. Not everybody grasps what I tell them. Many students perceive what I say as exercises in rhetoric, a kind of obsession with eloquence. The gates of their hearts are still shut for the truth. That's very regretful! They had just one more step to take to leave the path of their blind fate and follow the road of truth. It is useless to repeat what you heard in class, as if you were some kind of a clockwork doll – one must have moral principles. God only knows whether they will be able to take this decisive step!

We had an unexpected visitor at the Center: Kirill showed up again, supposedly, to pick up his belongings. At first he was quite friendly and even asked about our progress. He wanted to know, by the way, if we had changed our previous decision.

– Do you need to know because of some new circumstances? – I asked the demon, who was seeking our friendship.

– This may be the case, – he answered evasively.

– Have a seat then, – I invited him to start the negotiations.

– Sure, you have the right to feel offended but you have to understand: I have an agenda. I have to do what I'm told. But if you let me join you, I promise to be your most loyal and reliable slave.

– You can't be a slave because you are a lord, – I testily reminded Kirill of his recent claims to power.

– I underestimated you, – the demon admitted. – Now I am ready to accept any position you choose to offer me. You need me. It is far from being over.

– What is left? You have already lost the Armageddon.

– True, – Kirill concurred. – But we are talking about that other space. Here, on Earth, there is still somebody you will have to fight against.

– Interesting, – I agreed, realizing that the demon was telling the truth. – And who might this warrior be?

– The Angel of Darkness.

– Do you know him? Who does he resemble? – I asked my questions in such a manner that Kirill would not feel any hostility on my part. Let him brag about his omniscience, and I will heed his words with a show of the utmost respect.

With a sudden gesture, Kirill loosened the rubber band, which held his pony tail. His hair fell in a dark wave covering his face and shoulders.

I was stunned. I now saw a pretty young woman in front of me. Yes, this was a woman, not a boy who looked like a woman. How did he do it? This was pure magic. The demon performed such magic not in that non-physical space, where Igor and I could do something very similar, but here, in the material world, where he was instantly able to turn into a

155

totally different person.

– So it's a woman? – admiring my own naïve sagacity, I wanted to make sure I was right.

– Yes, – the beauty answered and then turned back to being Kirill, the boy.

– She will be very beautiful, intelligent and powerful, – Kirill threatened. – You'd be better off if I am close by when she shows up.

– You think we won't manage without you?

– It will be hard. She uses human wickedness as a source of her strength. Since people's wickedness is endless, her strength is limitless.

– Still, what if we manage?

– Then the one who is to come will come, – the boy spoke in puzzles.

– Do you know his name? – I assumed the role of an interrogator.

The demon smiled, gathered his hair in the back of his head and put it in a pony tail with the rubber band again.

–Who doesn't know his name? The one who is to come never concealed his name. Everybody listens to him saying it but nobody can hear it.

– You are becoming vague and mysterious again, – I pointed out, noticing the change in Kirill.

– Do you still think that I came from Mugen?

– And you? Do you really doubt that?

– My status is considerably higher, – Kirill answered somberly. – I am from the gods.

– With Mugen's seal in your pocket?

– You don't know anything about the situation and the disposition of forces. Besides, you have forgotten about the Confederation.

– Yea, sure… Suppurative appendicitis in the body of creation.

While I was cracking the joke, I noticed that Kirill was genuinely amazed.

– Who told you that?

I kept silent, hiding the fact that I actually didn't know it.

– How far did you manage to get? – the boy asked, clearly not expecting an answer.

As for me, I was proud that I succeeded in surprising him. It appeared that we, too, were good for something is this strange world of behind-the-looking-glass sciences.

* * *

It happened at night. I saw a man's huge body. He was suspended in the silence of the Cosmos – naked, with his hands stretched out to the sides, and a spiral-shaped energy vortex rose from his navel, like a giant funnel. The vortex was also similar to a galaxy with clearly visible sleeves.

For a while I watched from the sidelines, but then, obeying a vague hypnotic pull, I joined the spiral motion and began descending. The lower I descended, the more clearly I could see underneath a giant face that gazed back at me – good-naturedly studying me.

Then a voice emerged, and I recognized it. The voice said: "Once again you will embark on a journey. If you are asked, where you are from, you must answer: from the One, Who came from Himself. If they ask, who you are, you must answer: we are children of the Father. If they demand that you show them the sign of the Father, you should answer: it is in us."

The voice fell silent, and the vision melted away in the infinite darkness of the Cosmos. I was once again alone with boundless space and peace.

The next morning I told Igor about my nocturnal adventure.

– Something is going to happen, – he guessed. – Let's take a look.

We entered the Bardo channel and moved up to the platform. St. George was standing on the stairs next to his horse. He felt that we were close. The old warrior raised his gray head.

– Is there a cross on you? – he asked.

–Yes, there is, – we responded.

– Do you have the ring of the Lord?

– Yes, on the finger.

St. George nodded in approval.

– There will come a time when you'll need to use it. Don't forget about it. Faith, knowledge and the colors from the ring – that is your key.

He sighed, as if recalling something from long ago.

– "The Book of Life" – imagine what it will be like. What will its binding look like, its pages, its content, and when will you need to finish it? You should travel with this image on your mind. You will have to go far today. Take the life-giving cross with you from the levels. God speed!

We thanked St. George and turned around. He blessed us for a safe journey.

We took the cross along with us and imagined what the book will be like. Then we took off into the Cosmos from the levels. We saw a glowing trail of dust lining the path in space. We knew who it was intended for and moved boldly along it, flying through the Universe, with our hearts rejoicing.

Ten bright stars were shining on the black canvas of infinity. If you looked closely from the side, you could see: each star consisted of three disks sequentially connected to form a single structure. And each of these discs had a different color. These ten stellar spheres, joined together by beams into a variety of geometric shapes, beckoned and called to him. It was like a heavenly computer that controls all the processes in the Cosmos on the planes of material existence. It is thanks to this super-computer that everyone is free within the limits of their own imprisonment. Only knowledge can bring freedom to all.

This gigantic structure, which can't be seen in any terrestrial telescope, contains enormous amounts of knowledge. This knowledge can be obtained by building geometric links through manifested symbols in various combinations. All this, in turn, is associated with the billions of planetary levels of the Universe – the very same cones over the northern and southern hemispheres of the infinite number of planets that Igor and I refer to as the genie's bottle. From here, the dream counterbalances the forces of the day and night, and the spirit – both visible and invisible forms. This is the most important movie projector of the Universe, due to which you look in the mirror and see yourself, never realizing that your reflection blocks the view of the Universe. Because you behold what is real but not the truth. And they are as far apart, as the forms stolen by scientists from Nature and the essence that filled them.

Each of these glowing spheres is called Sephiroth – these are steps and phases in the development of consciousness. Thanks to them, people can rise to their Father and stand by His side.

Probably ancient mystics knew this path. In any case, the Kabbalistic term "Sephiroth" (or "Sephira") referred, in their interpretation, to the fields and spheres of the Spirit, Air, Water, Fire, four corners of the Earth, and height and depth.

However, some things have changed in Sephiroth over a thousand years. It is also possible that the ancient sages encrypted in their names some of their own knowledge, unfamiliar even to us. For instance, what is the difference in the meaning of "Crown" and "Kingdom"? Unfortunately, this isn't a good time to ponder about medieval scholasticism.

159

Igor and I looked at Sephiroth, glowing in dark infinity with the colorful radiance of their spheres, and as we watched this giant projection of the Universe, the knowledge hidden within us emerged of itself from the depths of memory. We could see a multitude of symbols in our mind's eye, and we knew how to use them to summon and utilize any powers at any given level. We knew that powers could be manifested not only in the present, but in the past and future as well, at the level of the physical Universe.

To enter any of Sephiroth, one must know the name of the Ruler and the image, that is, the geometric form that serves as the gateway. We were attracted to one of the spheres in the central triangle of forces, and we responded to its call. We entered the closest of Sephiroth: it was an entire world, infinite as the Cosmos. We were asked: "Where are you from? Who are you?" And we were told to demonstrate the sign of the Father.

A huge archangel appeared opposite us. His name was Zadkiel.

He asked us why we were here.

We placed the Cross next to us. We knew that through the Cross the Lord Himself was able to see what was going on with us.

– We came to receive knowledge according to the Father's wishes, – Igor answered.

– Are you surprised that you had no problem entering the Sephira? – the Archangel queried.

We kept silent and didn't respond. We could tell that the Archangel was going to explain everything himself.

– Those who come to the Earth from the Creator always possess knowledge of the soul. In the past such people were referred to as prophets. They showed the way to the light of absolute truth. People such as these are now called writers and scientists. But not all writers and scientists can be considered prophets but only those who oppose falsehood and aren't afraid to speak the absolute truth. You have now ventured on the spiral path which Christ showed to man, so you will come to Him. Don't look into the Abyss – it could pull you in from these three levels. If you feel its impact, you should imagine our Lord. Through Him you will overcome the forces of hypnosis and death.

Set your heart so that your years don't fly by too quickly. Remember, time here goes by in a totally different way. Set your other organs so that your health doesn't suffer. You will have to pass eight Sphinxes who are guarding the gates. Take along your Book, but in order to carry it you will need to create a form. This is the skeleton which will preserve its content. In the next Sephira you will fill the form with energy.

You are always welcome to call me for help. I will come. Don't forget to thank your teachers. You will soon find yourself in the Hod Sephira. It is the joy that accompanies victory. You will be greeted there by Archangel Mikhail. He will help you fill the Book with matter. Let the Lord protect you.

We were a bit taken aback to hear the name of the well-known Archangel pronounced as a foreign name. But you don't fly to Rome unless you are prepared to do what the Romans do.

The changing space was constantly busy building new decorations around us.

When the Archangel was through giving us his advice for the road, he asked:

– Would you like to see the one who always supported you and who is like a brother to you?

We answered in the affirmative. Instantly, we saw a familiar image appear before us: it was the one driving the chariot, who a while ago

161

helped Igor and me not to lose our way in the infinite vistas of the Universe. There was the sign of Jupiter glowing above his head. We dropped to our knees.

Of course, at that moment I couldn't think straight and was able to comprehend it only afterwards: Why was it Jupiter? Why was it the King of the gods of ancient Rome?

At some point in the past, I studied the history of world religions, so I know that "each time a nation changes the faith of their fathers for a new one, one and the same phenomenon can be observed: the gods of the old faith turn into demons of the new faith, whereas all the liturgical rites of the old faith become sorcery and witchcraft in the face of the new faith... In the eyes of the fathers of the Christian Church, the gods of ancient Greece and Rome turned into demons and evil spirits" (M. Orlov, "The History of People's Interactions with the Devil," St. Petersburg, 1904).

So why is the essence under the sign of Jupiter helping us? And what in general is the hierarchy of divine creatures that govern life in these multiple worlds? What are the actual relations between the old and the new gods? Or are these actually stages of human cognition? We've met with the Creator, with the Father, and we have His Ring, but who else sees Him as the Creator? Is there anyone above Him? Or His equal, at least? How do the spirals of evolution, the Sephiroth and the DNA correlate with each other?

There were a million questions such as these, and I decided to accept everything as it is without seeking answers. We were endowed with a special gift, and we must use it for the benefit of others. Isn't it enticing to find out things that aren't given to you yet?

– Get up, – said the ruler of the Sephira with the sign of Jupiter. – This house is all yours. You may use everything that belongs to me as though it were your own. But now, listen.

He leaned over to us slightly.

– Today, you will also have to pass through the entire triangle of the lower forces. When you get into the fifth Sephira, remember that it has two abysses. Be careful when you're between them. When you approach the Sephira, you ought to slow down. To avoid falling out of the flow, you should get into the center of the speed of light. Stay strictly in the center, – he reiterated. – If everything works out, come back here any time. There are infinite resources of knowledge and strength here. Take them. Speak the absolute truth to people but never try to prove anything. Why should you try to convince someone that the Sun exists? He is bound to understand that himself some day. Don't waste your efforts needlessly. Those who are given to understand shall hear you. Go with God, – he admonished, – just as God goes with you.

In the next Sephira we are greeted by two – Mars, the god of war, and Saturn, the god of the Golden Age and Jupiter's father!

The ancient god is magnificent and calm. He looks at us closely, waiting for us to ask questions. But Mars, it seems, is not as benevolent. His eyes sparkle fiercely and challengingly in the shade of the visor helmet. The challenge seems to be aimed directly at Igor. He puts his hand on the hilt of his sword, throwing back the fold of his fiery red cape, which slid from his shoulder, and then takes a step forward.

– Why are you here? – he asks aggressively.

Without turning to him, Saturn raises his hand and stops his militant ally.

– Those you are talking to, – Saturn says, still without looking back at his companion, – come from the center of the Sephira, from behind it and from the front. You can't destroy that which is nothing and is everything,

163

and can be found everywhere but cannot be given a name. So what, are you planning to fight against something like that?

We can hear a slightly taunting note in Saturn's question addressed to the warrior friend. Mars hears it too and stops. He is perplexed. He thinks.

– You want to fight against the space? And how will you be inside it then? – Saturn continues. – Go ahead, pick a fight – it is against you.

Mars lowers the hilt of his sword and retreats behind Saturn again.

Saturn says:

– This is your home. You can stay here as long as you wish under our protection. No one can disturb you here, or get in your way. All the knowledge and strength of the fifth Sephira are at your disposal. Here, any form can be filled with matter. After you pass through Sephira Tiferet and Sephira Hod, your way lies to Yesod. Don't stay there long. Look behind the glass, don't look in the mirror.

* * *

We advance to the next Sephiroth, where Christ welcomes us. Leaning on the rails, He sits on His throne, with the Sun shining brightly on its back. Next to Him are a lion and double-headed eagle.

– So you made it here, – Jesus says. – It means that everything has been connected. You have managed to unite the central Sephiroth .

We kneel before Him.

– O, Lord, have we done everything the right way? Do we deserve being next to You?

– Your efforts are very commendable. But be careful what you say.

This time Christ speaks to me directly. Apparently, He does that because He is aware that I am prone to sharing my newly acquired knowl-

164

edge right away with whomever I might meet, without accommodating it to a particular environment, and trying to persuade people who are not yet ready to trust what I am telling them.

He then addresses Igor:

– Don't be silent about what you see. The absolute truth is above truth and falsehood.

He looks at us attentively, empathizing with what awaits us ahead.

– Always accommodate your strength, your knowledge and your abilities. Help anybody who begs for your help. Don't deny anyone – regardless of whether he is rich or poor.

After a short pause he adds meaningfully:

– I mean, you should help those who deserve it. And punish those who blaspheme Me.

He falls silent again, closely examining our faces. We don't dare to interrupt His silence by asking a question. In truth, there is no need to ask any questions out loud. He reads them directly in our consciousness.

–You are currently at the learning stage. After that you will be ready to do good works. But first of all, obtain knowledge. Right now you mean a lot, and at the same time – nothing. Complete your learning. Knowledge is not something you can receive the way you are taking a pill when you are sick. Knowledge you have to earn.

– Thank you, oh Lord!

– You still have to go through the Sephiroth below. They are called Yesod and Malkuth. One of them is the foundation and the other is the Kingdom. This is the path of initial creation, the path from the light of Heaven to the Earth. When a person follows this path, he also brings light to the Earth, through the planetary spheres, and then he brings the Earth back to Heaven. You have to build your system. Don't be afraid of anything. I am always by your side, helping you in everything.

– Thank you, oh Lord! – We express our gratitude to the One, Who has redeemed the world from the control of the evil one with His suffering.

He permits us to kiss the cross on His chest, and then we continue our journey in the strange cosmic computer, inside its networks and programs. We know: one who learns how to work on this computer will accomplish any results, because it contains the control panel of the Universe, the Earth and Man. But before anything else, one has to study himself most thoroughly, to understand what it is that we have inside, and only after that we can attempt to control global processes. First, it is necessary to know, then – to develop necessary skills and finally – to act.

So we proceed on our strange journey along the spiral.

We take the Cross and fly through space. It is totally different here, among the Sephiroth. It can initially be empty, but will suddenly create an obstacle in the form of a mountain ridge or a dense forest surrounding you from all sides – how should we know where to go then? But something is guiding Igor and me, as if we have a compass built into our souls that shows us the right way.

As we were rightly warned, Archangel Michael welcomed us in the Sephira Hod. We immediately recognized him because we had met him before. He looked young and handsome, exactly the way he is portrayed on Russian icons when he is slaying the dragon with his spear.

We greet him and ask for help.

He draws a circle around us, which immediately makes us feel extremely comfortable and warm.

– Here you can be whoever you want, – he says. – You can become the sky, the air or a waterfall. Take the book into the circle I have just drawn. Here the force strengthens the form. The Lord has given you the

166

nine colors, just as He has given them to me. Learn how to use them. They possess great force. Also, beware of women's cunning, – Michael sees us off with words of warning. – When you approach the Sephira Yesod, turn the circle into a sphere. It will protect you. Remember, you are going to enter the world of the Moon. Who knows what kind of mood she might be in? Beware of hypnosis. But there can be something else there, not only hypnosis. It is difficult to foresee in what hypostasis the Mistress of the Moon might be. If you find yourself in danger, call for Archangel Gabriel.

We thank our host who was so gracious to us and continue on our way. Strangely enough, we know where to go.

At last, we approach the Sephira Yesod. We build our defense system – a double mirrored reflection. This is a double globe, and we are inside it. We put all its external shells into motion. They rotate facing each other and prevent anyone from reading our thoughts. We enter in Yesod, where we see the already familiar figure sitting on the throne, which looks as if it were made of sea shells. This is the sphere of the Moon. We already met with its mistress at the levels. She presented us with the Golden Fleece. She now smiles at us, but something really odd is going on around us... We see beautiful naked women dancing in the moonlight by the river. The images are in slow motion; they flow unhurriedly, as if time itself has slowed down. We guess that this is hypnosis, but the mirrored globes weaken its impact. Igor and I are barely affected by the charms – we smile calmly, and the goddess on the throne smiles back at us. Wearing a long Greek tunic, she looks very beautiful.

– You are lucky that you weren't met by the one, who is yet to come, – she sounds mysterious as she repeats the words uttered by Kirill, the demon. – Currently, he is there, on Earth. You may descend to the Sephira Malkuth, but be careful. Don't count too much on your

167

globe. There is a silver thread in the center of the channel, and you must hold on to it. Your faith is your main defense. Don't be in too much of a hurry to die. Whether you die heroically or not, it doesn't really matter. What matters to you now is to learn and to acquire knowledge. Seek the truth – you are capable of doing that. You will hear, see and find it. The Earth will be preserved. Everything is in your power, – the goddess concluded, as if she was emphasizing the main concern Igor and I expressed in our thoughts. Before our eyes, the Book that we carry through the Sephiroth, becomes filled up with thoughts, words and images.

– Anything you wish can be corrected here and made real, – the goddess laughs. – Come visit me again. It will be my pleasure. Keep in mind, though, I am not always that bright. I also have a dark side.

We thank her and leave the Abode of the Moon.

Holding onto the silver thread, we descend to the Kingdom of the Earth. As soon as we approach its surface, we are instantly hit by an energy torrent. The dark vortex of the funnel, crisscrossed by splashes of fire, sucked in the mirrored globe, but we could feel the powerful, unlimited force engulfing us even through its reflecting walls.

A minute later, everything calms down.

We are back on Earth again, without our protective sphere, standing on a road, which runs through an immense field stretching to infinity. A gentle breeze caresses our faces and delicately shakes the slim green tops of the grass. The Earth is beautiful and radiant with light! We feel that we are inside Pushkin's fairy tale about the Golden Cockerel:* to one side of us we see a sumptuous sharp-coned tent, and a beautiful young woman beckons us inside, waving her hand. It looks like she might break into

* Reference to Alexander Pushkin's 1834 poem "The Tale of the Golden Cockerel".

song any minute the way the treacherous Queen of Shemakhan sings in the opera: "My ornate tent is so dark, so tight; the ornate rug in it is so soft and warm." She reminds me of the woman I saw in that weird dream I had during my trip to Theodosia.

Next to the tent there is a table lined with delicious foods and drinks. Carpets, rugs, ottomans and pillows are strewn around, promising bliss and long-awaited rest.

– What's the matter, mighty warriors? Why aren't you in a hurry to join me? – the queen asks teasingly. – Are you afraid of me?

Igor makes a jittery gesture and squeezes my hand.

– We have to pass through and carry the Book of Life down to Earth, – he shouts. – Which way should we go?

– Come to me, – the queen taunts us. She tempts us with her lovely body, now exposing her legs, now turning sideways.

– Let's enact the love play! – she cries out to us. – You will have lots of fun. The Earth is like a very large theater! And people are such brilliant actors.

– We don't want the Earth to be like a theater, – I find the right moment to join the conversation, since I am on my turf when art is mentioned. – We are carrying the Book of Life there. Life is what everyone needs. And you need it, too.

However, my words, intended to appease her, produce quite the opposite effect. Suddenly, we see before us not a beautiful queen but an ugly old woman who looks like Death. Her toothless mouth is contorted in a grimace of hatred.

– I don't have a life because of you. Go ahead, drag your silly book down to the level of the Earth. These are still only words, though important ones. You think people will accept them? And what will Mother

Nature think of all this? Nobody knows whether she Will she agree to share her power with the male principle? No one knows that, not even the One Who protects you.

We turned away from this woman with many faces, who is both love and tenderness, and hatred and death. We walked along the road across the field, following the call of our souls.

– For thousands of years nobody cared about the Earth and look, now everybody needs it, – we heard the old woman's shrill voice.

We didn't even turn our heads. We were carrying the Book of Life. In a short while, it was lying on the office desk at my home.

This book contained words that could open up the souls of people. But those words were still to be connected with the voice of the heart. That was the only way they could become visible.

We had barely a minute to discuss what had happened to us when we were summoned again.

When we ascended to the Kingdom of Christ, we found a huge crowd of people right at the gates. They came here from various churches, various countries, and they were all seeking help. A man in light garments with a recognizable ring on his finger walked between the rows of people and sprinkled them with holy water. He stopped next to us.

– Yes, you have descended to Malkuth, – he says. – But this is not the entire path. Are you ready to ascend any further?

The way He posed the question clearly indicated that it would not be easier to ascend than to descend, in fact, it would be harder.

– Yes, we are ready, – we answer without hesitation. He makes the sign of the cross over us and sprinkles us with holy water.

– I believe it: you will make it to the gates of the Father. I personally will accompany you. Your efforts will be rewarded. The Energy of

170

the Absolute will pour into your souls. This is the purest energy. It gives health and radiant peace to those who are overwhelmed with feelings. Care for everybody who seeks help and take care of all the needy and sick. From now on the Gates of My Kingdom are always open for you. Many people wander right next to them, stretching out their hands in the pleas for help, but they don't even see where they are stretching them out. They don't know, Who they are asking for help.

There in the Sephiroth, if things get really tough, don't forget about the Lord's ring. You may look into it and come back any moment. You will just enter the ring and find yourself in My Kingdom. Here I am your protection.

He suddenly pulls two more crosses from somewhere and puts them on me and Igor, next to the ones we have always been wearing.

– Let my little cross defend and protect you, – Christ says. Go through My Kingdom. You will see a ladder, climb it, and you will find yourself in the right place.

We give the Lord a hug and break into tears. So we stand there, the three of us, feeling as though we are seeing each other for the last time. The Lord is comforting us.

– Don't be afraid of anything. Endure whatever comes your way before you use this ring as your last resort. Go ahead, don't be afraid. You are just wasting your energy which you will need badly.

We say farewell again and walk to the ladder.

We ascend to find huge gates in front of us. We are no bigger than ants if compared to them. But as soon as we touch them we immediately grow. We have the kind of strength we never felt before. We touch the leaves another time and the gates open.

There is a ladder in front of us. We climb up, and a heavenly view

171

unfolds before us. An archangel stands by the ladder, peering at us rather searchingly. Someone resembling an ancient king with a crown on his head is sitting by his side.

– What brings you here? – asks the archangel.

– We came for the word of the Father, – Igor replies.

– What is in it for you, in His word? – This question already comes from the one who looks like a king.

– There is nothing more important for us and for all the people, – Igor answers.

– Is it hard for you, warrior, to be surrounded by all these divine energies?

– It is not hard at all. I feel great here. This is the House of my Father, the One Who created everything in the world.

Suddenly, the boundary line, on which we were firmly standing, turned clockwise. Still, we kept our balance and didn't fall.

– Who sent you here? – asks the king.

– The Creator's Son.

– But you are ordinary people, – he says, and we can read between the lines that he is uncomfortable both with denying us entry and with allowing us in. "These people left the level of human consciousness and ascended here, where nobody has ever been. Moreover, the Son gave them the permission. What shall I do? Let them go farther but what if they die?"

He thought very seriously for a long time. Then he rose from his throne and began pacing, with his hands behind his back. Finally, he stopped.

– So, what kind of wealth do you possess that you were allowed to get here?

– It is our faith and the earth of the Father in our sack, – Igor answers.

– Also, the Spirit of our Father that nobody can destroy or take away from us.

The ruler of the Sephira loses himself in thought again. His face suddenly lightens up. He looks happy.

– Well, here is my blessing for you. Go to the left to your Mother's abode.

We thank him and go on. It doesn't take us long before we see another throne, from which a beautiful woman gazes at us with very kind eyes.

– Who you are looking for? – she asks.

– We are looking for our Mother, who is the Mother of our Lord, – this time I am the first to answer, not Igor.

– I know about you, – the Queen of Heaven says. Her voice tells us that She would have wanted to get up from Her throne and embrace Igor and me.

Her throne is surrounded by sadness, but it doesn't make us feel sad.

– I will not test you in anything, My children, – She promises, – because you have already experienced everything in your life – both grief and joy. I am happy to see you here. It will be easier for me now, more joyful. You are the first people who were able to touch the gates of the Heavenly Father with your hands.

After She made the sign of the cross over us, we find ourselves once again in the Kingdom of the Son. He is waiting for us and takes us to the gates. But this time the gates are already different. They open by themselves as He approaches.

– This is the Kingdom of My Father, – Jesus says, pointing with his hand to the infinite space around. – Study it and observe its laws. This is the road, and here is the Sun that is shining. It's warm there, pleasant and joyful. Go, go ahead.

The ladder is right under our feet. It isn't just any ladder: with every

173

step we take on this ladder, various questions appear inside our consciousness. Actually, only Igor can hear them. He is also the one who answers them. He is leading me by my hand, as if I were a child. Question – answer. The step on the ladder turns around, allowing us to climb up to the next one. There are 12 steps in the ladder and twelve corresponding questions. Very strong light is shining right into our eyes. Finally, we reach the last step.

We ascend it – and disappear. It feels as though our body and all its organs have fallen apart. We have no arms and legs, only thoughts and feelings remain. It is necessary to assemble ourselves now. But how is this done?

We pray, asking the Lord to strengthen our spirit and to grant us knowledge, which is the light of the soul. Miraculously, merely by the effort of our thought, all the body parts and organs start rebuilding themselves in the strict order, which we never thought we knew. Igor assembles himself first and helps me do the same. We look around and see the Creator standing next to Christ. We kneel before him.

– You studied the technology of immortality and resurrection right now, – the Father says. – The one who is capable of resurrecting himself will never die. People call it Doomsday. Did you feel that you were doomed?

– They had no time to get scared, Father, – Christ intervenes on our behalf. – You just saw how fast they assembled themselves.

– Your strength has multiplied, – the Creator says. – There are no obstacles for you now. Knowledge – that's all what you need. You probably thought that you've learned all that there is, but your learning has just begun. Each step in My Kingdom means greater knowledge and skills. I am pleased with you. Go now. I will summon you shortly.

We get up and thank the Father and the Son. When we get past the gates, we see nine colors around us, shining like the rainbow.

We descend to the levels and look at the Earth from the upper platform. It doesn't look anything like it did before. We are standing right above the solar plexus. We can see body parts, blood vessels, arms and legs. What is most amazing: the Earth-Man is standing on another Earth and looking down. This is the Earth's other state and its thinner body.

– Do you want to take a trip to India? – I ask Igor.

– Sure, why not? All the more so, since it will enable us to check out our new abilities. As far as I can guess, passing through the Sephiroth allows us to combine the informational and energy planes of the Cosmos and Earth. Is there anyone in particular we are planning to check out in India? – My friend asks this question in a business-like manner.

– It's Avatar Sai Baba, – I don't know why, but I switch topics from the Sephiroth to a perfectly real man, though he is one who is particularly famous for his miracles.

– Who is he?

– They say he is the reincarnation of god in a human form.

– And he is still alive? – Igor can't hide his surprise, apparently remembering how people usually express their gratitude to their Saviors.

– But we are talking about India. People there are known for their very special attitudes towards divine incarnations in human form. This is an entirely different culture with tolerance, understanding and confidence that such things are genuinely possible.

– Does he support his unusual claims with anything? – Igor asks. For one brief instant, I see the outlines of a police uniform hat on his head.

– That's the whole point. He supports it in a variety of ways. He is able to materialize objects. When hundreds of faithful come to him,

175

seeking his help, he passes them by, sprinkling them with vibhuti healing powder that comes straight from his fingers. This powder helps to cure many diseases. He is also capable of making sweets in the same way, and even diamonds.

– So, you would like to see how he does all this? Is that it? – Arepyev wants to make sure he understands my motives.

– Yes, I do, – I admit sincerely.

– Okay then, – Igor agrees.

We quickly find the place we need from the height of the levels. We see a man making his way through the crowd, his face surrounded with a huge black sphere of hair. He has so much hair that it makes his head look twice, even three times bigger than it is. This hair is what initially attracts attention, then the Indian guru's eyes and smiling lips. He walks through the crowd, and we actually see him sprinkling endless amounts of powder right from his hands. Then he enters a house where nobody is admitted. He sits down on the floor, all by himself, and starts meditating. He sits like this, motionless, for several hours, concentrating on his spiritual work. At night, when the town sleeps, Sai Baba comes out onto the balcony, stretches out his hands towards the houses and prays for the people of his town to be healthy. Many are healed in these hours before dawn.

– Let's see what he does with the powder, – I suggest to Igor.

We took another look at the image. When we slowed down the time, we were able to see how Sai Baba created a thought-form. He molded the future image by the sheer strength of his thought. He took this thought-form through the Sephiroth, through Yesod and Malkuth, and then it emerged at the planetary levels. Now it looks like a capsule, containing information about the events yet to come.

– Did you figure out what he has been doing? – I ask Igor nervously.

– What is there not to figure out?

– Let's create something ourselves then.

– Why not?

We instantly get back home, to my office from where we started our unusual journey.

– So what are we going to materialize? – Igor sounds business-like again. He is focused and aims for success.

– Let's make a ballpoint pen, – I suggest. – You know how much I have to write these days. Oh, yes, there should be as much ink in it as possible.

We create the informational skeleton of the pen – it's big, with a wide internal ink reservoir. We take it through the Sephiroth. Nobody interferes with our experiment. Here we go – the pen is already filled with energy, obtaining all its material features in Yesod. We lower it in Malkuth … and it disappears without a trace.

– What did we do wrong?

Igor scratches his head, deep in thought.

– Looks like this morning girl of yours isn't letting it in. We have to settle this somehow.

– What are you hinting at? – I ask suspiciously. Apparently, Igor is aware of my Theodosia problems with the mistress of the lower Sephira.

– There is no point pretending, – my friend reasons calmly. – I saw everything. She will continue to get in our way until we bow before her. And, of course, as soon as you bow, she will chop of your head with a scythe.

– Don't tell me that two strong men can't cope with one skinny woman?

– We'll see how it goes, – my friend agrees.

I have no objections.

– If we see, it means we're alive.

* * *

We had a meeting with Grabovoi scheduled for the following evening. As always, Igor and I tried to be precisely on time. It was not easy for Grigori Petrovich to find time in his extremely busy work schedule for a discussion of our current problems. Were these problems just ours, however? It seemed that the scale of events had begun to outgrow the boundaries of any personal destiny, even those of the country's borders.

As usual, there were crowds of people waiting in the reception area. Nobody here got into fights, or demanded that he or she be allowed to see the doctor immediately based on their high rank, important status or impressive position. Here, all are equal and no privileges apply. Everybody feels equally bad and all hope to find deliverance from their disease. As a rule, not without cause, because the statistics reflecting Grabovoi's successful performance is one hundred percent.

This time, too, we had to wait a lot longer than usual. Grigori Petrovich's secretary, Sasha, who knew about our special relationship with his boss, came up to Igor and me.

– You'll have to wait no less than an hour, – he said quietly. – He is taking care of something urgent. Someone in the government just called. He is now working.

– Does this happen frequently? – Igor asked.

– Very much so, – Sasha confirmed. After a brief pause, he added: – Actually, every day. I came to work here so I could learn these technologies. When is there time to study? There's a crowd of people waiting to see him all the while. He doesn't have one minute to spare the whole day.

Sasha is quite young, about twenty years old. We can tell that he is truly upset because he is unable to realize his dream. Igor suddenly suggests:

178

– Why don't you come to our Center? We will teach you.

The young man's face shows apparent dismay.

– Are you saying that you too can do these things?

– Our technologies are virtually identical. He simply started doing it before us. But we basically do the same things.

Sasha didn't have time to respond: he was summoned by Grabovoi. A minute later, Sasha called us.

– Grigori Petrovich asks you to come in, but he has very little time. Please try to be concise. He has to go to the Security Council in an hour.

Grigori Petrovich, as always, came from behind his desk to greet us. His face, indeed, seemed more concerned than usual.

I immediately began to update him on the latest developments of how Igor and I passed the various Sephiroth, and what trials we experienced along the way.

Grigori Petrovich was not aware of these events, which seemed puzzling to us. He was always aware of our adventures and proceeded to discuss them, without waiting for our report. But this time he examined what happened along with us.

Something had changed. And the change was dramatic. It seemed that Grigori Petrovich was equally perplexed by the fact that part of our work now escaped his psychic vision.

In the course of my story he asked for more precise details, seemed very tense and anxious, sometimes making important comments, especially about the Abyss. He knew about the Sephiroth and about the Path in general. But he didn't know – and it was quite obvious he didn't – how the two of us, Igor and I, covered the Path.

– I can only congratulate you with what happened, – he said when I finished my account. – People rarely succeed in doing what you have done. I will soon have nothing left to teach you, if you continue at such lightning speed.

– What should we do with the Queen of Malkuth? – I asked, suspecting that in the future it may turn out to be the most serious problem in our work.

– You have figured out her second incarnation correctly – it is Death. Tell me, what can conquer Death?

– Is it life?

–Yes, life, – Grigori Petrovich confirmed. – That's why you need to learn the practice of resurrection as quickly as possible. If you resurrect at least one person, Death will no longer be an obstacle in your way.

He checked the time on his watch.

– I have a little more time, and I'll tell you about some specific aspects of resurrection. Passing the Sephiroth allows you to utilize the third level of consciousness. This contains enormous power and might. Consciousness of the third level is able to compress time and space. What does it give you? Compression of space makes it possible to see the event at its initial stage, to work on the Sephiroth and take appropriate action. It is, of course, essential to develop practical skills. Theory alone is not enough, because much depends on the speed of interaction with the structures of the Universe.

He uttered these last words already while standing to leave. We understood how difficult it was for him to manage so much in so little time. And we tried not to linger too long saying our goodbyes.

* * *

The next day we began to see very serious complications in Marina Nikolayevna's condition. I already spoke about this woman in "Save Yourself", the first book of the trilogy. She suffers from radiation sickness and kidney cancer; her liver is badly scarred, while the heart is on the

180

verge of failing. Five months ago, when her husband came to us seeking help, the doctors said she had seven to ten days to live at the most. All this time we managed to achieve one victory after another in our efforts to combat the disease. Merely a month after we started working with her, she began to walk again and crave for food, even to read books. She was alive several months later, instead of having only a few days. Her hope for a cure strengthened so much that she began to make plans for the future. She called family and friends and told them that she was feeling much better, saying that she will soon go to stay at their summer house. And then everything changed.

We couldn't understand why it was happening. We saw that our program towards recovery was still active, but Marina Nikolayevna's consciousness was blocking its work.

The screen of inner vision shows us her strained conversation with some woman. The latter is clearly annoyed by our patient's plans for a healthy life. She gets angry and starts berating her companion: don't believe these fairy tales with psychics, no one else in the world has ever coped with such diseases; you've got to preserve your energy and not distract yourself with thoughts about work. As the sarcastic Ukrainian proverb goes: "My friend, don't waste your strength in vain, but descend to the grave without pain." What the woman said to her was monstrous – it killed her hope. The negative emotions caused by the conversation began to spread. Marina Nikolayevna started to have doubts and yield to despair. She became hesitant, remembered that no one indeed had ever been successful in curing radiation sickness at such an advanced stage. She resented allowing herself to hope, to believe in something that couldn't happen.

In fact, we were observing the negative influence public consciousness could have on the work of healers. It proclaims: "What you do is impossible in principle! It has never happened! Stop doing what is useless! A person's life is determined by his or her fate. By fate, not by man!" Regretfully, Marina Nikolayevna agreed with this negative attitude.

Of course, destiny is the flow and movement of Heaven, as the Chinese philosopher Zhu Xi maintained eight hundred years ago. So what? We were becoming increasingly convinced that the Soviet poet Ilya Selvinsky was closer to the truth when he said: "That fate of ours is less significant than we are; man is superior to his fate." Someone might say that these words were written in an era of mass heroism, which the circumstances imposed on the people. But the circumstances are manifestations of destiny. And if Leningrad during the Nazi siege and Stalingrad surrounded by German forces in World War II were able to resist these circumstances, what motivated people then? It was anything but resignation to their fate.

How many times was such perseverance demonstrated throughout Russia's history? In Europe, people never saw anything wrong in surrendering to superior forces of the enemy. Not so in Russia. Polish troops laid siege to Smolensk from September 1609 to June 1611. Over this period of nearly two years, the power in Moscow collapsed and the church freed all Russian citizens from their oath of loyalty to the deposed Tsar Vasili Shuisky. No one would have blamed the residents of Smolensk for surrendering their city. The number of inhabitants had decreased from 80,000 to 8,000, but they continued to hold their ground. In the end, they exhausted the Poles and gave Russia the heroic exploits of Minin and Pozharsky.* And what about the blazing fire that engulfed Moscow during Napoleon's invasion in 1812?

Below you will find some interesting data from American media

* Kuzma Minin and Count Dmitry Pozharsky became national heroes
after their army defeated Polish troops that occupied Moscow.

sources. In 1973, when physicians in Israel went on a month-long strike and the number of hospitalizations

fell by 85%, mortality rates in the country dropped by half, its lowest level during the state's entire existence. The previous significant reduction in mortality was observed twenty years earlier and, remarkably, it also occurred during a doctors' strike. One gets the impression that people do not survive because of, but despite the efforts of medics. And the old joke: "What do you say – should we treat him or let him live?" is not as far from the truth, as we used to think.

In 1976, during a similar strike in the United States, in Los Angeles County, mortality also fell by 20%.

How can this be explained? People recognized that they can rely only on themselves. They mobilized their spiritual resources, and half of them were able to overcome their ailments.

Nowadays, there is much discourse about the role Russia will play in the new century. Representatives of various faiths are saying that it is her finest hour. But the

things they see in their hazy image of future years, Igor and I know for certain already now. And we don't understand those who humbly refer to fate.

Fate, destiny – these are mediators between the Father and His children. But the Heavenly Father himself is eternal. He is not threatened by any illness or by death. So who placed this inevitable something called fate between man and his quest for the absolute truth? Who elevated fate, which leads man to certain death? And why is public opinion completely unaware of the possible and achievable unity of body and soul that cannot be destroyed, of non-dying and resurrection?

Igor and I are trying to give momentum to those segments of the soul

183

that have already left the body. It's hard. Marina Nikolayevna's soul is tired of suffering; it doesn't want to return to the earth plane and experience the same torment again. With great difficulty, we persuade her soul to stop the process of destruction of the body's physical structures and to continue performing its functions. Thus, we won a bit of extra time.

We must once again take a closer look at the levels of the planetary computer. Now that we have passed the Sephiroth of the Tree of Life, we must learn how to control the Earth's programs through them and to influence events towards positive change. Indeed, we now see the levels quite differently. We look at them from the platform above.

All the levels – at the top and at the bottom – are separated by the cross of the Bardo channel. Paradise opens up immediately in all its scope. It is small and huge at the same time. Its infinite vastness is determined by the additional coordinate of space and time compression. There are a lot of trees and flowers in Paradise. Armor, swords and chests filled with treasures are scattered everywhere. There is an apple with a bite taken out of it lying on a plate on a table. Apparently, this is a memory of how Adam and Eve had transgressed thousands of years ago. We see the five trees that have some special significance. They also have apples on them. As we look, we get the impression that

Earth itself is also an apple on the Tree of Life. There is a connection between what happens on Earth, and this place that people refer to as Paradise. But for some reason it looks like a holographic image. Actually, the word "image" is hardly appropriate here. It's more like a program of a giant supercomputer. Well, this isn't a precise analogy either.

From here, from the platform, we can see what is happening down below on Earth very well. We observe a derailed train: information about the recent event is expanding like a balloon or, more accurately, like a

184

mushroom, next to the wreckage of the train. Threads of information stretch out to different levels, including the ninth one, Paradise, towards the five trees. This is a global system of information interdependencies. And the "images" of the levels are not passive witnesses to the events, but active influences. We use the window of opportunity and effect positive change to the event before it has actually occurred.

Similar processes are taking place in the department of the planetary computer called Hell. It also has five trees. It's as though there are two different movie theaters next to one another – in the first one you feel good, free and joyful; in the second, quite the opposite – gloomy, oppressed and uncomfortable, even bad. Apart from their connection with the Earth, these two programs are also connected to each other, like communicating vessels. They maintain a constant balance, and, depending on this balance, someone on Earth is lucky enough to recover, but someone else, who is perfectly healthy, dies in an accident. All of this runs in automatic mode. True, it is possible to intervene. Those who are permitted can do that.

In these "movie theaters" each person sees his or her own specially designed film, with the meaningful title "My Life". Every action, every word, even every thought is subjected to self-analysis here and self–condemnation. The person examines absolutely everything he or she had done on Earth. He is his own prosecutor, defense attorney and judge. This is a thoroughly conducted trial, because every person has a certain program of incarnations and a set of qualities that he must test during his many lives.

He must be able to connect his initially disconnected components throughout a certain given number of incarnations. If he falls behind schedule, he should select such trials of life for himself that will make it possible for him to simultaneously pass two or three steps leading up Jacob's ladder within one life span. That's why they say that you can't really deceive yourself. As he enters a new incarnation, each individual must improve what has been achieved and earn himself those personal qualities that he hasn't previously acquired. If he fails to do so he will face new coils on the horizontal eight configuration of infinity, or worse, the rapid descent to the hellish structures of the underground levels.

We look at cities, factories and villages behind the looking glass. We can pierce the wall of their houses with our hands. But only we can do that. For them, this would be impossible. Their collective consciousness registers as indomitable reality what we perceive to be like a shadow theater, a virtual reality of holographic objects. True, they also perceive our world as a reflection of theirs. And it is unclear who is more correct. A world within a world... Who will cognize it? Who will understand? Who will be able to use what he guessed, and how?

A few days after Igor and I experienced the trial of Judgment Day, I came across a newspaper article, which described a totally amazing instance of resurrection after 26 hours of clinical death. This incident occurred with Dmitri Shulgin from the Ukrainian town of Enakievo.

Dmitri drowned on a cold January morning, the day after Christmas.* An hour later, a group of fishermen and the rescuers, whom they called in for help, were able to pull him out of the water. The young man's body was first placed in the hospital morgue and he was then taken home by his relatives, who started making preparations for the funeral. Suddenly, when the coffin and the wreaths were already brought into the house, and the death certificate issued, Dmitri came back to life. He was taken to the hospital again and discharged two weeks later with a "healthy" diagnosis. No brain damage was identified during testing.

*Russian Orthodox Christmas takes place on January 7th
(following the Gregorian Calendar, which corresponds to the 25th of December).

An absolutely fantastic event, though if all such cases were collected in a book, they would take up more than one volume. Why is it that people pay no attention to such signs?

Let us now give the floor to the "drowned" man himself and listen to what he remembers about the event:

"When the ice broke under me, I felt a powerful shock – my whole body instantly went numb. I had time to inhale just once and started sinking. Then I recovered slightly and began to surface. To my dismay, there was ice above. I hit my head against the wall of ice and lost consciousness...

I wake up and can't understand what is happening to me? I am rising above the Earth; there are houses and people below me. I don't see my body, but it doesn't scare me in the least. I feel an extraordinary lightness mixed with heavenly bliss. Then I am suddenly surrounded by extremely bright white light. Someone starts talking to me, and I somehow feel His immeasurable greatness and power. There is even brighter light ahead of me; it fills my soul with bliss.

This was the absolute Supreme Mind, and I spoke with it forever, but maybe just for a few moments. It had so much to tell me that I still continue to comprehend and process all this information. At the very end it showed me how the soul of the deceased is reborn in a new body. A ghostly whitish cloud rushed down, moaning and sighing, and I followed it. Down below, a woman was in labor at the hospital. When the baby emerged out of the mother's womb and uttered its first cry, the cloud merged with the infant and dissolved in it. At this very moment, as the Supreme Mind explained to me, all information about its former life is erased completely from the newly reborn soul. When the person dies, the soul will remember everything once again. It will wander in a disembodied state in the other world until it becomes embodied in a new human form. This cycle will continue endlessly, unless the person enters into a kind of Paradise, if he is able to fully get rid of all human vices. After his death, a person may spend years or even decades in a unique kingdom of shadows, observe what is happening on Earth, whether in bliss or in sadness, depending on what he deserves. Then he has to be embodied in a new-born baby once again. All his mistakes and all the evil he committed in a past life will come back to him like a boomerang. A villainous murderer will have to experience on his own skin what it feels like to be defenseless victim; an arrogant fat cat, who humiliated others will be reborn as a miserable slave. A person who committed suicide because of some stupid depression, or, say, because of foolishness typical of the young, may be reborn as a genuinely unhappy and unfortunate man – in this way God teaches us to love and value life. And, paradoxically, the person who ended his life so frivolously, when reincarnated into a half-blind cripple, for example, will as a rule really know the price of life in the end, and even begin to love it."

– What is the Supreme Mind? – journalist Alex Zagoryansky asked Dmitri during this interview.

– It's impossible to see and to know it. The power of the Supreme Mind extends not only to our planet Earth. It controls all global physical processes. By the way, the evolution theory is not at odds with religious beliefs about the creation of the world.

– Did you manage to enter the kingdom of shadows?

– I wasn't allowed there. I was told that it isn't time yet. The explanation I got was that I hadn't yet fulfilled my mission, so I will be sent back and will walk my life's path with dignity to its very end, living with goodness and creativity. By the way, the Creator is repulsed by unprincipled, primitive and stupid people who don't wish to develop their inherent potential for the sake of goodness and creativity. He turns away from people like that sooner or later... Here is how I came back. Suddenly, I flew towards the Earth very fast, and several moments later I recovered consciousness. I found myself under a blanket in my room. I was in pain and felt weak, and then I lost consciousness again, fully recovering my senses only in the hospital.

– Have you acquired any new abilities after your return from the afterlife?

– I respond to the world around me differently. I learned to enjoy simple and ordinary things, like the beauty of Nature, for example. At the same time I remain indifferent to everything that is superfluous and contrived, to all the garbage we people have created. I began to show a talent for painting and writing. My most important accomplishment, which is my life's purpose, lies ahead. I will do everything in my power not to be ashamed before the Creator later..."

That's the story – a concrete history of a particular individual. How should traditional science respond, when it encounters such things? Exactly the way it already does – by turning away and forgetting all about it.

Here is another phenomenon, this time from our southern provinces – Natasha Beketova, a nurse from Anapa, started talking when she was two months old. And she didn't speak only in Russian. She spoke in 120 languages of different language groups.

These are ancient languages often regarded as dead. Natasha speaks freely, reads and writes in all of them. The young woman confesses that she hasn't studied any of them.

An article about this sensational phenomenon by journalist Saveli Kashnitsky was published on March 30, 2001 in "Moskovsky Komsomolets".

"Oddly enough, Natasha did not know the Old Russian language. But

for some reason, she did know the Anglo-Celtic-Saxon language spoken in the 13th–14th centuries. The British do not understand her now, except for residents of Yorkshire, who speak a dialect more similar to the language of their ancestors than any other.

Hardly any Frenchman, except for a linguist perhaps, will understand Natasha, whose French sounds as if it was carried over from 16th century France. She will definitely find no one to talk to in Japan: the Japanese language has changed so much since the 12th century.

Sometimes, the young woman demonstrates such a profound knowledge of a language that it baffles scientists and experts. When she speaks in ancient Egyptian, for example, she clearly pronounces the vowel sounds, which to this day remain a mystery to Egyptologists. All deciphered papyri, inscriptions on stone reliefs and murals of the era of Pharaohs represent a set of consonants. No one knows how exactly the names of Ramses, Tutankhamen and Hatshepsut sounded in their time – that is why in different books one may come across a variety of options.

Incidentally, while reading the ancient texts of the Nile Valley, Natasha introduced a lot of corrections: the use of different vowels can, in fact, change the meaning of a word beyond recognition. Compare, for instance, such English words as "bed", "bid" and "bet". They mean totally different things. And if you write them down as "BD" or "BT" their true meaning may only be guessed from the context. Now imagine a text where there are several words with multiple versions of pronunciation standing next to each other...

I listened to Natasha Beketova along with two dozen scholars in the humanities. Of course, some of the things she said were checked for accuracy in a very subtle and inoffensive manner.

The young woman was asked to say something in Arabic. She spoke

190

at once, filling the room with guttural sounds, characteristic of languages throughout the Mediterranean world. Nikolai Nikolayevich Vashkevich, a prominent Arabic expert who attended the meeting, admitted that he understood only a small portion of the phrase. Quite possibly, Natasha said something in a dialect spoken by ancient herders even before the time of Prophet Muhammad.

One language scholar asked Natasha if she knew the tribal dialects of Southeast Asia.

She nodded modestly in response. These tribes, the linguist said, use certain words that sound identical, but denote different notions. Only the way they are intoned and their phonetic nuances allow one to determine exactly to what language these words belong. The Orientalist pronounced a short word in a particular way and asked Natasha to what language it belonged. She instantly gave the right answer. The linguist was amazed.

The journalist who wrote the essay also asked the hyperpolyglot a question:

– So you speak a certain language. But how could you possibly know that it is Chinese used in the fourteenth century before you discussed it with Sinologists?

– I don't know how. But I always know whose language it is and from what time period.

Pyotr Nikolayevich Andreyev reassured Natasha: she is not the only one in the world with similar abilities. In Guyana, a country located in northeastern South America, there are people who speak more than a hundred languages, some of them also remote in space and time.

Natasha was asked if there is any similarity between the languages she knows, and if they, perhaps, descended from a common proto-language. She replied quite logically, saying that not being a linguist she has no right to put forward her own hypothesis. But, in fact, she does detect a lot of common roots, say, in Russian and Sanskrit. Experts don't find this to be particularly surprising, but the similarities in the ancient Egyptian and Russian languages are, indeed, unexpected.

Still, which languages are descendants of a probable proto-language to the greatest extent? Natasha's response is certain to give linguists considerable food for thought. She suggested it is the Anglo-Celtic-Saxon, Turkish, Arabic and Russian languages.

And here is what occurred to me then. The semantic fields of languages so distant and different from one another should vary substantially. Since Natasha speaks all these languages, surely the Creator has placed much more than that in her subconscious mind. Therefore, in my opinion, Egyptologists can not only clarify the texts of translations done from the language of the Pharaohs, but find the answers to some secrets, which were revealed only to priests and scribes. That is why the phenomenon of Natasha Beketova should be studied not only by linguists and psychologists, but also by specialists in cultural studies, theologians and ethnology experts..."

These conclusions are quite logical. Do you think anyone will take the journalist's advice? I doubt it. Those people who have declared themselves to be the guardians and interpreters of the absolute truth are unlikely to listen to something that reminds them too obviously of God. They have their own god – their inflated Egos. And they do not want to know another.

No wonder one of the fathers of the idea of the "the retort baby" Robert Edwards announced the new era of genetic engineering with the following defiant slogan: "Ethics must adapt to science, not vice versa."

In fact, since the time a cloned lamb appeared before a group of photographers and journalists in the small Scottish village of Roslin, and the

192

"modest" bio-researcher Ian Wilmut credited himself as its creator, many experts decided that we have entered the era of "designed" humans. "Everything is now possible," – American biologist Lee Silver proclaimed in February 1997. British Nobel Peace Prize Winner Joseph Rotblat, on the contrary, publicly expressed his concern that "the future of humanity is at stake."

No sooner did a debate over the "rules for the human herd" begin to heat up in the media than a group of American biologists introduced their new lab creation: a mouse whose intelligence was increased with the help of gene technology. Weren't these new accomplishments the best motivator for a serious discussion about the future of biotechnology?

> Now a smile of knowing
> Lit the idiot's joyful face...

That is how the poet Yuri Kuznetsov responded to a similar experiment involving a frog about thirty years ago. And I can understand why. Rats and mice "breathe in the back" of Homo sapiens, based on their level of intelligence, so to say. If we should stumble on the twists of evolution, these rodents will grow up fast, learn to stand on their hind legs and replace us as leaders. So I dare you, scientific "geniuses", to expand their intellect, go ahead do it!

"Scientists played around at random with various methods of reproduction until they encroached in their efforts upon germ cells – the biological route transmitting the human heritage" ("Rossiyskaya Gazeta", October 29, 1999).

So far, genetics is a purely diagnostic discipline, which in clinical practice plays a rather auxiliary role. Still, modern medicine increasingly considers man as material for modeling. Surgeons and makers of artificial organs, producers of in-vitro babies and inventors of psycho pills – all of them are set on shaping our body and mind. They do not confine themselves to making man healthier; they want to create a more work efficient and even an overall happier individual. It turns out that Steve Hawking has many like-minded supporters.

Biotech labs are already growing skin and cartilage. Physicians use crushed bones to form human jaws and they mold ears out of discarded human cells. They make liver and connective tissues climb like wild ivy along subtly branching artificial skeletons and want to grow secondary organs for gravely ill patients out of embryonic stem cells.

It has become conventional in medical practice to directly influence consciousness itself: millions of over-active children consume pills which decrease their nervousness. Most people ignore warnings of experts that the drug has a serious side-effect: it undermines the individual's creative possibilities. Not hundreds, but hundreds of thousands of Americans artificially boost their mood by regularly taking special drugs. Hasn't pharmacology been creating a new type of modern individual for a long time by doing all this? Hasn't it been producing this happy person?

Reproductive medicine has made more advances than anyone on the way towards creating a new human being. The large directories of American seed banks offer women an extensive choice in finding a father for their child. They can choose whatever characteristics they like – the color of hair and skin, height, background and academic titles, including Nobel Prize winners. "In practice we are already engaged in selection," – says Detlef Linke, a neurologist at the University Hospital of Bonn, – the selection of sperm is now a reality that many consider unacceptable."

"We seize control of our own evolution," – echoes biophysicist Gregory Stock from the University of California at Los Angeles. And to prevent any misinterpretation, he immediately adds: "There is no way to hinder the development of this technology."

Nobody listens to lone voices of dissent. "Gene mapping will be a more significant accomplishment than splitting the atom, and a no less dangerous one," – warns the New York researcher, molecular biologist Liebe Cavalieri.

The newspaper "Sueddeutsche Zeitung" published the forecast of molecular biology expert Jens Reich from Berlin, "Not only man's life sources and physical well–being will be subject to manipulation by biotechnology, but also his path in life and potential longevity."

The well-known scholar Francis Fukuyama shares this view: "Mankind is at the culminating point of yet another technological revolution; it intends to 'create' a new human species."

In his book, Fukuyama provides readers with convincing proof that the technology of the future will make it possible "to grow less aggressive people", and he says that we cannot reject this opportunity. He was talking here about "Nietzsche's superman in a bottle" and about "post-human history." So why hasn't this work caused an uproar?

One gets the impression that man is overly fascinated with the role of King of Nature, although he has never been denied the part of the demiurge, and has even been given that role as a matter of course. All in good time, as the saying goes. Stalin and Hitler, as many others before them, also believed that they were ready to play the role of supreme rulers of the world. But if you examine these notorious characters more closely, you will see that they are distinguished, first and foremost, by their exaggerated rationalism. It is what we mean when we say about a person that he has no soul. This isn't at all a figure of speech, but a realistic assessment of the individual's personality. Because the soul is not ephemeral as those who don't have it would like us to believe. The SOUL is the foundation of the Universe; moreover, it is the main instrument of its creation. Opposing world forces fight for the possession of people's souls. The predominance of heartless people in positions of power leads mankind to a misunderstanding of its role in the evolutionary process and, consequently, to a distortion in its form of existence. All the troubles we have in our lives, in our health, and personal and interpersonal relationships are the consequence of a dysfunctional form of existence. Simply put, we are always in the wrong place, and always doing somebody else's job.

As a result, if we look only at the environmental aspect of our reality(and this is the slice of reality upon which our very existence depends), we will find out that: "Forests are shrinking by 27.2 million acres per year; the size of deserts increases by 14.8 million hectares; 26 billion tons of fertile soil is lost; one-fifth of all plant and animal species could disappear within the next 20 years; the ozone concentration has decreased by half over the past 20 years; mankind produces organic waste about 2,000 times faster than the entire biosphere. Due to the greenhouse effect, the average global temperature will increase by 1.5-4°C (34.7-39.2°F) by 2050, causing massive glacial melting and a 4.9 -8.2 feet rise in sea level.

"Over a short period time man has created a vast "dead" world. To begin with, it's tens of thousands of chemicals. Tremendous harm to all living things was done by pesticides and dioxins, which cause genetic abnormalities in an increasing number of people. Women in many regions are advised not to breastfeed because their milk has become poisonous. The semen volume in many men has decreased by half. It means that the stronger sex is losing its fertility. The inherent resilience, with which Nature endowed man, will no longer be capable of coping with the overload, and Homo sapiens will eventually disappear as a species" (Academician N. Moiseyev, "Izvestiya", November 9, 1999).

If I remember right, it was in Conan Doyle's short story "When the World Screamed" that mad scientists decided to drill a hole to the center of the Earth. Today, all the surrounding Nature is crying out in pain. The most sober-minded scientists warn us that the increasingly frequent natural disasters of recent years are nothing more than an effort on the part of what we call the ecosystem to defend itself from human abuse. But the desire for material comfort and an unruffled life of well-being are valued above all else by states and governments, and the majority of inhabitants.

The martyrology of the ecosystem which we inhabit can be continued. In our efforts to increase our daily comforts, we burn more than 4 billion tons of lignite and coal annually, more than 3.5 billion tons of oil and oil products, trillions of cubic meters of gas as well as enormous quantities of oil shale, peat and wood. As a result, many species of animals and plants disappear; we have poorer harvests and the quality of agricultural produce deteriorates; forests are dying and our ecosystem suffers. The properties of water and air are declining. The earth is polluted by lead, radioactive waste and the salts of heavy metals. People's deteriorating health is the consequence of these negative factors.

In Sweden, one of the world's most stable and prosperous countries, one in three adults suffers from some type of mental disorder. According to official data, only 18 percent of 40–50 year olds in Japan can be considered completely healthy. In Russia, 300 thousand mentally challenged children are born annually and a quarter of the children have some form of pathology before they enroll at primary school; among high school students, 80 % have some type of health disorder.

New drug-resistant viruses and bacteria have appeared (there used to

197

be three types of influenza, now there are more than 70; there were two types of hepatitis, now there are more than 20). It is increasingly difficult to control tuberculosis, despite the development of new drugs.

Various adverse anthropogenic impacts create favorable conditions for the origination and spread of AIDS, "the plague of the XX century".

More recently, mankind received yet another "present" – the Ebola virus, which kills nearly half of infected people almost instantly. AIDS compared to EBOV is more like a common cold.

All this testifies to dramatic harmful changes in the Earth's biosphere resulting from human activity. Because of this, many of the planet's bio systems have already reached that critical level where they start to rupture, dissolve and mutate.

Given man's low reproductive potential and the slow process of formation of his protective mechanisms compared to the exceptionally high rate of reproduction and adaptation of microorganisms, it is not hard to predict that the human species will lose in this war with Nature.

Hence, something is bound to happen to us and, possibly, already in the nearest future.

There is no way to escape the outlined dead-end within the framework of the technological culture and the prevailing world view. Modern industrial production technologies utilize no more than three percent of the produced substances and energy, doubling the amount of perilous emissions every ten years.

It took Nature billions of years to create the ozone layer and the planet's oxygen shell, before it permitted living organisms to colonize the land. The man's so-called rational activity destroyed almost thirty percent of the ozone layer of the ionosphere over just thirty years.

An old joke about two enthusiasts who are busy sawing a bomb comes to mind. "What are you doing? It's going to explode!" – "Don't worry, we have another one!" The point is, mankind does not have another planet Earth.

The world faces either a collapse of the entire global economy and all its life support systems as the result of a major environmental disaster, or a transformation in its overall path of development.

The homeostatic balance has been disrupted and that's a fact. However, as we are conducting a discussion about the problems of the ecosystem, we fail to realize that the greatest danger looming before us is the uncontrollable giant flow of information.

Mankind has created an entirely new living environment, and few people understand the situation we have presently found ourselves in. In the absence of defense measures and protective characteristics in relation to this new environment, we have become hostages of our own making.

All this is exacerbated by increasing problems within man's consciousness: his maladjustment to processing the necessary quality and volume of information, as well as creation of a state-of-the-art technology with the highest level of organization, which makes it difficult for the majority of the planet's population to interact with it. There is growing incompatibility between mankind and scientific and technological progress, leading to the falling apart of the various systems. Many scientists believe that this contributes to the maturation of global crises, to the appearance of "the society of loons" in the 21st century, who are unlikely to be able to continue the evolution of humans as an independent species.

In order to properly define their place in life and find their Path, people must first understand that humanity has appeared in space and in the depths of the biosphere not randomly, but as the result of the development by biological life of new areas and spaces. Through understanding, human beings can eventually comprehend the absolutely true world order, which clearly reveals before them the hierarchy of planes of life. They are numerous, and, having mainly the geometry of spheres, these planes are placed, depending on the subtleness of their bodies, one inside the other, like nesting dolls. Moreover, the material level has two main vectors of axial organization – in height and depth. Therefore, when a person is immersed in the core of his essence, cognizing it along the levels of its organization, he will inevitably reach the center of the moral law, where the infinitely large and infinitely small are linked together, as alpha and omega, as God and the individual ego. (Then people will acquire demiurgic abilities, because the infinitely dense on the inside and the infinitely subtle on the outside will obey his wishes, aspirations and dreams.) This will mark the achievement of real immortality and the happiness of infinite creative existence. It is that magical moment when the image of likeness becomes identical to God, the Creator, the Maker.

Chapter 4

The Book of Life that I am supposed to write gives me no rest. I think about it constantly, trying to imagine what it will be like. They brought the Book into the earthly plane through Yesod and Malkuth and wanted to start reading it immediately. But that wasn't possible. We can see through clairvoyance, its binding and pages, but the letters look liquid and blurry. As soon as we try to look at them closely, they lose their focus and begin to vibrate as though a powerful earthquake is rising from within the Book. We can guess as to why this happens – the pulsation of our consciousness does not yet coincide with the Book's text. We are not yet ready to read it

This means that we have to address, first and foremost, the root of the matter. Why is it that the onetime harmony on Earth has been disrupted? How did it happen that the Dark Ones attained such unlimited power on Earth? Did they decide on their own shamelessly to counter the plan of the Creator, or did they have secret accomplices?

We create in front of us a giant display and ask to see the events that led to this state of affairs, in which evil has so wantonly and so actively enslaved the Earth. And we are shown the battle once again. Again we see the thrones of Mugen, Satan, the devil, again the rows of Dark and Light warriors. And the burning circle in the center of the Bardo channel. We see the Black and White knights. The winged stallion – it's not me this time around. The rider is also someone else, not Igor, definitely not Igor. And it seems that this is a totally different day before the end, not the one in which we recently triumphed so brilliantly over the enemy.

The birds fought, and the eagle won. The wild beasts fought, and the lion won. The Black and White knights fought – Pegasus succeeded at remaining within the circle, but the White knight was thrown outside the field of battle. The levels flipped, and victory was proclaimed in favor of the Dark forces. This happened two thousand years ago. The figure 666 burned bright in the Bardo channel. From this moment forward, the Dark forces had the right not only to rule, but also to all knowledge, and all other power. They received the right freely to roam the Bardo channel and the Earth, to know what will happen in the future and to have power over the future. Their kingdom had come. But according to the laws of the Cosmos, the Earth was considered a child and could be redeemed. And Christ – the Son of the Creator – redeemed it.

He was to accept His Kingdom over the Earth, but ascended the cross instead of a throne. And, it seems, He fell prey to treachery. The Earthly gods, those who answered for the evolution of humanity, did not fulfill their duty before their Creator; they did not support his Son – they betrayed Him.

The screen went black. Now we knew what happened on Earth two thousand years ago. And why the Earth has for so long been under the yoke of the unholy one. We hadn't yet had a chance to discuss what was happening when the screen lit up again, and the familiar image of the Androgyn appeared before us. We heard his voice:

– The Lord with His power entrusts you with strength and possibility. Use them for good works. May you be free of greed and envy. May you escape the sin of pride, as we are all equal before the Lord, and we will all stand before His judgment seat for our deeds!

You were given the right to use nine colors, but it is easier to work with three. Remember how these rays work separately and in conjunction with one another.

Silver – this is the color of the Holy Spirit who helps people. It is the silver thread that leads a person to the place that has been allotted to him upon his death. This color has to be used very carefully, particularly in working with people who are weak in soul and in body. Use it with pin-point precision, on particular organs and parts of the body.

White – this is the color of the Son. It is the strength, but also the grace of the Lord. This is the color used to transform the unmanifested into the manifested.

Black – this is the color of the Father. It is used to drive out evil spirits, demons, the devil, Satan and the Anti-Christ by intoning: "In the name of the Father, the Son, and the Holy Ghost!" And you have to specify who must be expelled – the devil, the wicked one, a demon, or Dark essences. You must work from top to bottom three times or more, depending on the results and the strength of the one you are fighting.

Moreover...

The Androgyn grew silent, looking at us searchingly. He then resumed, as though he had assured himself that we would understand what he was about to say:

– The Sephiroth that you have passed are a dot in the center of circular motion And it is capable of changing, according to the environment in which it finds itself and also to change it. Be mindful in using this great power. The battle helped the Earth immensely. But now everything depends on people. We can banish death from the world, but it will secrete itself inside people. We can dispel evil, but it will hide inside people. Be cautious, but at the same time productive, inculcating Love and Goodness in those around you.

And also...

He was quiet once again, peering into our eyes.

–You know where the Kingdom of the Son is. There is a desert next to it. Tomorrow you will go there. And you will study there the way Jesus

203

studied.

The Androgyn smiled.

– What, it's been a while since you sat behind a desk? It's never too late to study, not at any age. And you should never be embarrassed. This should be an honor for you, not a punishment. Such knowledge as you are about to gain, only one man in the world before you was privy to.

He smiled again. And then burst into laughter – loud, rolling laughter for all the Cosmos to hear.

* * *

The desert is a space in which there is nothing, except for countless granules of the Universe, stones and sand, mirages, the merciless sun that incinerates all beneath it during the day and a nighttime darkness that pierces through you.

But is the desert really so empty? If you listen carefully to the silence, you can hear the voice of your own soul. If you peer closely into its openness, you can see how worlds are created from tiny particles. If you allow fear to creep inside you, demons are born. If you capture the connections and interdependencies around you, harmony will be the result. And if you are cognizant of all of this – knowledge is born. This is not the apple that grows in Paradise and that need only be picked off the tree and eaten to gain knowledge. In the desert, the knowledge is absolutely true, knowledge born out of emptiness, focused around the particles of the Universe, and around people. Here it is possible to know only by creating, through the creative process, even if this process is ignited only IN YOUR CONSCIOUSNESS, IN YOUR MIND. Reason, the will, and the dream will set in motion the images that are born, filling them with life, and will form the necessary space around them.

Igor and I are standing in the midst of a monotonous open landscape. We are perfectly still, stepping neither right, nor left, because this is a special place that can be encompassed only in thought. Here visions appear that lead to the one truth by way of the many truths of many people. This is our first class in the high school of the Universe, the class in which the Holy Son – Jesus – studied. And so we see, hear, learn...

We see the invisible, we hear the silent. But there is a limit, before which we must stop. Even if you know that God created the world, you are still like a knight at the crossroads. He who wants to live with God must allow God inside himself. He who wants to become God must immerse himself in God. He who wants to be Man must do both. Being Man is the hardest choice.

The light is unbearably bright; it is more blinding than the sun. It divides. That, which is behind it, is not known to anyone. Only the thought of Almighty, Him Who is bigger than the gods, becomes part of the world-creating fabric that we call the Universe. He who created the world cannot be divided, cannot be discovered, and cannot be known. But His thought can take any form and any content, and through division once again arrive at unity. And so it is divided. One becomes two. And each has a masculine and feminine name, although they were born of one – Cosmos and the Universe. Then the two gave birth to three. And in the word Christ we see the reflection of the Lord. The Autogeny created all things. In Him, the unmanifested was manifested, because He could be both One, and Part of One, as it was that time when He came into the world of people. And three were within Him alone. But the people did not know this. And that is why He could work miracles: see the invisible, heal that which cannot be cured, and bring back that which is beyond return. He contained within Him then what was the Father, what was the Holy Spirit, and what was the Son. He contained within him the external, and the internal, and this multiplied the strength of the three. Then those six forces converted into the twenty four that sat on their thrones next to the Father. And He contained within Him the structural, the organic and the plasma-like, and through the synthesis of all these the likeness, the image, the greatness were created that could not be limited in time – because it was infinite, and could not be measured – because it was immeasurable, and could not be comprehended – because it was inconceivable.

Stupefied by what we had seen, Igor and I stood in the middle of the desert. And once again, the Androgyn appeared before us and smiled, and began to speak:

– You knew the truth, but now you know the absolute truth. Now you see that the truth and the absolute truth are not the same thing – that they are divided by a boundary which separates the two.

And we saw that boundary that the Androgyn showed is. It was a line, and it was invisible.

– Stand on that line, – the Androgyn commanded.

We did as told and we turned, so that we could see around us. And the space became limitless, all-encompassing. And within the space, there were dots in constant motion.

– This is what information looks like, – the Androgyn said. – Each dot like this is minute on its own, but it is limitless for the one who desires to and knows how to create. In entering such a dot, one can see how the world works, one can understand it, and can learn that space and the soul are one. In space, with the aid of the soul, one can create any element of the world, any object of the world. And those who cognize them will acquire freedom of development and awareness to see the light that makes everything absolutely true.

– And the one absolute truth can be received from the soul and the world, – the Androgyn raised his voice. – Or, it can be received, as you received it – from the Heavenly Father, from the One True Man. His Absolute Truth is contained in the untranslatable word that signifies His Name, since the meaning of that word cannot be conveyed in any way. Even though, as you already know, the Creator has a physical body, which is real. It is real there and already real here. Because what was prophesied has become a reality: three were in one, and three were in three, and one became three. You see, the greatest thing that the Father created within Man – is His soul that can freely develop and create.

With thought, one can create the most effective technologies. But the human brain is almost inactive, swaddled in darkness. Free it from the chains, and give it freedom, light and a path to follow.

The Androgyn said this and disappeared. We were left standing in the midst of the desert, but now knowing about the boundary line, and about time, and about space, and about how one can connect them with the contours of the soul. Once again we directed our gaze into the past, in order to understand the history of people, to become cognizant of how the apple that man had tasted could lead to what we now see and have.

We looked searchingly into infinity, our gaze with the help of intuition choosing one of the endless dots of information, and we entered it.

This is heaven, but the one that lies below. It is the reflection and the opposite of the one true Paradise. In its very center stands the Tree of Knowledge, and Adam is frozen in contemplation before it. The serpent glides up and down its trunk, whispering to Eve that she should tempt

Adam to eat the apple.

There is a massive island in the ocean, big as a continent. It is a very powerful state named Atlantis. Its inhabitants could raise giant stone blocks merely with the force of their minds. With the help of tornados, they transposed the sand in the desert and moved large volumes of water onto specially designated lands. New cities and gardens came into being. The energies of the Cosmos bowed before the Atlantians, and they turned their increasingly more belligerent thoughts towards challenging the Heavens, where they saw as their competition the One, Who was responsible for the creation of the Universe. They refused to recognize the Almighty and served only their own dark masters, those kings and gods who joined forces with them.

With their thoughts and actions, the people of Atlantis so inverted consciousness that the Holy Spirit could not remain inside them. Their souls darkened and their reason was distorted. In addition, the servants of the king of Darkness purposefully gave heavenly names to everything that they created themselves so as to fully confuse people, and in order to take under their own control, from the beginning of days until the end of time, all that the Creator had made. And that is why the ancients gave different names to the very same things.

It was impossible to improve or correct anything under these circumstances. And so the events that everyone knows about came to pass – the Earth was cleansed with water, for water was perilous only to the chamber of the body and not to the light of the soul.

We turn on the boundary line and look up, into the Cosmos. We see how constellations, even entire galaxies, reorganize themselves to form the image of a giant person. The whole Cosmos is that person. But notwithstanding his massive size, he is a child. He is only twelve billion years

208

old. He is but a toddler as compared to the eternity that begat him. He doesn't sleep. He looks at us.

He has light skin, and we can see his chakras. There are seven of them. They rotate clockwise. The lowest chakra is red, and the uppermost, in his head, is white. His throat is a vortex of dark blue energy, and in his heart the green color is visible. His solar plexus is yellow energy, and just below that, the energy is orange. In his forehead there is a slow rotation of different colors. This is the chakra of consciousness, and no one can influence it.

Around these energy whirlwinds, the colors of the aura are visible in layers – red, orange, yellow, green, light and dark blue, violet (which blends into other colors), and white. Informational spirals hover overhead, documenting future events. If one directs one's consciousness towards this child, he responds, turning his head and smiling.

– You saw everything right, – he says. – The Cosmos, the Son, is here. There, behind the strobes of light, is the Absolute, the Father. The boundary line between us is the Holy Spirit. No one can remain upon this boundary line except for the three.

Soon, you will be tasked with reading the book of the Father. There are seven seals on it, in front – seven icon lamps, behind the icon lamps – seven riders on horseback, behind them – seven corners, behind the corners – seven religions. This is knowledge. Be careful. Before you, two people tried to open the book without the Father's permission. They were eradicated with fire and drowned in water. No one has heretofore succeeded in doing what you have been destined to do.

I wish you luck, my brothers. In two thousand years, you are the second to find yourselves in this desert.

He disappears, but he does not leave us alone. A giant person in dark

209

garb appears; he is wearing a hood on his head. The Cosmos has melted around us. We are standing, all three of us, in the sand, and there is a door before us, leading into the unknown.

– You must enter, – he says.

We push the door with the full force of our arms, but it does not give.

– You need the key, – the Teacher hints to us.

Igor looks at me, perplexed.

– We ourselves are the key, – I proclaim, surprising even myself. But Igor understands, and the door opens before us. We step over the threshold and hurtle down into the Cosmos. The Teacher catches us upon his outstretched arms and holds us over the abyss.

– You must think of something, – he commands us. – I can't hold onto you forever.

We unite our own consciousness with the collective consciousness of mankind, its collective energy and soul. With the help of these ties, we create a bridge under our legs. Below us are the abyss, stars, and tornados. But we have already moved onto solid ground, and we are smiling.

The Teacher asks:

– Can I let you go now?

– Yes, – we confirm.

We get onto the bridge we created with our own thoughts. The Teacher is also with us.

– Let's go, – he invites us.

He takes two steps, we take three.

The Teacher stops.

– No one could take these three steps but you. To think but a moment ago you could have fallen into the abyss. I have more information and greater knowledge, but I could take only two steps. It's interesting to be

210

with you. Well, shall we continue further over the Universe? Truth be told, though, I cannot go so fast, I fall behind.

We will always extend a helping hand to you, – I respond, my voice resounding with gratitude for his rescuing us over the abyss.

But the Teacher harshly remonstrates:

– Never make such promises to anyone in advance. No one knows what I will ask for later, and you won't be unable to refuse. I am part of the Dark forces, but am in the Kingdom of Heaven. And this is my class – the thirteenth. So as to your promise, let's imagine that it was just small talk. There is so much behind one's word: energy, consciousness, and the soul. Don't throw words around.

Thus he speaks, and in the meantime, we walk over the Universe. But it is getting harder and harder to move. Some kind of resistance is growing before us.

– It is too far to go back, but the goal is quite close, – the old man explains with a hint. – Too bad the energy is blocking the way. It's just ten more steps to go. However, the decision is yours.

We continue on our path – a step, a second, a third. The old man is struggling to walk. We give him our hands to hold, and we drag him along. Another step, and another one ... and then, the energy's resistance suddenly disappears.

– Everything is as it should be, – the Teacher says. – The appropriate consciousness causes the resistance in the path to disappear. To control events one needs to give due consideration to global situations.

The bridge dissolves beneath our feet, but we do not fall.

– Christ also walked on water, – the old man reminds us. – He knows the laws, he knows how to pacify the elements, and he is always holding you by the hand.

We are happy and we laugh.

211

−Seek harmony is everything, – the Teacher instructs us in parting. – There can't be a single big plus or a single big minus. You three must hold each other by the hand, and the good work will follow.

We glance at each other. We know who the third one is.

* * *

For the first time in five years of managing the "KhudLit" publishing house, I received the bonus that was part of my contract. The objective reason for it, the publishing house's statistics, had been in place for a year and a half already. But the ministry ignored this, quite contrary to the terms of the contract. Finally, the facts began to speak to eloquently that it would have been outrageous to ignore them: 1.1 billion in profits for the third quarter, in other words twice the profit projected for all of 2000. The size of the bonus was determined according to the specified formula – twenty-four thousand rubles. The documents were drawn up. But at the last moment, when all the visas had already been assembled, someone, with a mere exercise of his will, cut the bonus to a mere third of its allotted size.

For me, this has meaning only as a symbol, a signifier, information. And such information speaks volumes. Well, as they say in such cases, at least it is mutual. There is something pleasurable in being disliked by such unpleasant people.

The most intriguing piece in the whole story is that fact that the team of Lesin, our minister, and I didn't really know each other; in other words, we had never met in person. But as the Lord said: "You will know them by their fruits."

I walked into the office of my deputy, Sergei Georgievich Kolesnikov,

212

to discuss the situation. But there was a woman in his office. I had seen her before. She was the head of a company that specializes in delivering commercial freight cars for Ministry of Railways. She looked exhausted, her face barely concealing a grimace of pain.

Sergei was delighted to see me.

– Nadezhda Anatolyevna and I were just talking about you.

It was good that he reminded me of the name. Her last name, I think, is Stadnik.

– How did I become the subject of your conversation?

– Nadezhda Anatolyevna is in dire straits. She has just received a telegram from her home town in the Poltava area, – Sergei explained, – her father is on his death bed. He has cancer, and is in the hospital. As they say in such cases, it can happen at any minute. Nadezhda Anatolyevna bought a ticket. Her train departs from the Kursk Railway Station after dinner. But she herself has been so worried, she developed an ulcer. She is hemorrhaging blood, she is in pain, and the doctors are insisting on surgery right way. And so I told her: go talk to Arkady. No one else can help in such a situation.

As Sergei delivers this monologue, the woman, barely able to conceal her suffering, looks at me searchingly.

– Do you understand that we help, but we don't treat? In other words, what we do is not like the doctors?

– Sergei Georgievich talked to me about you for an hour, – she answered. – I couldn't understand a word he said. But the position I am in is so desperate that I am ready to entrust myself to anyone. I just want to leave today to go see my father.

– Then, I invite you to the Center.

At the Center, I call upon Igor and another one of our specialists. The three of us sit down and we begin to examine her.

We are shown the family tree – a very ancient one. (Of course, all lines are equally ancient, we all descend "from Adam and Eve". It's just that some people only know their grandparents, while others have dug more deeply into their family lineage. This patient is from the latter group. And we, of course, are looking through the prism of her consciousness.) There are only two dark fruits on this tree, Nadezhda Anatolyevna herself, and her father. They are the last in the line. Blood streams down the trunk of the family tree. Why?

Igor explains what we are seeing. The woman looks at us in bewilderment. She does not understand anything.

To some extent, she was prepared for the fact that there are people who, with the help of clairvoyance, can see a person's internal organs, as if he had an x-ray, and even somehow influence the body's internal functioning. But she was evidently unprepared for talk of family trees.

– We will work on the ulcer now, – Igor timely changes the subject. – Listen to what is happening inside your body.

He substitutes the information from the past, a time when the illness was only just beginning. We combine this new information with the future, in which the disease is already gone.

– Quickly, register this, – I urge my friend.

And he registers the information about the ulcer's absence in the present.

The result is instantaneous. We never had such success before.

The patient straightens in her chair. Her eyes are wide with surprise and fear.

– Nothing hurts, – she states, bewildered.

214

She listens closely, as though searching within her for the pain that had tormented her over the last few days. But there is no pain. It is gone, and wasn't coming back.

We ourselves were surprised at the result. In the past, in order to achieve the same we had needed weeks or even months.

Nadezhda Anatolyevna, her face now free of the pain that had haunted her, suddenly implored.

– My father is dying. Our family consists of just the two of us. Please, do something. Please save him.

It seemed that she decided we could do anything.

– Please save my father. I would give up everything for this. I am willing to give anything. Just save him. You need not save me. He is the one.

We look again. We see a big two-story house with a large garden and a lake nearby. In the garden, in the midst of flowering trees, a pool of blood is forming. Igor tells her what he sees and I ask to clarify:

– Do you have a two-story white house in your home town? It's big and stately.

Nadezhda Anatolyevna grows even paler, although it seemed she was already white as a sheet.

– We had such a house, a very long time ago. It was taken from us in the thirties, – she explains. – Now, there are only the remains of walls. There is no roof. All that's left is the ruins.

– Is there a garden around the house?

– There used to be a very big garden. An apple orchard, really. They say that my family's treasure is buried there. But I don't know where.

– What about a lake nearby?

– Yes, there is a lake. A very beautiful one.

Now, she is even more persuaded that she is in the company of very unusual people.

– I beg you, – she says, tears streaming from her eyes, – please save my father.

– He won't die, – Igor says. Then he repeats, – his death passes through you. And you are alright now. Go home, talk to him, try to understand what is happening and why. There is nothing more we can do. It is not in our power.

We say goodbye, and the woman leaves. But our work continues. We now focus on an autistic boy by the name of Michael (I recounted this boy's story in my first book, "Save Yourself"). He is not with us in our office, but that doesn't make any difference. We observe his situation. It is as though a net is pulled over his head. It is thinner than hair and colored red. This net is the informational plan of his illness. It explains why his nerve endings are partially dead, and control signals are unable to get through. We don't yet know how to remove this net. But each time, when we look at Michael, we discover new details that had previously escaped our attention. There is a pattern in this. Only the one who makes an effort to attain something, does; he who doesn't want to stay forever in one spot, moves forward. The dynamic of leaning gently transforms into the dynamic of healing. This doesn't happen right away, but it happens inevitably.

* * *

One day we received an unexpected visit to our Center from Gleb, the General Director of one of the largest new publishing houses in Russia. Gleb was in terrible shape. The neurons in his brain were starting to fail. This was hardly coincidental: as soon as Igor and I began to study neu-

216

rons, many people with related ailments began to approach us. This was so even though we didn't advertise anywhere.

I've known Gleb for a long time. He is a smart, tactful guy, always conscientious in his relationships with other people. It was with him that "KhudLit" put out a compilation of the works of several classics a few years ago, and it immediately became a huge success. In other words, we had an even-keel collegial relationship, which is why I was especially sympathetic to his plight.

Gleb was fully aware of his current situation.

– I went to the States for treatment. I spent a truckload of money there, but the only thing I accomplished was finality. I was told: this is untreatable. And I have very little time, – he added, laconically. – I never believed in any extrasensory treatment methods, but I've heard incredible things about you. And so I have a request: if you could somehow give me another year or year and a half to live, I would be satisfied. I just have to close out some financial matters, so that I know my family is provided for.

Gleb spoke evenly and calmly. It was clear that he had already accepted the inevitable and had determined what he wanted to accomplish in life during that one remaining year.

– And how was it in America? – I inquired in passing.

– It's a huge electoral circus, – Gleb answered. – They beat the drums, they play the fanfares. But my brain is out of commission. I forgot all foreign languages, even though I used to know six. My right hand stopped obeying me: I can't even sign documents anymore. When I walked down your hallway, I was reeling from wall to wall. So what do I care right now about Gore or Bush.

– Do you think those two are better off? – I asked Gleb, surprising even myself.

– Well, they are not doing any worse, I can tell you that.

– Not so fast, – I disagreed. –You will be fine in the end, but I don't envy Bush. All American presidents elected in years ending with zero, in other words under the signs of Jupiter and Saturn, got into very tough scrapes. They got into trouble both at the level of government and in their personal lives. Their lives, as a rule, ended in tragedy. So an auspicious beginning gives no guarantee that there will not be a bad ending.

– But what about me? – Gleb pulled me back from my imaginary voyage across the ocean.

– Have you ever heard about extrasensory killers?

– I have to admit, I've been quite far from such subjects. There are so many other things to deal with in life, no time for the exotic.

– Let me explain then. There are certain informational constructs that can invade the energy informational matrix of a person, leading to a rapid deterioration in health and then to death.

– Are you saying that this is what I have? – Gleb asked and looked quizzically into my eyes.

– You were very recently a healthy man, weren't you? You are young, and athletic.

– Yes, I am active in sports, a sub-master athlete.

– And then, all of a sudden, you fall prey to a strange, inexplicable illness. Did the physicians at least give you a diagnosis?

– They said one thing in the States, something else in France, and a third thing in Russia. But they were all unanimous in their prognosis – I won't be suffering much longer.

– In the old days, this would have been called placing a curse on someone, – Igor continued. – There are many methods, but the one used on you

218

is very serious. These people know molecular genetics and genetic engineering. This is not the work of a local magician. Expects of such caliber must belong to some organization. They have a laboratory, means, and access to scientific resources.

– It's like some kind of a horror movie, – Gleb shrugged his shoulders. Evidently, he hadn't really believed us.

– A little over a year ago, did you get a threatening letter? – Igor suddenly asked. He had hooked onto a piece of information and was trying to unravel that particular thread from a billion others.

Gleb was visibly shocked by the question.

– I received an anonymous letter with the words: "You will die soon."

– These words were a code that set into motion a program that was already previously installed in your energy informational matrix, – I explained, while Igor continued to pull on the thread of long-ago events.

– Do you have a business partner with a foreign last name, not a Russian one? I think it starts with the letter "F"? – Igor asked.

Gleb became even tenser.

–Yes, I do. He was a partner of mine in a very substantial project. But we broke up as enemies.

– Well, he asked two extrasensory experts, who work in some top secret laboratory, to take a homework assignment. And he paid a lot of money for it. You are a valuable asset, Gleb, if someone was willing to pay suitcases of cash for you.

– So what can be done about it? – Gleb asked, quite logically.

– We can take apart the nasty program. But not right away, over a few sessions, – I promised.

The construction that attacked Gleb looks like a snowflake. Its foundation is six intersecting little sticks. These sticks fall from the informational space periodically onto a predetermined object. When such a snowflake reaches the neurons of the brain, it falls apart into six fragments, each of which penetrates the brain cells, where global information about the individual and humanity is written on the walls of the neurons. And this is what the deconstructed snowflakes target and destroy.

As a result, the person first loses his talents and abilities, then his health, and then his life.

Cutting off such a "snowflake storm" is not easy. The people who set it in motion have perfected their craft over time. They may not know anything otherwise about the properties and the structure of the informational space as a whole, but what they learned, they learned to do well. It's like a boxer who spends years training to perfect one particular punch. It may be that everything else he does no better than the rest. But that crown hit brings him victory time and time again.

– When do we start? – Gleb hurried us along.

– We already have, – I answered, watching how Igor cleared away certain fragments of the informational construction.

– Their program will continue to exert its effects on you, but not as strongly as before, – I explained to Gleb. – You will come here from time to time, and we will try to deconstruct it completely. But as of now, it already does not pose a danger to your life. After a couple of weeks, you will start feeling better.

A week later, Gleb was fully able to control his right hand. After two, he took off on a trip abroad to manage his projects.

He seemed to have forgotten that we never promised him full recovery after just one session.

* * *

"Not the flesh but that spirit of ours has decayed in our days," – the poet Fyodor Tyutchev wrote, distinguishing between the two. Gleb's story quite clearly indicated that the world we live in is quickly and dangerously changing. Many people are starting to acquaint themselves with bio-informational technologies and, unfortunately, they don't always use them to the benefit of those around them. Time and again, we see the same situation repeating itself: a discovery that could, in theory, redound to the benefit of all humanity and radically change the way we solve our problems is turned, first and foremost, against people. The secret extrasensory killers, who installed the lethal informational construct in Gleb's mind; Lapshin, who created his global "spider web", activated by information energy deformations in space – all these were extraordinary, worrisome signals of what lay ahead. To fail to notice them is to place oneself and one's future at the mercy of people who are not burdened with the yokes of conscience or morality.

Lapshin's "spider web" is particularly dangerous. Everyone is familiar with the insect described by the English word "spider". Except, in contrast to that small blood-sucking creature, which has its own legitimate role to play in Nature's niche, a human magician taking over this ominous position is far more perilous. When this energy web is fully woven and occupies a significant space, the magician creates a spiral movement of low frequency energy at its center, a drain of sorts, using people who are programmed to be bio-informational donors. This, in turn, causes the space to seek to right the energy imbalance, and so the bio-energy of people, who are ensnared in the web, is directed towards the center of the vortex. And energy gives might and power. Any system will fight for it. Thus, some

221

lose it, and others appropriate it undetected. There is only one way to withstand such an onslaught: to acquire knowledge and to remove the shroud of secrecy from that, which can be used to the detriment of mankind.

The light of absolute truth – this is a powerful tool against those who seek to use secret advantages to enslave their own kind. Another powerful weapon is the Lord, because sooner or later, having fully drunk their fill of power on Earth, these people will stand before Him, the One Who is always bigger, mightier and stronger than they are. But even here on Earth, any person who masters clairvoyance will counteract the deception, the dishonesty and the treachery, will help in curing people of illnesses and even help them achieve immortality. Immortality forms the gates that take us to the Creator, leading the children to their Father.

But we are getting ahead of ourselves... First, we must understand: any thought, good or bad, immediately creates an embodiment of its presence in matter and begins to influence other beings in Nature and the Cosmos, in proportion to the strength and power that created it. That is why the path to the Father is so tough, and that is why it is so important to experience on one's own skin, what are good and bad, what are Light and Darkness, love and hatred, friendship and betrayal, a mistake and the price you pay for it. You see, as we enter the era of immortality, we must become the master of these entities – our own shadows. Otherwise, they will become the source of all sorts of troubles in our lives, and at that point we will find it very difficult to defend ourselves against them.

The psyche, consciousness and our will power – all of these are not only structures of your body, but also integral components of the entire Cosmos, the whole Universe. That is because the bio-field of each individual contains within it an original set of programs that determine his relationship with the entire Universe around him. God created man, and

222

man reciprocated. And this isn't really a joke. The Father created an extension of Himself in the form of the Son, and the Son, having attained immortality, returned it to the Father. Thus, the cycle of eternity manifests itself, set into motion by the power of love; thus the eternal resurrection of spirit in flesh and flesh in spirit is attained.

Life is a great mystery. He who passes its rituals and its trials with dignity becomes unchained and acquires freedom. All the rest is an illusion: the might of kings and the captivity of slaves, the pride of learned fools and the self-inhibiting doubts of those who genuinely hear the voice of the absolute truth. All these things are merely unwanted intermediaries between the Son and the Father. And the most dangerous of them is learned ignorance – one of the worst afflictions known to man. The lie is deliberately concealed and confused. It is also especially proud of its artificially bloated meaning. The absolute truth is always simple and open. One must only want to see it and not be afraid of the judgment of others...

Nadezhda Anatolyevna Stadnik returned from Ukraine. There was no longer any talk of the bleeding stomach ulcer, with which she appeared at our Center only ten days before.

– I forgot all about it, – Nadezhda Anatolyevna commented briefly.

Her eyes were alight with a feverish spark. In her elation, she brought a cake – a hint at drinking tea together and an excuse for an unhurried and frank discussion. If I never saw one of these cakes again, that would be too soon – people bring them to the Center several times a day.

But we never manage to escape these desserts. It seems that this is my karma. We sit down, the three of us, and Nadezhda Anatolyevna tells us unbelievable things, things that just a year earlier would have perplexed even me. When she was sitting in our office ten days earlier and we worked on her bleeding ulcer, she was begging us to help her father. At that point,

223

we told her that his life depended on her own well-being, that now she and her father were like two communicating vessels. Imagine her great surprise when, upon returning to her home town a day later, Nadezhda Anatolyevna found her father not dying, as she had been told, but smoking on the sly outside his apartment. He explained to her that precisely at the moment when she was in our office in Moscow, he suddenly began to feel so much better that he changed his mind about dying altogether. Looking ahead just a little, I can tell you that half a year later, she brought him to Moscow to try to cure him of alcoholism. (He is still alive today, several years later).

This fact on its own was astounding. If a person is inclined to look at such situations critically, he could dismiss it as one of those very rare happy coincidences. Nevertheless, we cannot forget that Nadezhda Anatolyevna's father had a diagnosis of cancer that isn't known for its generous offering of happy coincidences.

But the most surprising part was yet to come. Nadezhda Anatolyevna recounted to her father what we had seen: the house, the lake, the orchard and the pool of blood among the fruit trees. And the father suddenly confessed to her: in 1932, there was a terrible famine raging in the Ukraine. It was then that a woman was killed and eaten in their orchard, precisely in the place that we had indicated. This horrible case of cannibalism ultimately led to the disintegration of a once large family, to its demise. Leaving behind no progeny, its members died, and the family line was cut off, preventing it from continuing the process of reincarnation. The father and daughter were the last in their line. And now we knew why.

* * *

We were once again in the desert. Our Teacher was lecturing us in his dark garb. Like a mirage, we saw before us what he was describing. And he was describing resurrection.

– Here is a person who died ten years ago. What is left? Only his skeleton and a layer of earth above it. There is no consciousness, no soul and no energy. The natural laws of your three dimensional space do not allow for even conceiving of the possibility that he may be brought back to life. But the laws discovered by your science are very superficial. These are the laws of a sphere bordered by reflective mirrors. Those who find themselves inside the sphere, in essence, are studying the laws of reflection in funhouse mirrors. They see themselves and what happens to them, and ask one another: is it true that this fat person is so thin? And everyone around them is ready to confirm it. In order to revive a person, one doesn't need any special instruments. The best instrument is your own consciousness. Except one must act from its highest rung, from the fourth dimension. And who has that? – he queried, a light irony in his voice. – What's more: The Kingdom of Heaven is itself that highest state of consciousness.

He paused so that we could grasp the import of what he had said.

– For instance, now, on your Earth, people have gone so far that they would like to clone one another. But why don't any of these experts speak of the soul, consciousness and harmony. It looks like all they want to do is assemble arms, legs, internal organs and see what happens. There are events, there is desire – but will there be any happiness as a result? Once again someone has dreamed of playing the role of the Creator without having resolved the most fundamental problem, the problem of one's personal spirituality. Still, we must resurrect the dead. And, of course, we won't do it the way your genetics' experts propose.

– First of all, only those who are permitted access to this kind of work are allowed to do it. You already know how the energy informational contour is created. For this you need to use the most powerful instrument of creation – your own mind. Basically, one can assemble a person in an instant, but that's still a ways out. For now, we will have to ascend step by step. Before you can create the contour, you must think about the consciousness, energy and the soul. Where do we find them? – he asked and then answered himself: – The third level, on the right. And what if you look for them on the left? – he continued. – It doesn't have to be that there are only bad people of the left. Perhaps for some of them, only one fragment out of their ten lives was bad. How will you assess that? Does this mean that the one bad life outweighs the ten good ones? Don't always look on the right side. On the left, there are also those who yearn and who seek. They study the mistakes of their prior lives. You can also see the life of those you want to resurrect. But you don't need to look through every year – just look at them as a whole. You need to consider balanced situations – the bad as well as the good. Do you agree?

– Agreed, – we confirmed.

– Good. The person on the right, who we will be working on, died ten years ago. Let's take the consciousness, the soul and the energy. The soul begins to build the contour and the person stands up out of the grave. Let's fill him with energy. Then we start growing his cellular tissue. Make a note: at the beginning, the cells are bigger than normal, they look either inflated or stretched out. The latter is, perhaps, the more accurate description, because the cell was actually stretched out by the forces between the Earth and the third level. Later, it will assume its regular shape.

But this is not yet the end of our work. You have to build the causal connection between events, in which one follows from the other. That is because the person, having passed on from this life, did something else in the other world. In your world, there is a gap in events. You must fill it

226

with information both about what has been and what will be. Information about the future is life-shaping. It must be drawn up as a scenario of the person's destiny. Set the goals, the aims and the aspirations. All the rest, the person will build himself.

The most important thing is to show him the way to harmony, to creativity and to an adequate perception of the world around him. He must understand that life is unceasing creation. Why do you think the Creator is eternal?

The Teacher looked at us, his gaze full of expectation, and we tried not to disappoint him.

–That is because he is constantly in the process of creating, – we responded in unison, pleased with our own astuteness.

–Those, who you will resurrect, shall not reenter the physical world with their memories erased, as others have done. They will bring tremendous knowledge to the Earth, gained through the process of their reincarnations. But, most importantly, they will have mastered the technology of immortality and they will share this with other people. Why die, if the Creator never created death? The long battle for people's right to immortality is over. Ahead is the wondrous time of creation. At the same time, much of what your enemies have hatched to hamper this right to immortality will continue to stand in the way. Although they have been ousted from the informational plane, they remain active in the energy plane. And, most importantly, they can act freely among people.

He fell silent again, looking probingly into our faces.

– You are surprised that even though I belong to the Dark forces, I am telling you all this about the Kingdom of Heaven?

It was true that when he brought this up, Igor and I were surprised, although this idiosyncratic situation hadn't caught our attention before. If the Lord gave us this particular Teacher at this stage, then this is the way it was supposed to be. But now he himself decided to underscore the point for us. And we froze in anticipation, understanding that it was exclusively up to him to decide whether he would elucidate for us this surface incompatibility between the instruction and the subject being covered.

– On the Heavenly Father's staff, there are three rings of different colors: black, white and silver. They contain great power and great sovereignty within them, and they are capable of various deeds, depending on the Creator's will. They have one aspect that is uniquely dear to my heart. In part, they embody peace, agreement and creation. There exist Dark forces, with which I do not agree, and there are also Light forces, whose opinions I do not share. But peace, agreement, creation – I understand what these are, what stands behind them, and where they lead. That is why I find myself at the Creator's side and why today I am teaching you about creation and resurrection.

You have great talent; that is why you were chosen. You passed through thousands of years of incarnations, and you were not tarnished. Indeed, you are learning again. You must remember what you already know. There will soon be an armed conflict that will escalate to a nuclear confrontation, and you will have to intervene. The years 2002, 2003 and 2004 are decisive. The situation can be resolved by peaceful means. There is still time. But the work will be difficult. There is chaos and uncertainty in the world when it comes to both energy and information. Now, after you have emerged victorious at Armageddon, all can be set straight. There are millions of sick people! And sick people represent a sick Universe! You can see the gravity of the global problems before us. We must resolve everything, stabilize everything. The time that has passed and the time to come are no obstacle to us. Man stands at the center of time. Both past and future coalesce within him. He is the center of matter, energy, information. Who can prevent Man who has mastered the technology of the Creator and who stands by the Creator's side from achieving anything he wishes? Show me someone so powerful – I am unaware of his existence.

Energy, matter, information – we must reflect on this!

Energy and matter equals result. We must reflect on this!

Time equals result. We must reflect on this!

Energy, matter, chromosomes equal illness and healing. We must reflect on this!

You can see that in the next dimension there is no production of houses, clothing, food. There are no slaves or machines. Everything is created through thought. This is a different kind of development, a different consciousness, a different way of thinking. We must aspire towards this, strive towards it. If you cease striving, if you stop – then... Remember about the last line of defense. What happens next is called precisely that – the last line of defense.

What benefits does your new position have when it comes to work? The ability to do the main part through your thoughts. Do you remember when we walked through the door and you fell into the Abyss, what did you use to build the bridge underneath you? No matter how hard it was, you had to do it, and not just for yourselves but for everyone else as well. You need only to try it once, and it is already there with you. You need only succeed once, and you will succeed always. Is everything clear, or is there something else you wish to know?

Igor looked indecisive. I could guess what he wanted to ask about. Recently, he had been very interested in the technology of materialization. This was indeed what he asked about.

– Everything begins with a point and ends with a point, – the Teacher

229

explained enigmatically. – Look around. The desert around us suddenly compressed into a single point. There was no more sand or stones – not to the right, not to the left, and not beneath our feet. Let us look at the desert from the position of the absolute truth – there is no desert, there is only a point. Let us enter it.

We enter the point following the Teacher, and we see the holographic image of the desert unfurl itself around us once more.

– That's it, – says the Teacher. – The technology is as simple as can be, just from a different vantage point of consciousness. This is the crux of the problem – to have the right vantage point of consciousness. There is the world within you. There is the world around. There is an invisible world that nevertheless exists. In any of these spaces, you can have individual qualities. Or even in all of them at once. Try it yourselves. What will you do?

– I will try to materialize a big pen for Arkady, – Igor says.

– Very well, – the Teacher agrees.

Igor takes the point, and makes the contour of the pen out of it. He fills it in with white. It hangs in the air like a balloon.

– The coating looks good, – the Teacher confirms. – This is the volume of the space and the time of its passing by means of an impulse. But the form must still be filled in with its contents. And the contents must be the right one. The way you did it, a real pen will not appear here for another ten years. Are you planning to wait?

Igor is uncertain. He scratches his head. He understands that we don't look particularly victorious right now. He doesn't even look at me. He knows that I am far from overflowing with knowledge to be shared.

Suddenly, we find ourselves again in the open Cosmos. Two heralds appear and announce that the Creator will be here soon. Then He appears with staff in hand.

– Well, well, My children, – He speaks to us tenderly. – This is the Cosmos. Come in. You can touch it with your hand. It is the real thing, not a hologram as your desert was. Here, everything is real.

Chalices, candles, icons appear nearby. The Father explains: "We will need them soon."

He takes a paintbrush, dips it in the chalice and draws crosses on our heads, necks, chests, arms, stomachs and legs.

– You were just anointed by God, – the Father explains. – You were anointed by Me personally in the Kingdom of My Son, and in the future you will also be anointed personally.

He smiles.

– Do you think this is unreal, a dream? Look behind you? What do you see?

– Shadows, – Igor answers.

– And so, there are shadows behind you. This means that you are as real here as you were there. I am teaching you now, but in My class there are no desks and no computers. In order for those to appear, you need only think. The same is true of the pen. You must think, and it will come down through the layers that you have already mastered. Then, you will be free in your actions and you will no longer need intermediaries named Fate and Death. There is much evil and injustice on Earth, but is it not you, the people, who are responsible for creating them? The man retains his free will. He himself invents all the terrors that then come back to haunt him. Do you think this is what I wanted? Take a look.

The body of a person appears before us in space. He is well-balanced, middle-aged, and he radiates well-being and good health. He is an idealized human being. Suspended before us in space horizontally,

231

he does not move.

– Enter him one by one, and understand what inside you is not the way I wanted it to be, – the Father commands.

We enter this exemplary man, and lie down inside him. First Igor, then me.

I compare the organs. The first thing that occurs to me is this: "Three buckets of fat, what do we need them for?" Then, the head attracts my attention. Here, everything is out of order – the brain's neurons are asleep, and those that are working are out of sync with one another. There is chaos and lack of coordination. This is the source of irregularities in thinking. The left hemisphere is fully open for cooperation with the Cosmos, but the right hemisphere and the sphere of the third eye are closed off by a film. This barrier prevents them from cooperating with the internal space, the external space, and the space in which we live. And there is also the gall bladder, the appendix, the kidneys.

– Your barrier is no longer dark, it is transparent, – I hear the voice of the Father. – You can see through it, but it still gets in the way of action. But it is the right hemisphere that links one to the collective consciousness, soul, energy. How can you transform or materialize anything through this barrier? As your Teacher has told you, it will take ten years for the wonderful pen you are making for Arkady to use at work to materialize in the earthly plane. There is no magic – there is only knowledge and cognition, which consist of three component parts: illusion, truth and the absolute truth. But the problem is that people often confuse them and take one for the other, confounding, for instance, the truth with the absolute truth. But these are not the same things. Come on out. Let us try to make the pen once more.

Again, we stood off to the side, and the exemplary man disappeared.

232

– The first time you created the pen in the form of a hologram, but it did not materialize. What does this tell us? It tells us that there was a weak impulse or that some knowledge was missing. Try it again.

We make the pen. It immediately shrivels into a point.

– Let's increase the impulse carefully, – the Father helps us along. – Give it a frequency, and holding it constant, lower it through the Sephiroth onto the layers.

We do as the Father commands us. We increase the impulse, but is it enough? We assign the frequency, but how? Our long-awaited pen floats through the Sephiroth, enters the Malkuth. We see it on the layers, where it unexpectedly loses its color and then disappears.

The Lord smiles. For some reason, I think about the Queen of the Earth. We had already lost one holographic pen before!

* * *

She came during the night. And this time, the Queen of the Earth was clearly spoiling for a fight. This was no dream. The vivid nature of the image bespoke the reality of what was happening. Strange names reverberated through my consciousness when she began to speak, and once again I had the sensation that this had happened before, although this time, someone had lightly edited the events.

The Queen of the Earth was wearing a long gown, whose transparency was so indecent she might as well have been naked. A lightly shimmering haze didn't conceal much.

– We have to talk, – she said in a manner that did not require a response. Even without my affirmation, it was clear the conversation would happen. She had decided on it. I listened to her voice and heard the names Fate and

233

Destiny rustling ominously inside me.

– Am I in this deep? – I asked the Queen, whom for some reason I felt like designating as IT.

– Deep enough, – she confirmed, looking at me curiously, but there were no notes of victory in her voice.

– Here is my surprise, – the Queen announced suddenly. – Allow me to introduce you to my friend Kali, the goddess of death and destruction.

The Queen's gaze shone with satisfaction when she saw my bewilderment. I found next to me a three-eyed, four-armed goddess, who looked as though she was cast in gold. Not a single muscle twitched on her dispassionate face. Her eyes looked at me steadfastly, and they seemed to be penetrating into the depths of my very essence. She held two of her arms before her. They were encircled, as if by bracelets, by the coils of snakes, which were slithering up and down her body.

– I have heard much about you, – she intoned without smiling and touched my palms. – Do not be afraid of me. I have extended my motherly arms towards you.

– Kali is the goddess not only of death but also of motherhood, – the Queen felt it necessary to explain. – Two of her arms destroy, the other two protect.

The snakes were sliding up and down the goddess' body unceasingly, hissing loudly, intertwining and threatening. Their eyes burned with the gloomy fire of death, and their forked tongues struck out like lightning from their mouths.

– Don't these accessories make you a bit uncomfortable, Kali? – I forced myself to say something, barely suppressing my disgust.

– Every goddess wants to stand out in some way, – Kali answered, studying me coldly. – I am glad that you, the young gods, recognize this.

234

– Her upper lip lifted slightly, revealing sharp, even teeth. Now I knew for sure that I had heard these words before, but at the same time something had changed. The past and the future, in touching, had made certain edits in the present.

– First of all, I am a man, not a god. And second...

– Are you consistent in this hypostasis? – Kali interrupted.

– That is my belief, – I explained curtly.

Kali seemed perplexed.

– You cannot have just one of the polarities in a pure form for yourself. This does not correspond with the Primordial Forces. That is how the Universe works. And we, being a bulwark of the Universe, must have many visages in our hypostases and must correspond to both Light and Darkness, – she said, and the snakes lifted their heads, listening to what Kali was saying. – Excessive Light and excessive Darkness blind equally.

– It all comes down to conviction, – I stubbornly maintained my point. – I do as I believe necessary, because I am convinced I am right, although, in my opinion, there is some element of truth in what you said about excessiveness.

– But do you know how dangerous it is to be right? – the Queen asked and suddenly inclined her head towards me. The sharp thorns of her crown touched my forehead. – It is better to serve only one's own desires, caprices, fantasies. This frees you from inner discord.

– You are hurting me, – I cringed when the thorns of her crown pierced my skin.

– Bear it or lose your mind, – the Queen advised.

I moved away.

– You see, – she said, admiringly, – there is yet another opportunity to get what you want. Now, you aren't in pain, right? Don't forget that what you were shown in the crypt and what you were shown in Theodosia were real versions of the way events may unfold. Which will you choose?

– The third.

– I don't believe I offered you a third.

– No. I will create it myself.

– How?

– With my will and my thoughts.

The Queen turned, whipping my face with her raincoat, and melted into the impenetrable darkness of night.

This strange dream, this secret page from a life unknown to me, provoked a flurry of emotions and thoughts as I tried to analyze what had happened.

That this scenario had already unfolded before was beyond any doubt. Yet some corrections to it had been made. At first, these seemed fairly insignificant. But, at bottom, they were quite important.

It follows that there are some secret caches of information inside me, or points of archiving, in the phrase preferred by Grigori Petrovich. By some method that I am not aware of, they can be activated at any moment, and transferred from the passive state of pure potential into the active and real state. In other words, on the one hand, this is something akin to genetic memory, which archives events, and not only those in this space. On the other hand, the mechanism of creating reality – the world in which we live – turns on in conjunction with new vectors for the development of the future.

What I was shown represented part of the labyrinth. The point of archiving, connected by the invisible ray of all-powerful psychic energy with the Sephira Malkuth – the Kingdom of Matter – catalyzed a series of events in which I was to play a given role, that in turn determined the

236

passage of events in the present. Not a single detail in what went on was happenstance. Everything counted, everything had significance.

The Queen had invited me to participate in negotiations. It followed therefore that the process had its subjects and that there existed some topic in the controversy, about which we were to agree.

The nighttime scenario was unquestionably an original form of the negotiating protocol. Enjoyable forms of traditional sexual diversions were presented to me with an unclear division of roles as events unfolded further. There was blackmail and a veiled attempt to frighten me with the Queen's friendship with Kali – the goddess of death and motherhood on the energy plane.

I analyzed once more in my memory the minutes of my encounter with Kali, her gaze that searched and appraised me, and the calm that I maintained even in the face of the snakes that slithered over her arms. Now I was sure that it was precisely this internal calm that caused the terrible goddess to extend her maternal arms towards me. Out of the two potential versions, the better one was implemented. It could have been otherwise.

The great secret of existence was contained precisely in that "could have been". I felt that I had come very close to that sacred treasure of the Universe – the individual's possibility of affirmatively governing events. Had I made a mistake when I first met Kali or reacted aggressively to the Queen's provocation when she pierced my forehead with the thorns of her crown, everything could have developed completely differently. But I did not cede the territory I had previously won and succeeded in getting Kali to offer collaboration, by extending towards me her maternal arms.

And how priceless was that inconspicuous, fleeting: "you, young gods." Was this dubious compliment addressed to me personally? In fact, any new god would be but an infant before Kali on the earthly plane: she has so many years behind her, you couldn't count them all. And still today the only vestiges of her former reign are the city of Calcutta and a few sects.

As for me, I have no desire to be a god. But what if I'd agreed? It is entirely possible that the ancient goddess would have handed over her power to me, just like the fabled warrior Svyatogor shared his power with Ilya Muromets.*

And what would have happened to me if my consciousness responded to the veiled bribe with sweet surrender? The thin boundary line of absolute truth that divides Light from Darkness is not all that harmless. At times, it is a sharp razor. Who can stay on it without a clear understanding of good and evil?

When I described to him the details of my encounter with the Queen and Kali, Igor approved of my behavior.

– Everything was proper, – he concluded. – You did not violate any diplomatic protocols. We gave nothing away and comported ourselves in a way that fit the circumstances. Congratulations.

* * *

I have noticed time and again that when I find myself confronted with a choice, the events that unfold afterward depend firmly on the values I professed in that moment of trial. Igor and I are ordinary earthly people, burdened with our share of life's baggage of problems – financial, family and social. But for some reason, we consistently make choices that correspond to some ideal rather than those that will most concretely aid in the resolution of our problems. And, by the way, in our real everyday lives, we

*Ilya Muromets is a celebrated epic hero of medieval Kievan Russ.

never encounter the ideal (that's why it is an ideal), but still we stubbornly follow it as our north star. How many times have we refused money or strength, which immediately turned out to mean power and might here in our actual lives, to say nothing of so many other temptations? At the same time, we were fully cognizant of the connection between what

was happening on the information plane and in our physical world. What we chose, as a

rule, led us not to additional opportunities to benefit from our victories but to even more hard work on the earthly plane and to trials of increasing levels of complexity on the information one.

I must admit that temptations and provocations are always abundantly available, at times with the most benign of intentions. One of my friends, for instance, often quotes Omar Khayyam* to me:

> If grace should choose you as someone blessed,
> In search of truth forsake whatever you possessed,
> But never question a good man's name in vain
> If he fears that seeking truth might cause him pain.

I am not a magician – I am still only an apprentice. But if you look at it from another perspective – what are our efforts worth? I've had to write numerous times that from the point of view of official medicine, we fall somewhere between ignorance and quackery. Nor did the new bureaucrats at my ministry particularly see eye to eye with me. Other examples abound.

Our dream lies elsewhere – in going to the end, striving to suppress all the doubts within us, not letting fear influence us in any significant

* This is an original translation.

239

way. The path we are following will be accessible to many tomorrow. And thanks to our efforts, that path will be an easier one for others to follow. They will see and understand that one can follow the path and overcome the obstacles it presents.

Once again, after the negotiating process in the Sephira Malkuth, we put something into motion in the secret mechanism of the Universe. And that something, having taken shape, offered us the opportunity to stand behind the values we espouse by fighting quite concretely for their reprogramming on the energy information plane and then their embodiment on the earthly one.

* * *

As soon as Igor and I entered the Bardo channel in the levels to work with those who were ailing, we were immediately sucked into a tunnel, as though with a giant vacuum. We were carried in the torrent, and we could clearly discern its vibrations. After some time, the tunnel spat us out into the Cosmos. After tumbling through it for some distance, we found ourselves sucked into a torrent again and pulled into the hot space of a new tunnel. For a few minutes, we were tossed around from wall to wall, and then spat out onto the Sun itself. If this was the physical plane of the heavenly body, we would of course have burned alive. But fortunately for us, this was a different space that ordinarily no one sees – it was the unmanifested Universe. And after our significant training over the preceding year, we feel fairly comfortable in it. The giant surface of the Sun, boiling with volcanoes of molten plasma, didn't cause Igor or me to heat up in any way. We calmly stood on some surface and looked around us.

Suddenly, a host of silhouettes appeared right out of the boiling space.

They came out of the fire and stood opposite us – the Heavenly Father, the Holy Spirit, Christ, a very beautiful woman in ancient Russian garb, saints, warriors, sages, angels and archangels. We dropped to our knees before this greatness, but the woman who came out of the Sun raised us again to our feet. She looked at us with such love and affection as only a mother could bestow upon her children.

Igor and I knew that this is the energy information plane. But here is what was strange – the woman, when she raised us up, did not seem a phantom. Her arm was strong and firm, her clothes smelled of some fresh, springtime grasses. She was in every way identical to us and unquestionably existed in reality. She was no more a phantom than any of the other characters that played a role in our drama, and indeed in past events as well. No, the Black Knight and Dragon Gorynych were no illusion. And the same is true of all who in one way or another participated in events both in the space that is not manifested and on the earthly plane.

The woman is silent. But how is she silent? We are not just random people to her. She has known us for a long time. This we can easily discern both from her joyous smile, darkened from time to time with the shadow of concern, and by the tender way she looks at us, barely constraining her desire to run towards us. Likewise, the knowing silence betrays the uniqueness, the significance of our encounter.

And this woman did, indeed, almost rush to embrace us, but at the last second the Creator, with a light touch of his hand, stopped her impulse, which was otherwise becoming uncontrollable.

– My children, – she intoned quietly. – I have waited for this day, and I have feared it. You will have to go below, to where the Sun-two is. No one can be sure right now how this will end. Your success will depend both

241

on your knowledge and on luck. You were sheltered on Earth until the last possible instant. Those who searched for St. George presumptuously believed that there was no time to prepare strong duelists before Armageddon. Only after they narrowed the contours of their search were we able to return your clairvoyant powers to you.

She sighed and her glance, full of sad tenderness, once again ran over our figures.

– I will give you two small suns to help you. You will see that they are tiny, and they hang on chains made out of wheat grains, – she warned us. – But they contain great power.

Someone from the side handed her the amulets, made to look like golden suns with rays. And she hung these on our necks. These golden suns only shone for an instant on our chests. Then, they flashed and disappeared deep inside, where the heart is, where the soul is.

Everyone was praying around us.

– Do not be afraid of anything, – the Father said. – When you need to, you will remember everything.

Other women appeared and began to tie wool threads of different colors around our arms, legs and waist.

These are protections – red, light blue, green, golden.

Christ was praying next to us that not a single joint, or vein, or organ of ours be harmed.

The sages approached us and put sweet communion bread into our mouths and something like church wine on a spoon. They put dots on our heads where the third eye should be.

This is some kind of new ritual as compared to those we had seen before. They were sanctifying us, giving parting words of advice, wishing us luck. The Father, the Holy Spirit and Christ were crossing themselves

242

and blessing our journey.

They saw us off, and we instantaneously found ourselves in the Bardo channel where a pentagram was burning instead of a cross. We stood in the center of the mystical sign and everything around us started changing quickly – the Sun, the Moon, day, night, light and its reflection.

"Why reflection?" – the question reverberates through our consciousness. It appears in an instant and tries to melt just as quickly in the depths of our memories, but we are able to grasp its alarming essence. And we see that there is a large mirror on the left. It is the archetype of that which divides the left and right hemispheres in the consciousness of man. It is a distortion purposefully interposed between the Creator and people. We would have to search for the authors of this distortion below. Using an impulse of our consciousness, we compress the mirror and take it with us. We figure it would come in handy below. As soon as we removed the mirror, a cross appeared again in the center of the Bardo channel.

Now, we could descend. We were entering enemy territory, going inside the layers of the structure of Hell. Devils and demons gape at us in shock. They don't know what to do – whether to attack us, like last time, or leave us alone. They remember the consequences of the recent fight. It was good to see that they were contemplating the matter. It meant that in principle some evolution was possible even for these hopeless, infinitely evil creatures. Still, they were crowding together and not letting us pass.

Suddenly, two heralds of the Creator appear next to us and without indulging the shaggy population of the lower layers in too much ceremony, order them to get out of the way. And what is most surprising – the Dark ones obey, although they pucker their pig-like snouts in a show of animal fury.

We begin to descend again, and find a new obstacle before us. This

243

time, a Titan blocks our path – one of the ancient gods of the Earth. He is much bigger than Igor and me, but we know full well that in this world, it is not size that matters but the knowledge that one possesses. We ourselves are uncertain about the amount of knowledge we possess although we sense that a great power is either still dormant within us or is just beginning to awaken.

The Titan is truly colossal. He is the kind who could put you on one palm, slap with the other and leave nothing but a damp spot. He is fully aware of the impression he can produce, so he tries to inspire even greater fear in us with the animal-like expression on his face and the bristling of his red beard.

– I can crush you into the ground with my mere thought, – his growl thunders.

This is not mere bragging. He is truly exerting such pressure on Igor and myself with his thought that we sink up to our waists into the ground.

And here something awakens inside us that we ourselves were not aware of but that the Father hinted at to us. Igor and I simultaneously broaden our consciousness almost to infinity and encompass the thoughts of the Titan within it.

Our spirit is stronger. It presses, bends and compresses the psyche of the ancient god practically down to the size of a pea. The Titan grabs his head. It looks as though he has a migraine. In the meantime, we clamber back out of the ground. The Titan is still not in his element. His eyes are bugging out, and he is far from spoiling for a fight.

– You cannot do anything to us, – Igor says. – Five seals from the thoughts of the Holy Spirit protect us in the water's mirror. We came to take what is ours and to give you back what is yours.

The giant tries to do something inside himself, but we chase his thoughts back into his consciousness shrunk down to the size of a pea.

– Fine, you can go to the left, – the Titan agrees. – Perhaps, you will come back out, and then I will allow you to go down.

We walk to the left, into their hellish paradise, and we see apple trees. Next to them are five saucers on pedestals, all of different colors, and there is also a dry tree.

We hearken to the voice of our intuition and pull off one particular apple, putting it on the black saucer. The apple falls apart immediately, which means that evil begets only evil and is not capable of creation.

We take another apple from another tree and put it on the white saucer. The apple was black but turned to red. It is the apple of life. Notwithstanding its original deceptive color, we were right to reunite it with the white saucer. We have connected the creative and harmonizing forces.

We approach the Tree of Knowledge. The saucer is turned over. These are select, ripe apples. But somewhere deep in the thick of branches, we spy some leftover scraps of apple. For some reason, we pull those scraps off the tree and put them on the saucer. The scraps immediately regenerate on the saucer because they contain knowledge. What's more, it is not important who obtained the knowledge and how, even though it may have been through deception or evil. Knowledge is a good thing in and of itself and remembers that it carries light within it.

The fourth apple tree is truly enchanted: its fruit has a top but no bottom.

The fifth one is reversed – it has bottoms but no tops. And the pedestals with saucers are somehow sliced in half. We pull the halves from different trees and join them in a single apple. We move the pedestals together and put the fruit on the saucer. For now, this apple will be more than enough for everyone, but when there are more people with knowledge, they will

245

come here to continue our work, and place a new apple on the saucer.

As soon as we finished our work, a light shone from above and illuminated their paradise.

The Titan stuck his head into the layer and saw that the trees were green, the plates were whole, the apples properly distributed. He waved his head.

– Go that way. There is a prize.

We went, and found a room carved into the wall and around it chests with precious stones and untold amounts of gold. Suddenly, a wrought iron lattice plopped down behind us and locked us in with all this wealth.

– Take whatever you like. Then you can move along, – the Titan cried out.

– We don't need anything here. Whoever collected all this weight of responsibility for himself, let him carry it on his coffin to the Last Judgment.

No sooner had we yelled this than the lattice dissolved into thin air. We came out. The Titan silently got out of our way. He didn't strike us as loquacious in the first place, and after the migraine, the last thing he wanted to do was even look at us anymore.

We came out onto a platform and saw their local saint, meaning their greatest specialist in dirty tricks. He looks at us amicably, radiating affected kindness.

– Yes, – he muses over the facts. – Your power is unusual. We haven't seen any like this here in a long time. That's why I will not lead you to the left or the right. It is apparent that you can choose your own way without wavering.

–Why would we waver? We can illuminate the road with our cross from anywhere at all.

– True enough, – the dark old man agreed. – When you have a cross, you can light your path. But try and help the people here. This leper here, for instance.

No sooner did he say this than a skeleton appeared next to us, barely covered in skin and shabbily dressed. Little bells jingled on his rotten tattered rags.

– If you hail from God – heal him.

– We do hail from God, – Igor agreed. – But he is a disguised demon. And this is not his disease.

Instantaneously, a different personage appeared next to us, all twisted with his internal organs covered in lesions.

– Then heal him.

We take a look. In order to heal him, we must banish the devil that has taken up residence inside, crystallizing into dark energy and destroying the internal organs.

We put pressure on him with the Holy Spirit, and the Dark one jumps right out as though he has been scalded with boiling water.

And the man he jumped out of starts begging us:

– Heal me, heal me.

But how can we heal him if he has no soul, not a single ray of light energy? How can we do that if he doesn't know the truth, much less the absolute truth?

– We can't heal you, – Igor proclaims. – You do not have that which a man needs. You have no soul.

– Then please give me a soul, – he whimpers insistently. – A man came here once before you who could provide a soul.

– God gives the soul, and we bring the Lord's word, – Igor rejects the man's claims.

And he falls into a meaningful silence for a long time, and I together with him. What is there to add to these words?..

– Well then, – the dark old man admits, – I am obligated to give you the key and show you the door you were searching for. Here it is in our

Sun that warms the body of the Earth. Here, our civilization was born and our desire to obtain everything. Much of what people are proud of today first appeared in our subterranean cities and laboratories. Even the flat screen TV that Americans and the Japanese are so fond of nowadays. So, too, with the ultramodern computers, robots and cyborgs who free you from hard work. A little more, and man wouldn't have to do anything at all, just entertain himself and enjoy life. Robots specially created for sexual diversions could enact any fantasy. And all of this is being destroyed because of you. Take the keys. The King of Darkness awaits you.

– We don't need your keys. We can open any door with our thoughts, – Igor says.

– And we don't need your dolls for entertainment either, – I add. – We will manage fine on our own. It is interesting to ponder what would become of man, if robots did indeed do everything for him?

The creature is silent. He has his own thoughts and his own goals. He knows that if a man does not bother to become a man, his place can be taken by one who is more competent. He doesn't want a man looking in the mirror to see the limitless Universe, not himself, and for the Universe to see the man. But with our thoughts, we open a passage into their false Sun and we carry into that passage their damaging mirror.

Inside the subterranean Sun, Mugen sits on the thrown in a giant hall, he who once called himself "the only zealous god". For some reason he is jealous, but of whom would he be jealous if he was higher than the highest? He had countless names, changed his image countless times. We look at him in wonder: he is a man but not a man, a demon but not a demon. He is something incomprehensible and in-between.

He looks at us too and studies us. We see that he doesn't like us. He asks:

248

– Why did you bring the mirror here?

– Take the mirror. It is yours, – Igor says.

– But why? Three own that mirror, and two of the three are the two of you. So drag it back.

– We don't need your wily mirror that shows lies instead of the absolute truth.

– Well then, I guess I lost the battle, and according to the rules, I cannot object to you. Put the mirror in the corner.

He looks askance at us with a stupefied expression as we turn the mirror with its reflective side facing the wall. Then he suddenly becomes agitated, entreating us to be careful and not to break it.

– This is no mirror, – I challenge him. – It is a superstition, a lie, a hoax. Trick yourself with it and enjoy.

– I just want to stay here, and I will not get in your way. Just ask your Father to let me at least have my Sun.

– Ask Him yourself, – we answer without any sympathy for his pathetic situation. – And free all the layers of your shaggy guards. Your reign is over. Now sit here with all that you had conceived for others. All of it will come back to you now.

We leave. As we walk across the layers, we see them become light and fill with energy and information. Now the left hand will know what the right one is doing. A shadow has appeared on the layers – it's neither long, nor short, but precisely the size that corresponds to mankind's present knowledge. As a result, man can establish an appropriate connection between the left and right hemispheres of his brain and understand that which only very recently he had no desire to understand, to believe that which is worthy of belief, and to perceive the absolute truth. From now on, what the heart desires and what the brain seeks is free from the distorting mirror of a one-sided perception of reality and it is capable once again of harmony and integration. Neither a science-centrist platform nor church dogmatism will henceforth pull apart the united whole that is man. No preconceived notions will again absolutely and unquestionably govern over his freedom to strive to attain the limitless knowledge of the Creator.

This knowledge is already harmoniously arrayed in rows of interdependencies and therefore harmless and capable of creation. The absolute nature of this knowledge is determined by the very existence of the Universe. Scientific-technical progress in its contemporary form is no more than a mass of dangerous discoveries and technologies. The world is not a workshop, nor a temple in and of themselves. It is both one and the other, and in it the creative process must be illuminated with the sublime light of moral guidance of the Lord's revelation.

You can see that not one of nature's laws works in isolation from the others; multiple factors invariably influence an occurrence or event, and it is hard to imagine that anyone could enumerate them all, both the significant ones and the minute ones that are most often ignored.

Legend tells us that Newton invented the formula for the universal law of gravitation after a falling apple hit him on the head. But the formula is abstract, good only for the textbooks. Let's imagine that the apple did not fall from the tree but that Galileo dropped it from the tower of Pisa while studying the laws of falling objects. And if the apple "wanted" to fall no place other than on the genius' head, it "had to" take into consideration not only its own mass and the gravitational constant but also other influences: the strength of the wind, the condition of the branch from which it had to detach, the density and the humidity of air, and even the condition of the philosopher himself. To be sure, there were other factors we are not aware of. Newton and Galileo were approaching different problems and thus made different calculations.

The parachute jumper, by contrast, does not need to know the law of gravity in order to land on the tiny pre-designated patch of land. His many years of practice determine his success, forming knowledge of a different kind at the level of intuition. Experience and habit replace theory. And who will judge which form of knowledge is closer to the absolute truth?

I am more and more convinced that for the moment the essence of the Universe, Nature and therefore the Creator's plan are inaccessible to most people. Very well then, we will master thousands of new worlds, layers, forms of being, and man will become immortal. Then what? And for what purpose? Thousands of children in the nursing school we call Earth will become the new creators and will create new worlds in the infinite Universe. But the questions remain the same – what for? What next? What I know now the old man Hegel would have called senseless infinity. It discomforts a restless soul. Even the greatest and most learned man can do but one thing: with humility do the Father's bidding. St. George the Great Martyr said: "Prattling, as best we can, we give but an echo to the secrets of Divinity that surpass us." Man forces his way towards the absolute truth by means of trial and error, and only a few have the gift to know a bit more than the rest. But even they are far from the absolute, perfect truth. Perhaps someday humanity will gain the truth through pain like a mother who gives birth to a child. But for now our task is to fulfill God's commandments, to widen their reach in the personal plane, and to work out for ourselves and others such rules of life as are most conducive to the best implementation of the principles and laws of the Universe.

Chapter 5

At the end of November 2000 the next World Informationalogical Forum (WIF-2000) was held at the Kremlin Palace of Congresses. I was offered to present a report. It was called "System for Developing Super Abilities in a Person. Effect of Inner Vision, Controlled Clairvoyance, and the Energy Information Matrix."

After receiving the text, the organizational committee published it in the collection of the most important forum presentations. The report was also published as a separate booklet.

Igor and I both arrived to participate in the Kremlin forum. The huge hall was packed. No less than two thousand people from dozens of countries came to Moscow for these several days to discuss mankind's informationalogical problems in the next millennium. The event was conducted under the auspices of the United Nations and UNESCO, one of its agencies, which enabled such broad-based participation. Representatives of these organizations were directly involved in the work of the forum and its committees. World-famous scientists, including Nobel Prize winners, statesmen and public figures, ambassadors of foreign states, governors (not only from Russia but also from the U.S. and Canada), senators (again, not only Russian ones), elected members of governing bodies and city mayors gave what was happening at the gathering great prominence.

It was fertile ground for generating ideas of a new vision about the organization of the Universe, in which information was to return to its rightful position as one of the fundamental constants in creating the world. Here, fresh ideas had the greatest chance to be heard and understood. All the more so, since the President of the Moscow Aviation Institute (MAI) Ivan Iosifovich Yuzvishin was directly working on issues related to the theory and practice of information and intellectual development of human society. The presentation of his latest major work "Fundamentals of Informationology", summarizing the conceptual essence of this science, as well as questions concerning the biosphere, the social sphere and even global space systems, was held in the foyer of the forum.

It is, indeed, a really important work. Its substantially developed theoretical part will be of great help to researchers. For in the beginning was the Word. And the word is information. "Through him all things were made... The Word became flesh..." (John 1: 3, 14).

When Igor started flipping through Yuzvishin's book, he almost jumped for joy.

– Look how profoundly he covers the subject. If scientists have taken up information so seriously, it must mean that soon the curtain of the Temple will be spread apart.

Ivan Yuzvishin's book, using the language of mathematical formulas, suggests a new approach to the science of the Universe. It actually speaks about the very things, which Igor and I learned only recently – about the informational foundation of the World, about God and the personal Creator, through which all things exist in this world. The point is that the greatest mystery of space and time lies in the fact that these two are, essentially, a reproduction of reality in thought. But in whose thinking does it happen? Perhaps that first person, Whom we call the Creator, is simultaneously the entire outer and inner world of the Universe? Who then are we in this world, we, created in the image and likeness of God?

We had seats in one of the front rows during the forum. A little farther behind us sat a group of leading experts from Lapshin's Academy. They scanned Igor's mind and mine very hard in the hopes of accessing at least some information about our current situation. It was an entirely hopeless undertaking. The information plane, where we are now able to work, was totally beyond their reach.

Probably they don't even know about the recent extremely important developments that have occurred in their own world, where Satan and the devil no longer enjoyed any of their former greatness and neither did the King of Darkness Mugen. The empty thrones at the bottom platform near their underground Sun are the last remaining vestiges of their bygone power.

New presentations distract us from these thoughts. Congratulatory messages to the forum from heads of foreign governments are read, followed by more words of recognition and more presentations. Many of the reports are very interesting. There are some, where the topic of society's spiritual development sounds as it never did before – powerful, convincing and with a view toward the future. If this is such an urgent issue and one discussed at the level of the scientific elite, it means that the Creator has designed everything presently happening with us. Hence, the priorities of social development have been outlined.

This was also indicated in my report, where I emphasized that it was time for a new understanding of man – his psycho-physical structure and personality. I said that the situation, where each science had its "own" vision of man as the object of study could hardly be useful or productive.

In this hall I was not alone in this vision of the organization of the Universe. I did not want to create the false impression that we, at our Center for Bio-information Technology, have discovered something totally unknown to mankind.

"We do not deny that our system of developing super abilities has synthesized the diverse experience of ancient teachings, but not only that. The issue is that we perceive the teachings on the nature of the self, soul

and spirit, not as abstract disciplines, but as a real opportunity for
to rise to a new stage of evolution. I repeat, a real physical oppoиш
rise, finding already at the Soma level possibilities for self-healing, s
regulation, and even the ability to influence physical processes."

* * *

The days spent at the forum added to the number of my friends and like-minded colleagues. We exchanged information about our work and guided each other in finding the right approaches. The forum helped us establish useful relationships with a number of reputable foreign scientists.

Then the forum was over, and we were back doing our usual routine. The work of the Center was, of course, our primary responsibility. There we practiced and perfected the new bio-information technologies – these were technologies directly from the Creator. And the more we worked, the more precise and efficient were our psycho-physical effects. We were now able to obtain faster and more powerful results.

The purpose of this book is not only to narrate the events of my life and destiny, but also to uncover some specific methods and techniques for working in such an exotic field as controlled clairvoyance. I will, specifi-cally, present here a transcript of a tape recording – the document which we usually use to test our research.

Two patients are involved. One is a young woman with serious com-plications after an abortion. The other has ovary cysts. I believe that this practice session may be helpful for those who begin to explore the tech-nology of controlled clairvoyance.

"Arepyev: Let's begin by looking at the girl's leader cell. Do you see how this fluid it entering it through the outer shell?

Petrov: Yes, from all sides. Nothing prevents it from entering the cell. This is the physical plane. What if we look at the information plane?

Arepyev: Let's do it on the physical, information and energy planes all at the same time. It will be easier that way.

Petrov: What we see looks like a mini-factory with different shops and production facilities. There are six shops on either side of the nucleus. The process in each of them follows a horizontal eight.

Arepyev: It's all due to the pressure. Impulse and pressure – and the fluid enters the cell. It is immediately stretched out along the eight. This starts a sequence of chemical reactions. The fluid is charged with energy. And energy – that's life. Various processes continue in each shop.

Petrov: The components are being mixed in certain proportions. Control is maintained from the nucleus. You see glowing threads, bright like neon, which stretch from the shops to the nucleus. No electronic microscope would give you such an image. Everything there would look different. These glowing threads, they are stretching already at the energy information level. It has a nucleus, DNA strands, ribosomes, mitochondria. And these processes of interaction, control and what specific information is recorded on the DNA, these problems in the information chain – all of this isn't visible on the physical plane.

Arepyev: Even if they could see it, then what? Information on recovery should be introduced into these abnormalities, into these problems – that's what. But who can do it?

Petrov: Look, the information chains are very similar to those painted in the Chinese Book of Changes.* Remember, I told you about it. The ancient clairvoyants defined information as a distortion of space. Suppose we take these broken lines, which we now see in the DNA strands, as

*The Book of Changes, or I Ching is one of the oldest Chinese classical texts.

256

something that separates two information spaces, Light and Darkness, for instance. Then active interaction will be initiated between these two warring beginnings of the Universe at the place where there is a rupture in the line. So, if Darkness penetrates into this rupture, it starts some pathology, disease and other negative events. If Light penetrates the rupture – the process is reversed. But apart from all this, these ruptures are manifestations of the personal will given to humans. What his future holds in store for him depends on how the person will cover the gap from the rupture to the next strictly delineated interval of life.

Arepyev: Exactly. This is the dividing line between the manifested and unmanifested worlds. And the battlefield is man.

Petrov: He doesn't participate in this battle himself, as a rule. Others do the fighting, but we, people, get the punches.

Arepyev: How would man get into the fray anyway? What weapon does he have? This is a typical situation: when two are fighting, the third better stay out of it.

Petrov: I agree. Don't get involved, if you have nothing to fight with. But if you know how to fill the gap with information, the body becomes healthy and the disease is gone. Then what?

Arepyev: Perhaps we weren't able to attain the sought result in the past because we were trying to squash the illness at the energy and physical levels, and negative events continued to penetrate these ruptures right here at the information level.

Petrov: We can now see and understand it. Why couldn't we see it before?

Arepyev: It means we weren't ready yet. If you try to jump over too many steps at a time, you may rip your pants, you know.

Petrov: The nucleus has a very strong influence on the work of the mini-shop. Here's the spiral – it contains information. We now know what to do. Let's initiate the process of division: we will need it for the regeneration of organs. Let's take a look at how the process goes. We also need the cells right now to correct the damage to the walls of the uterus. See those incisions left by surgical instruments? Like butchers, they scraped off living tissue with these iron tools of theirs.

Arepyev: All the walls are damaged. Scars everywhere. It looks as if they used some kind of a tool with beveled edges. It's like they plowed ditches or trenches. After that you can expect anything to grow here – from fibroids to tumors. All the cells are mutilated, the walls are broken, and the fluid has oozed out of many of the cells. Start the momentum for division. I will follow.

Petrov: I am writing down the information into the DNA right now on this semblance of tape: the disease is not there and is not expected to strike; the phase of the body's positive development has been initiated. I'm now initiating the impulse into the nucleus.

Arepyev: One more time. It's got to be stronger.

Petrov: Good. I'll do it again.

Arepyev: There's energy deep in the nucleus. And your impulse is like a laser beam. Powerful pressure is formed inside the nucleus. Energy and information radiate from the spiral. They are building a new mini-cell inside the mother cell. This cell is expelled from the mother cell by the excess pressure. But there's something else: tiny rays radiate in every direction from the nucleus of the activated cell. And now the other cells that we pierced with one of the tiny rays also begin to actively divide. It is turning into an avalanche process. Just look how the trenches and ditches that the kind people in white coats left behind have healed.

Petrov: They are doing the best they can. They don't have any other knowledge. I will now get back into the cell and look inside. It seems as though something like spikes is sticking out of the nucleus on both sides. Discharges of energy are shooting and branching off in all directions from these spikes. This is the energy plane. Now I am going to one of the shops on the physical plane. Everything inside is also divided. Dark on the left and Light on the right. The fluid enters the shop, moves into the eight, and an electrolyte is emitted. I just move with the flow together with the electrolyte. We reach the nucleus. A passage opens up. Inside there's some light yellow, lumpy jelly. That's where most of the energy is stored. Its reserve is large enough to last for thousands of years of the cell's functioning. Why then is our life so short? Why do we constantly fall ill in this short span of time we're given?

Arepyev: Because we don't know how to record information about our healthy condition and physical well-being in the gaps of this unique tape called the DNA.

Petrov: It appears then that a man's destiny is partly predetermined. But if he can write down this information in these gaps, he becomes free of any sort of predestination. And to receive the right to record this information, he has to spend some serious time running around the other world, as the two of us did.

Arepyev: We're completely done with the girl. The scars are fully healed, in just a few minutes. In several days all this will move to the energy plane, then to the physical. Even ultrasound won't detect any problems here.

Petrov: And before, do you remember how many times we would have to sweat over a similar problem, adjusting the impact this way and that? One time we would win, killing the disease, another time the disease would be the winner. And it was all because we didn't support the bio-energy impact with the information one. Scientists are playing around with the human genome to control intracellular processes. We, in fact, are doing just that right now. Controlling it and achieving results. The girl will recover and forget how ill she had felt. That's all there is to it. We have already helped hundreds of people, not in theory but in reality, relieving them of their ailments. Maybe this is how it's meant to be. After all, titles and honors were invented by people. God never asked the Nobel Prize committee for a reward. He has another slogan: knowledge and work.

Arepyev: Well, let's continue then."

We pick up the medical history of the second woman and the results of our preliminary diagnosis. This is sufficient to establish visual contact through clairvoyance.

"Petrov: I can see the ovaries. They are dark in color and practically non-functional. There are cysts on the ovaries, like two clusters of grapes. In the left ovary, I see a small dirty yellowish stone. Ovarian function is virtually paralyzed.

Arepyev: Why am I not surprised? That's why the doctors refused to operate on her. Let's act the same way we did in the first case: give an impetus for the recovery of organs, and remove the cysts with the help of the excess pressure in their nuclei.

Petrov: What about the stone?

Arepyev: We'll remove it along with the cysts. Go ahead. I'll track the process as I have last time.

Petrov: I give the impetus with two beams simultaneously on the two ovaries.

Arepyev: You're doing everything right. But you must act faster. You

260

see, we have your impulse for the recovery, and right next to it is the impulse for the disease. It feels your influence some way and tries to get ahead of you, to move into the future along the information network and arrive at the zone where it would be out of reach. Once it's there, it will fill the gap on the tape of DNA. Anyway, your impulse is more powerful, but now it needs to be a bit more nimble. It is necessary to put a bridle on that brisk impulse for the disease. So let's give it another try, but a bit livelier. No need to examine how and what it's like out there. Initiate a quick, powerful impulse with the information on the future installed in it. There's no ovarian disease in the future, no cysts and no stone, and that's that. Let's have another impulse.

Petrov: Like the two laser beams you can see?

Arepyev: Yes, now it's fine. The concentration is very good. It smashes the cyst cells into smithereens. They simply blow up from within. The cells in the ovaries themselves have become very active. Both the plasma and the energy have become activated. The series of events are lined up along the tape of DNA. Continue to hold the two beams for now. It's like holding a hose when you are watering the vegetable bed. The energy there is now flowing powerfully to the diseased organs and with it comes life. Everything is beginning to look lighter."

The way we directly interacted this time with the information plane of the damaged organ immediately yielded positive results. The following day both of our patients told us that they clearly sensed how we were working with them. They said that immediately after our mental and physical impact they felt much better. They hadn't felt that way in a long time, they added.

What was characteristic of work with one organ is unquestionably also

261

typical of work with the whole body. Global information on human health has to be stored somewhere. It became clear to us as never before that disease is mainly caused by field deformations, the incompatibility of the characteristics of human bio-structures and the matrices in the information fields of the Earth and the Universe. Each negative action, or vice versa – a good one, any thought or emotion, form some hernia-like protrusions on the boundary line between information energy structures. In other words, negative or positive information is squeezed out in one direction or another. (That is how the soccer match for the future of the Earth is manifested in our everyday life.)

In the afore-mentioned gaps, which are, incidentally, pre-programmed, man himself records the expression of his will. Life stinks, one person says, I am in constant pain, no one loves me and everyone is just out to get me. Things happen exactly as he promised himself. That is why I am asking you, my dear fellow-earthlings, please understand: your psyche, personality and ability to react appropriately to the circumstances of your life – all these are elements of the encoding of your destiny. Each person's bio-field contains a set of programs, which outline, but don't define with certainty, his or her relationship with the rest of the world. Such emotions as love, hatred, resentment, which we all feel toward each other, are, in fact, the tool which fills the information gaps in the tape recording of your existence. Fill them with goodness. Remember, if once you are able to show restraint, not let your feelings boil over, and you solve the problem with the help of thought – you will overpower your destiny, and this concept will no longer have any relevance for you. You will simply have a life, and it will be far more enjoyable than you ever expected.

* * *

It turned out that we were not the only ones to enjoy working with these two women. The next time we entered that other space we were met by the Creator. Then maybe we went there exactly because He was waiting for us?

We hadn't seen Him looking so happy and content in a long time.

– You finally did everything right. I have long dreamed of this hour. Now you know: if the horizon is in front of you, don't think that it's far away. Think that it's close by.

The Father said these words pacing in space, as if it were the street pavement. And we tried to walk by His side, without falling behind, heeding His every word. His speech was accompanied by images appearing in space.

– You see the forest over there, the lake and the river. Behind them is the horizon – a line beyond which you can't see. But you have the ability to think at your disposal. Zoom in the horizon with an impulse of thought. Have you moved it close enough? What's behind it now? A mountain, another mountain, then a mountain range. And nothing prevents you any more from seeing what you want. With the help of thought and consciousness, you have crossed the line of the horizon. You succeeded in doing it, although many others would never allow themselves even to imagine that it is possible to see that way. In this context it's important to understand what kinds of reality people live in. You live in that one: you move the horizon, like a ruler on your desk.

Let's now take the gallbladder, with which Arkady had such a hard time. What did you use? You used levels. The consciousness resisted and didn't produce a true impulse. Such a consciousness is impenetrable like a

263

лı. How to get around it? By working on your own, without any levels. You must cause cell division to fill the contours of the gallbladder. Initiate an impulse directly at the cell and it will be restored. You don't need any structures acting as intermediaries for that, or any levels. After all, who knows about them, except for clairvoyants? Collective consciousness is also a horizon. It's impossible to get it to move since it doesn't suspect that it can move. So we circumvent the obstacle and work directly with the cell. Cells are everywhere. This is common knowledge, a fact everyone accepts, including the collective consciousness. Therefore, in this case we shouldn't expect any resistance from the collective consciousness. To conclude: we deal with the cell and the impulse. The organ is restored. Information about its recovery is recorded on the tape of life and destiny. No instruments or devices are used, but the work gets done.

The world of space and the soul are one. If this is understood, it becomes possible to understand the essence of man, his soul, to create any of the world's elements, which are simultaneously also objects in the world. With understanding and awareness there comes instant resurrection, and the gift of freedom in both development and comprehension.

You can obtain information from the soul and the world. You can also get it from the Heavenly Father, that is from Me. While in space, you almost have a physical body and can unravel any object of information. Consciousness and the soul are your only supporters in understanding the world and harmony.

The manifested and unmanifested worlds are the same. And they also have the same harmony. In space you understand the degree of freedom of the soul. It builds the body. It is the world's eternal element, which can develop freely, endlessly and have its individual personality. You can communicate with it through symbolized information and through the voice.

The soul develops the body and is responsible for revealing the physical in the physical, and the material in the material. The greatest thing that a man has is his soul, which is free to develop and create.

Everything in the world contains information. You can take it and give it a positive direction. Then the world will change, change for the better. But people don't know how to use information, how to view it. The key to understanding is actually through consciousness. Understanding what is in the world, what is in man's physical body, and how the two are interconnected.

The grandeur and diversity of the world and of space start with creation. And I hereby give you the right to create and create.

I will now show you some instances from an evaluating standpoint...

When the Father spoke these words, the space and the soul moved even closer to us.

The Father said: you have now arrived at a point where the line between black and white no longer plays a role. It's because you came to infinity. It contains every kind of information – be it positive or negative. But the farther you move away from the Earth – the less the information.

The future, like space, is infinite. If a positive future is linked with the present, the space and the future will move close to us. We don't move toward it, but the other way around.

The more you create, the more information you get and the more you are able to control.

As for reading the book – we now look from a vantage point, where information is distributed to the entire space, to the whole world, to all of Earth.

What for is the text, what is its meaning, and why does it have an effect on everyone and for all time? You have to understand all the principles of the world in order to create more profoundly and more substantially.

I have been creating and I have created an archival point, from which a great amount of positive information is derived. This second book will also heal. You must create an archival point based on this book. You should know how to do it, how it can be created, where and what parameters to build it on. Information and support should be given to everyone. Such archival points exist and you must enter your own parameters into them.

You can enter infinity. There anything can be created. You can also help people and cover everything here on Earth.

Choose the position that you are most comfortable with and create.

I created this world without any computers and devices. Don't waste your time for nothing – go ahead, create. Work is moving upon you. What about you?

He stopped, looking at us.

– Will I hurt your feelings if I say something not particularly pleasant?

– No, we won't feel hurt, – we assured Him boisterously. Actually, we had a sinking feeling that we'd done something wrong again and slipped up.

But the Father read our thoughts instantly and smiled.

– Don't worry, you haven't slipped up this time. But remember how it used to be? It's not the first time the two of you get together with Grigori Petrovich. Twice already you've failed to execute your life's plan at these levels. The first time it was the reincarnated dragon. He fell into Daath later on. The Dark forces used him, remember? The second time there was a different construct. Let me tell you how I see your earthly rigmarole. Grigori Petrovich is assembling a bicycle. Two other guys come up to him: one of them picks up the wheel, the other takes the keys. According-ing to their life's path, that's exactly how it should be – one should get

266

the wheel, the other – the keys. What then should the three of them do together, in what order?

If they get into a fight, one will take the wheel and leave, the other will grab the keys. How can the bike be assembled now? How will the three of them be able to ride on it? Who will turn the steering wheel? Who will show the way while sitting on the frame? There's a pretty pickle for you. Arkady is ready to let go of the wheel, but Igor wants to keep the keys. He is holding them in his hand and won't give them away.

Sometime before, the three of you were unable to come to an agreement that same way. And no one went anywhere, though the opportunities were there. Igor had two hundred grievances. He is the youngest of the three. His two adult brothers could assemble the bike and leave. What would he do then? They could also place him in the rear seat, and he could fall down. So he doesn't give them the keys, he thinks instead. It is hard for a threesome with no consensus of opinion on where to go and how, to win the race on the spiral of evolution riding one bike. Especially if one of the three is the path, the second – power, and the third knows how to operate the device, i.e., is the bearer of knowledge.

You must agree among yourselves, finally, who is responsible for what. I'm not always so generous, not always.

He wags his finger and disappears.

We stand there, scratching our heads.

– Why won't you give us the keys?

– Do you know where we're going?

– No. Kirill said he did.

– I don't need Kirill. That's a good enough reason to be thoughtful.

– The threesome, all three of you, must decide everything together, – we hear the Father's voice nearby, though there seems to be no one around.

267

Confused, we look back. It looks as though our confusion has prompted the Father to meet up with us once again. He materialized beside us, holding a staff in his hand. The austerity written on his face is barely able to hold back his smile.

– Let's continue with the lesson. The soul is the Cosmos. It is alive. The spirit is present in the soul and produces movement. It is the force within the force. Consciousness is the control system. It defines the reality. She, he, it – that's how we get the trinity.

With this unity you can control information, receive an impulse or produce an impulse. So we get hold of information, decode it, and create some object with the help of matter. It can be a pen, for example. One of My sons – and we already know that son – has tried many times to create a pen for his older brother. To create something like that, it's necessary to influence through the soul by means of an expanded consciousness. You

can create anything you want that way, really. Not to transfer it through the levels from one world to another, but create it on-site with the help of information. It can be found

everywhere – it is mobile, pliable and very handy. If you insert matter into information, you can create any object through the soul. There is just one problem here: does the one who is creating have the soul and consciousness that are required – not the usual, but the extended kind? Does he have more knowledge, more skills and something else that you will find out about later? All of this should be received through information, because it is the world's living substance.

When you are helping people, keep in mind: any human cell interacts not only with the entire body, but also with the entire world. It might seem so small, while the world is so big, and yet one can't be without the other. Therefore, if you want to have something big, think small.

These processes are controlled by consciousness. And consciousness is controlled by what is above this world. To control means to see the whole machinery of the world. Let's take cancer. It's a deranged cell, not wishing to be managed by the control system. As a result, the body dies, and with it the cells which went out of control. Man is also a cell of the Universe. Thus, if something in him or he himself no longer obeys the control system, they will need repair. This is exactly what you did yesterday: initiated an impulse toward the ovaries and the cyst, and thereby restored the function of the organ within the world's substance.

The possibility of creation within the world's substance is infinite. This is achieved by shifting space and time. Yesterday Igor remarked very astutely that the disease intended to escape into the future. But you overtook it with the impulse and not only left it behind but also erased any memories of it. How did you do it? In reality, you accomplished it by means of shifting space and time. In other words, by using the dynamics and not the statics, which is an attribute of eternity. This is also some information for you to sleep on: eternity has static structure. Why should this fact be given special consideration? It's because the time is near when you will be resurrecting people, those who have departed today from your world. They will come back viewing space as an absolute, perceiving it as some structure that can't be transformed. Though, in fact, this is not true. You already know that space can be controlled. But those who are resurrected were unable to move for quite some time. They were at some point in space, which had internal expansion. At this point everything remains static with the exception of spiritual processes taking place due to the collective consciousness.

Those who have been returned will need time to reverse from static processes to dynamic ones. It won't happen immediately. They should be

269

helped. They will have to be taught how to live in a changeable world. It is necessary to explain to them that even if they were static for some time, the information following them as objects of creation was dynamic. As we know, information is the world's mobile, flexible, living substance.

How do you create the impulse to cure, to resurrect? You compress space or time, cause them to contract, and then expel them, already in a compressed state, toward the object you are trying to revive. You do it through the soul, because the soul is the regenerating organ. As for consciousness, it is the organ that regulates the interaction with the surrounding world.

All the cells and organs of the body are created with the help of the soul, created from a single cell. Just one cell is needed to create everything. And even if this cell is not there, though it always is – we still have all the necessary information at hand about this cell, the data bank. We can use it as well.

The Father stopped and turned to face us. A multicolored radiance blazed on the rings of his staff.

– So, let's summarize. The soul is a bridge, a rainbow through different spaces. Then with the help of the impulse we initiate motion. This is already power. Power within power, and you know who I am talking about. Besides, there is the function of control in this world. And again you know who I am talking about. This trinity in unity reflects the entire reality of the world, in any space, in any time. It is originally developed by the soul, then by the spiritual structure and the body.

The cell, the most complicated structure of the Universe, reflects the reality of the world. A human cell produces only humans. Your scientists are busy counting the genes in the chromosomes. They are surprised that there are relatively few of them. The alphabet doesn't have too many let-

270

ters, either. But look what you can create by using these letters. The world, in the course of its development, develops consciousness. Consciousness, while expanding, makes it possible to compress space and time, to reduce them to the point of concentration, to initiate an impulse. Expanded consciousness is statics. Concentration is reality. The impulse is the ultimate truth. That is how the world can be created, My children. That is how it can be constantly improved. Everything may be changed and created infinitely. God has more than enough days, doesn't He?

The Father looked at me and smiled.

– The days represent time. And time represents the perception of an object at the moment of cognizing it. So cognize the world as soon as possible, don't comfort yourself with lulling proverbs. Nobody until now had such an opportunity as you do. You have a lot of work to do. It is necessary to make everything the way it was before. Man has to be in God, and God has to be in man. And you still continue to monkey around with your bike.

The Creator's last words betrayed his grief, which he had apparently been hiding from us for a long time. The Universe and a bike are clearly incomparable in scale.

– Let's take a broader look at this matter, – the Father suggested.

At these words three enormous factories emerged in front of us.

– Look, one factory is up and running at full capacity. This factory belongs to Grigori Petrovich. He is very knowledgeable. He is creating a new science for mankind. Let's assume that his product is a large, beautiful mainframe computer, which is able to solve all human problems related to health, and many other things. This computer is even capable of preventing global disasters.

There are two other factories next to the first one. They are standing idle. These are your factories. What are you planning to create here? You

271

don't know? You own two factories of Cosmic scale, and you know nothing about their production. Perhaps you should simply take Grigori Petrovich's drawings and expand his production of computers?

Let's face the reality: Grigori Petrovich created a mainframe computer, while you created nothing. Instead of looking ahead, you look under your feet. It could have been worse of course. You could have broken your brother's machine, the way you did before. Now you just looked at it and put it back.

What can you demonstrate to Grigori Petrovich? Tell him you added a case and a pen to his machine?

You have two factories of your own. It depends on you how they will develop. So let's go see your facilities. We will start with Arkady's.

He walks briskly toward the factory management located in an attractive large building, where everything starts. We ascend to the director's office. There's nobody inside. All we see is a desk with the pages from my novel "Eldibor" laid out on it. The Creator comes up to the desk, randomly takes one of the pages.

– The drawing is brilliant. Nobody on Earth is presently able to understand this book in the right way – too bad, because it describes the computer of the future. This machine will work. But cognition and understanding are essential for that. The design of this work is brilliant, – the Creator emphasizes once again.

This praise from the highest authority eventually fills me with joy, though I continue to feel anxious.

– A totally different technology is used here, – the Father points out. – It has no mechanical parts. The product is created solely by thought.

To be able to start your own production you learned the mechanical part from Grigori Petrovich. You learned it so well, as though you created it yourself. But your factories need to start to produce and they continue to stand idle.

You need tools? But you already have them. By the way, they are perfect: soul, spirit, consciousness, energy and information. What else do you need to start working not in your brother's shops, but in your own? You could create everything necessary in any point in space. Not only is it convenient but it's perfect. I like this technology.

At this point, I couldn't keep silent any more. I respond to the Father in a rapid childish chatter:

– We can create new technologies and explain to people that these technologies can be controlled by thought alone.

The Creator's face lightens up with a smile.

– I like this. I will take it. It pleases me. What remains is presenting the results. How are you going to achieve them?

– Using the consciousness, the soul and energy will enable us to generate the impulse to restore, resurrect, and transfer events from one point to another in any time and space. The goal is to bring people back to health, – I hurriedly blurted out my sudden revelation.

– Alright, let's go to the shop now, – the Father agrees.

We enter a large, empty space without any trace of equipment or production lines.

– Let's take the cell and work on it, – the Father suggests. – This cell might grow to become double, triple, or ill. We are able to cure it. A cell is concentration of consciousness, the way to regeneration and rejuvenation of organs. It is the path to immortality. The Sun itself has a shell and a nucleus. Let your consciousness help you reach the Sun without getting burned. If you do, you will stand next to Me. The fourth substance of consciousness is the point from where you can acquire information in the form of the solar energy. The one who gets control over it will be able to shift the Earth with its impulse and see other Galaxies and other Universes. After that you can put your work on a conveyor implementing whatever you have set out to achieve.

The Creator turns to me.

– Do you need any equipment?

– No, thank you, I use only thought.

– That's the right thing to do, – He commends me. – Thought technology is more powerful, more global, reaching its goal through the substance of the world. Also, imagine how much better the ecology of your world shall be if you use only your thoughts in production instead of depleting the riches of the Earth. How are you going to start?

– To control the substance of the world, I have to establish connections.

– Go on, – the Father says reassuringly.

– One such connection has already been established by the Cosmos. It is the connection with the world we live in.

– That's correct, – the Father approves once again.

– We establish the second connection using our consciousness, and by condensing it we suck in and compress the space of the Universe. Then we send an impulse toward the point in the circle.

– Great, – the Creator praises me. – Thus, using thought and consciousness you are able to connect with the substance of the world from the Earth. This is not magic. This is the technology of the Cosmos. I occasionally use it myself when necessary. First I wrote down the script, the one you call the Bible, in which everything that is to take place on the Earth is encoded. Nobody is able to read my script until his level of consciousness reaches the fourth substance. After you initiate the impulse, the energy of the spirit and the knowledge of the soul enter the cell. This impulse helps us to restore the cell, to divide it and remove the tumors. The energy also kills the bad cells. The only thing that changes is the information in the point – our inner world. Here is an example. Say, you are restoring a kidney: there is a growth on it that has to be removed. So it is removed both physically inside the human body and also above, in the Cosmos, where information about it is removed. This information is in the world around us. But in the world where you, people, live you can have an ultrasound as confirmation that the growth on the kidney is gone. That's the way work has to be done.

I look around and see a group of people in my recently empty work shop. Not that many, something like twelve-fifteen people. A column of energy over the shop signals that the connection between the Cosmos and the Earth has been established. The shop immediately becomes operational – we are able to restore human organs and regenerate tissues.

We proceed to the neighboring facility, where Igor is in charge of all production. True, there is actually nothing to manage right now – the shops are empty exactly the way they were at my factory minutes ago.

– What is your plan of actions? – the Father asks. – You are the power within the power. Because of you everything lives. If you left, not a single organism would be able to function.

– I can remove the lower level of consciousness, which is not motivated to perfect itself, – Igor replies.

– This was already done before, – the Creator reminds us, hinting at something we don't have a clue about. – First it was a little dragon of some sort made by someone you might know; then this someone started reinventing the bike.

While the Father is speaking, vague recollections begin to stir in our

275

memory – about something we did wrong a while ago, something rather embarrassing.

– Yes, it's true, – the Father confirms. – You are thinking in the right direction. First the three of you had to discuss everything, come to an agreement, and then to start acting. It's true that the Earth is like a kindergarten for future Creators, but still, you shouldn't behave there the way kids do at a playground. You have to think about the consequences of your actions.

He was silent for a short while, giving us time to absorb what we just heard. Then He went on.

– The Spirit abides in the soul and it produces motion. So what will you do?

– I can compress the space to a small size – to the point, where the new dimension contained within will be infinite, – Igor explains.

– What about time?

– Time can be stopped or slowed down. We can also speed it up. Further, we have to determine the coordinates of our position. Then we must figure out the coordinates of the object at which we will direct our impulse.

– What is in the point, into which you have folded the space of your thought and consciousness?

– Information about the planned events.

– That's right, time to start acting. Do you remember how the nucleus of the leading cell triggered the process of division in other cells with its tiny rays and how it launched the process of regeneration? You can activate the process the same way, and it will be controlled by the power of your thought for as long as needed.

There were now people at Igor's factory as well. A similar energy column pierced the space in the shop, above it, and beneath.

– Congratulations! – the Father smiles. – Your factories have been put into operation. You are granted the right to restore, regenerate and resurrect.

Then He adds with a tender smile:

– Who else on the Earth has ever been given such rights, My children? Who else had such opportunities? As for the Heavenly Kingdom every-body is looking for, it is inside you. Because there is a tiny part of Me within each of you. The Temple is not a structure of stones placed in rows – it is man himself. You are the Temple. That's what My Son preached when He came to the Earth two thousand years ago.

* * *

Already on the day following these events a disabled young woman by the name of Marina Vladimirovna was brought to the Pushkin branch of our Center. Twenty years ago, she lost both of her legs after she fell onto the track and was hit by a train. The legs were severed altogether; all she had left were two short stumps. She spent half her life in a wheelchair. She developed many concomitant diseases: problems with her liver, kidneys, heart and eyes. She had hypertension and, worst of all, diabetes.

Her turning to us for help was no accident, of course. She came to the Center after our encounter with the Creator, when He authorized our right to engage in regeneration.

Marina tells us about herself, about her life, her suffering and hope. It is terrible to watch a beautiful young woman bound to a wheelchair, look-ing so tiny without her legs.

We begin to work on her diagnosis. We see energy blockage in the shape of a line at the place where wheels of the train cut the legs off. This is the aura, which short circuited in area of the legs. On the physical plane, many cells are already dead. We instantly exchange ideas on how this skin can be used: most likely, for the souls of the feet.

Marina reacts to what is happening calmly. It feels as though someone has internally already prepared her to think that she will grow legs again. She believes in it. She had a dream that she will soon be able to stand on her own feet and will have none of her other diseases. Moreover, she saw Igor and me in her sleep long before we met. All of this is, indeed, astonishing and inexplicable. But more importantly, her inner readiness to our regeneration efforts helps us to do our work now.

We find the leader cell in the stump. Its nucleus contains information about the contours of the amputated legs and their structure. We are offered a clear plan of the structure, where each cell, obeying the program, will initiate the mechanism of division and, bit by bit, will reconstruct the bones, veins, skin and connective tissue.

Then we come up with an estimate of how the living substance, both the field and the information plane, will respond to our impulse. We send away everyone crowding around the room, all the employees and those who came to assist us. The thoughts in their minds are now in chaos. They create static with their confused thoughts and feelings, and they interfere with our work.

We prepare to start the impulse. We compress the space into a point and record the information toward recovery into the DNA, confirming that in the future Marina has no diseases of any kind, and that the terrible event resulting in the amputation of both legs has been erased completely from her medical history. We initiate a fast and abrupt energy release directed at the nucleus of the leader cell. And the cell instantly produces its own impulses to start the process. We see how a hologram unfolds in the empty space where her legs should be. In the place where we could previously see a pale white line of collapsed aura, there is now a powerful glow, resembling that of the plasma during welding. The cells of bones, muscles, veins, arteries, nerve endings and skin have become activated and begin the process of division. The most amazing thing is that Marina also sees what is happening. Right here, in this room, her clairvoyant abilities were unlocked. The process has begun. This historic event took place modestly, as an unremarkable routine. There were no media representatives or medical professionals. It looked as though no one was really interested, except for a small group of our employees and the patients crowding in the hallway.

Yes, the country continued to live its usual life. Someone was scheming how he could grab even more to what he had already grabbed. Someone else had pangs of jealousy thinking about the lucky ones who were at the right time and at the right place to hog the most. Still others woke up in the morning, drank a quart of moonshine and fell asleep again, waiting for a brighter future.

After the session, we called Marina regularly. Immediately, after a brief "Hello", we would ask the inevitable question:

– Are the legs growing?

– Yes, they're growing, – Marina reported gleefully.

– By how much?

– Over half an inch in a week.

Our hearts missed a beat with happiness when she said these simple and at the same time very unusual words: "Over half an inch."

Over the first month Marina's legs grew more than two and a half inches. Olga Ivanovna Koekina paid her a visit from the Institute of Traditional Medicine. After many exclamations of surprise, she asked Marina numerous questions and measured the grown tissue with a ruler. The new tissue differed sharply from the rest of the stump – it was young and resilient, like a young girl's.

– It's unbelievable, – said Olga Ivanovna. – But it must be registered in an entirely different way. No one will ever believe you or me that something like this could happen at all.

– So they believe a lizard, when it grows back its tail, – I said mockingly. – But if one day a legless person should walk from his house on his own two feet – they won't believe it.

– They won't, – confirmed Koekina. And I don't argue about this anymore. I can now understand her.

Marina kept a diary of the things that were happening to her. Not everything in the process of regeneration went smoothly. The new cells required a certain number of biochemical reactions, and depleted the patient's already exhausted body of the nutrients necessary for their growth. The process of growth sometimes stalled for weeks or even months. Let's listen to the voice of Marina herself, as she shares how she experienced the entire process:

December 22

I had to call a physician. Got a bad case of pneumonia. He prescribed three types of shots, medicinal candles and herbs. I need more treatments again. The immune system is very weak. But I don't feel despair. There is only a desire to pass this hard and complicated time as fast as possible to become healthy. My most difficult experiences have to do with my vision – this is not easy for me. But after talking with Arkady Naumovich and Igor – and they assured me that I'll see well again – I've become more optimistic and confident about the future. This was the only thing that bothered me and undermined my confidence. For some reason, I'm not

worried about anything else related to my health. I know that I will over-
come these problems.

Actually, it sometimes seems to me that there is a high fence around
me, consisting of all my illnesses. And it is growing higher and higher. It
seems impossible to jump over it, there's just absolutely no strength for
that. Then, as a rule, I get myself together to continue fighting and trying
to find a way out. Of course, my situation is now much better compared
to what it was before, but I haven't gotten rid of all my problems. It takes
time, effort and patience to be reborn again and become healthy. I will be
able to do it. God and the people who help me will not leave me alone. I
believe that. But I, too, will make every effort for my legs to grow, and for
all my organs to recover and function properly. That's my goal.

December 23

Despite all my illnesses, I feel uplifted in spirit again today. The future
seems perfect. I did my workout with zeal as I used to and not out of neces-
sity. After dinner I called Zinaida Ivnovna. God, she is completely dispir-
ited and wishes to die; she doesn't want to fight for her life. Over the 5
years that I know her, it has been her resentment, lack of faith, not just her
diseases that have slowly been killing her. I feel so sorry for her and would
like so much to help. But without her desire to get better it is practically
impossible. I'm not even sure that she listens to my words. Of course, she's
having a hard time: she suffers from diabetes, her leg is in a bad shape
and they may soon have to amputate it; also, her son visits her vary rarely.
In the past, everything was different in her life: she was a senior nurse
working for the hospital emergency department, with many friends and a
sense of joy and satisfaction, because she did something people needed.
But the disease got the better of her. How many other people also suffer,

281

are tormented with pain and see no way out of their desperate position. Such feelings are so familiar to me and so understandable. I know very well the meaning of pain and tears, when you're alone with nobody but yourself and your suffering. I should call her more often, talk and try to cheer her up. I want so much for diseases not to kill people.

I remember an episode I once experienced: after another stressful day, it seemed to me that all human the pain and agony were centered in me. My soul felt extremely heavy. I wanted to do something for this weight to go away. Only I didn't know then how. Now I do. I can help people, make their pain at least a bit less. Igor and Arkady Naumovich said that it is possible, that I will be able to heal people. But right now I should focus on fighting with my own diseases. I will be able to realize my dream only after I am healed. My pressure is 180 to 100. Insulin: 10 long-acting units, 8 short-acting ones. The liver responds very little to my statements, my tests are bad and there aren't any improvements with my eyes. What I do have is a strong desire to overcome all of this. Oh yes, I forgot to mention that I asked my guardian angel if what I have is pneumonia or a tumor. And I understood that it is an inflammation. My doctor confirmed this. I was pleased that I actually have contact with my guardian angel.

December 24

I practiced for two hours. I've started doing the exercises in new ways. For example, I do the flushing of the small and large circle by imagining each time that a golden balloon, or a golden stream, or even a small white ball or a tightly compressed energy flow are moving across my body and, incidentally, I have from him a strong sense of my body filling with energy. Training has become even more interesting, I detect a more active movement of the cells in the legs. I think that the more I exercise, the faster my legs will grow. But now too I have little reason to complain because I constantly feel surging and small wave fluctuations on the ends of my legs (I don't like the word "stump" and always call them "legs").

Otherwise, nothing much has changed...

December 26

Yesterday I felt very sick. Perhaps it was because of the magnetic storms, or maybe the shots that I am getting against pneumonia. I wasn't myself the whole day, and I couldn't force myself to exercise or type. I had no strength left, and felt down in the mouth. I even cried a little. Yes, it won't be easy to pass through this complex maze of my various problems and illnesses. I collected myself as well as I could, then I prayed and felt better. This may be the most difficult period in my life (I am referring to my diseases: my health isn't improving at all; my high blood pressure is torturing me horribly), but at the same time there is a foretaste that everything is going to be fine; my legs will grow and I will be in good health, against all odds. This hope helps me to have faith and endure all the problems associated with my health. I promised myself that I will endure. Why the tears then? Even very strong people cry, they just don't show their tears in public and cry when left alone. Many people consider me a strong person. I don't think of myself as strong. I'm an ordinary woman who's been on a painful quest for a way out of this situation for many years – through trials and errors, and numerous failures. I think that my natural optimism helps me to part, as my intuition and, of course, my mom. Now I can also think about my future, which I find to be very interesting.

My brother and his wife came over yesterday. We're making preparations for the New Year, buying the produce we'll need and discussing the menu. Then, as we were drinking tea, the conversation once again turned

283

to my health, and they asked me about my vision. I said that everything will normalize in the following year; that my pancreas has begun to function, but my liver refuses to absorb the body's insulin and I need to talk to it and persuade it to abandon its dependence on artificial insulin. The guys gave me a strange look and said nothing. I don't blame them and don't try to prove anything. It's simply that they don't yet understand and don't believe that the treatment I get at the Center will help me restore my health. Let time pass, let my legs grow, and then they will look at me with different eyes.

My brother doesn't believe any of it in general. I'm not even talking here about my legs growing back. If I so much as hinted at that, he wouldn't just give me that look, he would most likely twirl his finger at his temple. I am talking here about his mistrust of the Center and my training there. He said that I am being hoodwinked, and how do they dare take money for all this nonsense. But nobody is taking any money from me. And I am not upset with him for saying all this. Time will tell that he was wrong.

When he says such things, he is not alone. I am now so convinced of this that I practically stopped talking to anyone about my training, except my mother, of course. She fully supports me. So I take those rare moments when I have a chance to contact Igor and Arkady Naumovich and talk with them, both as education and as confirmation of my own thoughts. I still have a lot of unanswered questions.

Today, I was already better. I did some exercises. When my mom was flushing my eyes, I heard the light sound of tingling metal for some reason. I even laughed, saying that my head was now made of iron. I think that my liver has begun to respond slightly to my conversations with it. I reduced the dose by 2 units of short acting insulin and am now doing 8 long and 6 short acting units. And this despite the fact that yesterday I eat some

284

chocolate. This is a small joyful event. As for the rest, everything remains almost all the same. My legs were measured, and the numbers haven't changed: the right is a little less than 12 inches, and the left is a tiny bit shorter. The sensations of surging, small wave fluctuations and tingling is almost constantly present, but it isn't as strong as it was before. My blood pressure is 180 to 100.

December 28

Mom is decorating the Christmas tree. Yesterday, she hung colorful shiny garlands on it. In a few days, it will be the New Year, and the start of a new century and new millennium. I am waiting impatiently for the old year to end. I've even started counting the days. This year was quite a difficult one for many people. Many people I know lost their family members. My friend Tatiana lost her mother. Too many losses. My mother and I lost our pet, little Pusya.

This small cat brightened my life. I love cats, but for some reason they don't do too well at our place. Pusya lived with us for three years. The other cats we had either ran away or died, from the rats in the basement, or from the dogs. Pusya never left the house or tried to run away, but it so happened that he developed urolithiasis. We found that out a little late, and by the time we called the veterinarian, nothing could be done. He died painfully and suffered for a long time.

I was in grief, because when somebody dies it doesn't matter, whether it's a person or an animal. We love and get attached to both. When my mother went to bury Pusya, I told her that he had taken with him all the dark, bad things. When I later talked about it at the Center with Amir Fuatovich, he confirmed my words. He said that dogs and cats, who live in the house with their masters, take away with them all the evil when they fall

285

seriously ill, often dying because of it.

The same thing happened to my cat. Probably that's why I can't help thinking about him. I remember, during the celebration of the year of the red cat, when the chimes began to strike at 12 o'clock, Pusya jumped on the back of my wheelchair and started kissing me, as if he wanted to wish me a Happy New Year.

There were still some bad things in my life. Some people don't wish me well, to put it mildly. I had a series of dreams in which I saw poisonous snakes, then some creature resembling a huge poisonous spider or scorpion. I constantly struggled with them. True, I won in the end or managed to run away from them.

This went on for quite a while, with some small intervals in-between or even months. I was becoming increasingly sicker, sometimes getting better, so that it seemed that everything was getting back to normal and I would begin to recover, but then my state deteriorated again. This went on for a number of years. Sometimes I felt as though I was bewitched. Losing my sight was especially hard. I tried everything I could to prevent it: I got eye shots and used drops; I experimented in various ways and stayed at hospitals too. But the result was always the same – after a short period of improvement it always got worse. I became depressed and cried my eyes out. I tried to convince myself that I must learn to live with the vision I had, just as I learned to live without legs, but I couldn't. This period, starting in 1996, was the most difficult challenge in my life. I could no longer work, my personal life was in shambles. My illnesses tormented me every day. At times it became unbearable. I had different thoughts, even including thoughts about suicide. I even considered taking some pills to forget it all. In the end, I couldn't do it because of my mother: how would she be without me? She needed me even in my sorry state. She lived for me. And there was something else – maybe a ray of hope or faith in a miracle, and, of course, my optimism.

After all is said and done, I am a big optimist in life and a romantic. I love dreaming, and always believe and hope for the best. And I once solemnly promised myself that under no circumstances would I stop fighting, start drinking, or using drugs, no matter how difficult it was or how much I was in pain. Even if I go completely blind, I will still continue to live and try to be happy. It was by no means easy to give such promises. And of course there is no limit to the gratitude I feel to my mother, who carries this cross with me. I am very fortunate to have a mom like that and thank God for giving her to me. Her support has always been very important to me. Now, as I recall everything, I begin crying. Tears keep dripping from my eyes. I am a very sentimental person, after all. After Pusya died, I stopped having my nightmares. I believe that animals were created to help people and they are sent to us. And they help us, even at the price of their lives.

I will no doubt remember the past year for the rest of my life. After all, I went to study at the Centre, where I met with wonderful people; my consciousness was unlocked and my legs began to grow. So apart from the difficult and bad parts, there were things that were good – it was the beginning of my revival. I started my new life.

I called Arkady Naumovich and wished him a Happy New Year. He says that in the New Year everything is really going to be different and that there is a reason why I am waiting for it so impatiently.

December 29
They probably changed their phone number at the Center, I can't get through. It's such a pity: I wanted to personally congratulate Tamara Afanasyevna, Amir Fuatovich and Boris Mikhailovich. I hope that I will have

better luck next year.

My mother is baking a cake – or rather, the basic part, to which we will add the filling tomorrow. She refused my offer of help, saying that she would do everything herself. I have to accept it and just whip the cream tomorrow and place the filling inside the cake. It's some kind of special cake with cherry filling, called the "Monastic cottage". We already baked one like it, but without the cherries and with another cream.

So what has changed in my health? It seems that there is somehow greater light in my eyes, and I have begun to see things a bit more vividly. My legs continue to grow, but the tremors and the surging have become weak. Arkady Naumovich said this about it yesterday: "Slowly but surely." The main thing is that I'm in a good mood and my faith in the future is big – very big.

December 31

It's the last day of 2000, the last day of the century and millennium. Tomorrow we'll have another year, another century. We will be able to say that we lived in the past century or millennium. When I was in third grade and we lived in Ukraine in the city of Khmelnitsky, our homeroom teacher, looking at us when we raised a ruckus in class, said that we will all live in the third millennium. At one time, I refused to return home myself. It was after the injury. We were then living in Dmitrov District not far from Moscow. I thought with horror about how I would return to Ukraine with no legs, and I said that I wanted to stay in the Moscow Region. That was the way I made my choice, which, in effect, predetermined my fate. If we returned to Ukraine, it is unlikely there was such a center there, so I probably would have never met these people who are helping me become healthy again and have my legs back.

288

Now a few words about how I feel. In the last few days I began to feel that my sugar is reaching the normal. I think my conversations with the liver are beginning to have their effect. I feel better, though my blood pressure doesn't go down, it's always high. But that, too, will get back to normal, I believe it. Over the past 2 months my legs have grown by more than 3.5 inches, but I went through a crisis, which prevented them from growing even more. Things will be different next year. I will do everything I possibly can.

January 3, 2001

The New Year I was waiting for has arrived. There were so many tasty dishes and delicacies on the table, and I ate everything without taking Festal, which I usually used when eating fish, meat, etc. I really felt that things were starting to improve.

My legs are growing very slowly, I hardly feel it at all, but the truth is I have not been exercising this week. I decided that I'll start doing all the things I need to properly after January 8, after Christmas. I even told my mom what I feel: right after Christmas everything will begin to improve. I don't know why, but that's how I feel.

January 8

Yesterday we celebrated a wonderful holiday – Christmas.

Today, at 12 p.m. I suddenly felt some sort of internal tremor and a slight surge. Immediately after, I felt small shocks and surging at the end of my legs. The surging sensation was quite strong, especially compared to the last 2 weeks. I thought then: Igor and Arkady Naumovich had been working with me.

I'll be sure to ask them about it later. They work with me at a distance,

289

and by phone. As I am writing about this, there is constant surging in my legs. I exercised quite well again. I began to work on myself very actively, just as I promised I would.

January 10

I was finally able to get through to the Center. Tamara Afanasyevna answered the phone. We congratulated each other with the past holidays. Amir Fuatovich was also there and sent me his best wishes. I briefly told Tamara Afanasyevna how I was doing, about my health. Compared to last month, I really feel a lot better. The liver doesn't bother me and my pancreas, too, behaves well. I've stopped taking Festal. Right now they are dealing with my organs in their work, so my legs are growing very slowly. All the energy and the work have been focused on my internal organs and my eyes."

* * *

That's the whole story. Somebody may find it to be very insignificant in the scale of global events. But in the personal world of Marina Vladimirovna there is presently nothing more important than this creative process – form, matter, life. The process of regeneration we launched (one in which an active impulse penetrates passive material) has given meaning to her personal existence. She discovered in it her own hope for recovery, and it opened before her the horizons of creative existence (do you recall how she envisions her own useful work as a healer?). It helped her see the essence of life and understand its meaning. This event, taking place in the secluded space of our Center and at Marina's apartment does not belong to the present time any more. It belongs to the future and can be compared to the Renaissance, where a personal problem of a single individual, cutting through the levels of space, becomes the starting point, radiating new immortal existence for all of mankind.

In January, several relatives of our former student (let's call her Irina) came to the Pushkin branch of the Center. The visitors told us that Irina has been diagnosed with a very unusual blood disease. Her condition is so critical that she was denied admission to a hospital.

"She will not live long with this disease, – doctors told them. – It all might end by tomorrow."

Irina's family chose not to reveal to us the name of her illness. They persistently avoided answering any clarifying questions. Meanwhile, the woman was dying. Her fever soared to over 38°C (100°F).

They soon brought Irina to the Center. She was semi-delirious. When asked questions, she grunted something incoherent in response. Igor Arepyev and I started examining her. In fact, there was something very unusual in her blood.

We never saw anything like it before. We had the feeling, as if we were in the middle of a new episode taken from the Star Wars. Weird hexahedrons resembling giant spaceships were traveling through the blood system of our patient. Certainly, their huge size was very relative, since we were observing them at the information plane. But in the scale of the information microcosm of a human being, their parameters were, indeed, striking. New groups of cells – lymphocytes and other protecting cells – emerge and multiply opposite them, forming defense squads. They attack the enemy, next to which they seem small and weak, yet they are completely fearless. But the situation is not in their favor. A medieval knight is very unlikely to be capable of stopping a modern tank.

The group of the hexahedrons somehow creates in front of it a space

291

distortion, which, like a mirror, reflects the "who-are-you query" for "friend-enemy" analysis of lymphocytes, and they thus manage to mislead the latter for a while. Then a powerful vacuum funnel (by the standards of what is going on) emerges in front of the perpetrators. This funnel sucks in the defenders of the body, lymphocytes, erasing their antivirus program. The hexahedrons destroy those cells that didn't end up in the funnel by using energy beams. The road is cleared, and they advance.

All human organs contain so-called maternal cells, which are responsible for the proper functioning of each organ. They set the correct frequency of functioning and existence of the cells mass, like a resonator. So the hexahedrons move precisely toward the radiation of the maternal cells.

When they reach them, they perform the following maneuver. One of the hexahedrons splits into six small sticks, each of them sticking to the DNA of the six chromosomes of the maternal cell. Now, the virus controls the cell's work, and the virus decides which resonance frequency to set for the cell mass of any particular organ.

One gets the feeling as if this grime has intellect, not just a program of action. Now it can hide somewhere in the body for a while, waiting for an opportune moment.

In this particular case, the virus is already in its active, aggressive stage, not up to waiting any longer. It multiplies rapidly, intruding into a growing number of the body's cells. It looks as if the cells are exploding from within. Meanwhile, viral particles attack new defender cells, penetrating them and blowing them up. Nothing stands in their way, since the leader cells are taken under control.

Igor and I try to assess the situation. Certainly, this virus looks much scarier than the cancer cells we already know how to fight.

We begin to transform the virus. Unfortunately, its program envisaged such a turn of events. There is an energy jelly inside capable of destroying human DNA.

It looks like before eliminating this grime it is necessary to get inside it. We enter and here is what we find out: each of the six sticks forming the information structure of the virus contains a program. We instantly figure out what we are dealing with. This is the virus of AIDS.

The first wall contains information aimed at destroying the six principal organs – heart, kidneys, liver, stomach, spleen and thyroid.

The second wall contains information targeting the cells and blocking the brain. We look at how it actually works. The virus climbs to the brain up the spinal column. Strangely enough, once it gets closer to the brain, the AIDS virus stops. Somebody or something has managed to stop it. The intellect of the brain did it! It is superior to the intellect of the AIDS virus, and this determines the outcome. The grime will not be able to penetrate the brain.

Now the jelly of the AIDS virus is also a form of consciousness. It communicates with the grey matter of the brain. The two intellects collide.

The jelly forms geometric shapes – a circle, a triangle, a square. The information is transformed into various shapes. But how could the primitive organism of a virus be capable of forming such complicated shapes? It must be connected to something. The information field of the Earth helps the AIDS virus to form the shapes. In other words, it sets the parameters of its intellect, memorizing its information.

Now why would the planetary field do something like that?

We read the information: this is the response to human actions directed against Nature. Nature, in its turn, perceives humans as a virus that destroys her body. Nature protects itself from man. What we consider to be a virus for our human body, Nature considers to be immune resistance for her own body.

We erase the information on AIDs and burn the virus. It dies almost instantly, without any complications for the human body. That's the right way to fight it! But who is able to fight it this way, considering that one has to enter the virus through the vacuum and then erase the information?

Igor is now chasing the hexahedrons across the entire body. They blow up and burn. Now blood will carry and easily expel the harmless remains of foreign organic pathology. Those who created this virus counted on its insurmountable might. But if a stronger opponent confronts the virus, it will be easier to defeat it than the flu. The problem is that those able to crush the AIDS virus are still in very low numbers. On top of it, in order to get help from them, people have to break through the barriers set up by the Health Ministry, which directs crowds of patients suffering from this terrible disease right to the cemetery.

Already next morning, Irina felt much better. The fever was going down.

The day after, she called me up herself. Before she had time to say something, I surprised her with my guess:

– So your temperature is almost normal and you no longer wish to die?

– Exactly, – she confirmed.

– Well, tomorrow your temperature will be perfect.

I instructed her to do another blood test in a couple of days.

A week later she came to our Center herself, letting us know that she intended to go back to work. Her test results were good.

As for us, we started analyzing what had happened.

AIDS penetrates the body sexually or through injected drugs.

Main goal: To get to the brain neurons, destroying the body or placing it under control.

To gain control of the neurons is tantamount to capturing the microcosm. The brain contains the most important information, which is why the AIDS virus is trying to capture it. That will make it possible to reconstruct the parasitic system and make it more sophisticated.

And it's not just at the micro level. There is a rule of negative systems. If the leading system breaks the defenses of the human body, the one following it will be even more powerful and resistant. On the contrary, if it is defeated, the one following it will lose certain advantages.

Tactical goal: To bring the parasitic cell to the organ, where it will multiply.

In the physical plane the AIDS virus is microscopic. In the information plane it is gigantic. Nothing can be compared to it. This virus looks like a hexahedron in the information plane with somewhat uneven and rounded junctions. On the outside, it has dark blue or purple color. From the inside, parallel to the outer sides, there are six sticks, which contain information. These sticks are in some kind of lumpy jelly of yellow color. This is the energy battery of the virus.

Capturing the brain neurons is the most difficult part in this fight, because the color of the energy information tracks linking the neurons is the same (dark blue or purple) as the color of the aura of AIDS viruses. There is no way, either empirically or practically, to set a trap for the defender cells in this identical purple environment. Besides, the density of information in the neurons of the brain is so high that it makes it extremely difficult to influence it from outside. The AIDS virus cannot get through this dense information and become integrated into it.

The walls of the AIDS virus have the entire history of the fight against

AIDS recorded on them. Because of this, the virus makes its attack system even more sophisticated and more dangerous. All the efforts by our physicians have actually helped the virus to perfect itself. Approximately 40% of the world's population could be infected already in the nearest future. However, all this can be changed now.

Strategies to fight AIDs. The methods of controlled clairvoyance make it possible to erase the information of the virus' leader cell and destroy its consciousness. This is not at all difficult. That would prevent the virus from multiplying and existing. Therefore, AIDS would fail to fulfill its goals.

A simultaneous attack is launched at the structures, which form the cell of the AIDS virus, and it is filled with information. Thus, the virus' local defeats are translated into the global defeat of AIDS. When certain regional statistic data confirms the success of the fight against AIDS, the disease will retreat in all the countries, even without any special measures against it.

The consciousness of AIDS is not significant at all! When information about it is erased, it immediately becomes destroyed!

Interestingly, when we launch our attacks at the cells of the AIDS virus, they squeak like mice. Later, a friend of mine told me that when the computer virus is detected and destroyed by an antivirus program, it also produces a sound resembling the squeak of mice at the moment when its information is being erased. Obviously, in this instance it happens because of the special computer program. Still, there is ironic symbolism to it, isn't that so?

* * *

Soon after that we had to deal with another illness considered to be

296

incurable, the symptoms of which were very similar to those of AIDS.

A physician by name of Lyudmila Mikhailovna Litovchenko asked our Center to help an acquaintance of hers, Ms. Caroline Bonzraye, a British citizen.

This case presents special interest because we had to work on it from a distance, using nothing but photos.

Caroline works as a manager at an office design company and she resides in Gilford. Preliminary diagnosis: alopecia areata. Physicians came to this conclusion based on the tests performed in Britain. According to Caroline, she has this problem since February 2001, when during a routine visit to a beauty salon, her hair stylist discovered bold spots on her scalp. Caroline hurried to take the necessary tests, after which she was given the above diagnosis. She was denied treatment because this rather rare disorder is qualified as incurable.

The virus affects blood in such a way that red and white blood cells become incompatible. British physicians warned Caroline that she would lose all her hair. Then her teeth will fall out, followed by damage to the entire spinal column, tendons, and destruction of joints. She was offered space in a hospice facility.

After the first session we succeeded in reaching Caroline by phone. During the session she experienced sensations of heat on her head. The bold spots were red, sweaty and hot to the touch. After that Igor worked with her individually. The patient had the same sensation of flushes of heat on her head. She felt this way in the course of the whole week. Unfortunately, the anticipated result of her hair growing back did not happen by the end of the week, and Caroline got depressed. Experts from the Center monitored her photos on a daily basis, which showed that her hair loss continued to progress.

Nevertheless, the treatment went on. On April 10, we had a call from

Gilford. The report was very optimistic: Caroline's hair started growing back, mainly in the spots where it initially began falling out. It is worth pointing out that her hair loss did not stop but became less intense, whereas Caroline's new hair, on the contrary, grows rapidly.

Anyhow, this record shows what exactly we did in this case.

Protocol

of treatment in abstentia based on the patient's photos

City of Moscow   *March 2, 2001*

Time 5.10 p.m.-6.40 p.m.

Present:

1. (P:) Petrov Arkady Naumovich – Academician of the Moscow Aviation Institute (MAI), President of the Center of Bio-informational Technologies.

2. (A:) Arepyev Igor Vitalyevich – chief expert of the Center of Bio-informational Technologies.

3. (L:) Litovchenko Lyudmila Mikhailovna – primary physician representing the patient.

4. (S:) Sergei – student at the Center of Bio-informational Technologies.

5. (G:) Guldin Alexander Nikolayevich – Vice President of the "Severyanin Charity Fund".

Litovchenko – the patient's representative, delivers a summary of the problem

298

L: Caroline, a close friend of my children's, has been experiencing hair loss on her entire body. She resides in England, her diagnosis is alopecia areata. She was refused medical treatment in Great Britain. Medics say that this illness cannot be cured in their country. This disorder belongs to a series of neurodermal diseases, which are characterized by the incompatibility of red and white blood cells. Caroline has spots on her body that look like bruises. All the hair on her head has fallen out, and so have her eyebrows and lashes.

(The Center's staff establishes contact with Caroline and her information energy system, using her photos).

A: Indeed, very unusual dark cells can be seen in her blood formula. What I find strange is that the damage goes right to the head. There are 2-3 formations that would seem typical for the AIDS hexahedrons when viewed on the informational plane but, strangely enough, their color is not dark purple but rather lead-grey. However, the leader cells are not affected yet.

P: Possibly, we are dealing with AIDS in its new, third version. The hexahedrons of previous versions could not penetrate the head. Frankly, these ones are not that active, either. Apparently, they are lying low for the time being.

A: This is a cover up. The virus can start destroying information. There are some shells of dead cells in the blood. We'll soon observe some manifestations of changes in perception, mood swings. There is no apparent memory loss yet. I can see a white spot in the middle of the hexahedron; the connections are colored dark purple with a black haze around them. The neuron is not transmitting anything.

P: We cannot wait any longer with the treatment. Additional tests are essential:

1) Thyroid ultrasound;

299

2) Cerebral tomography (though the picture won't depict the damaged area accurately)

3) Advanced blood analysis – scrupulous analysis of the blood should reveal what is left of the destroyed structures.

If we are successful in getting test results by Monday we will be able to conduct the treatment session on Monday. We are dealing with a new virus. I don't exclude the possibility that it has readapted and learned to spread by airborne droplets.

L: *I will call England today and tomorrow, asking them to be ready with the tests ASAP. If you think the treatment is possible we can arrange Caroline's flight to Russia.*

P: *Distance is not a factor. We have established the connection, so we can go ahead with the treatment without Caroline necessarily being present. We can cure her illness.*

L: *Caroline is a very active, positive, responsive person. If you think you are able to help her, do so without any delays.*

P: *Yes, we can cure her but without the tests we might confront difficulties in securing the fact of healing. Igor, what shall we do?*

A: *I would remove it right now, while the virus in the brain is still inactive. I see ties with the past. The cause of this illness – contacts with an underground storage of radioactive material. Very hard radiation: 3-4 different components, rapid particles in the soil, the container for the source of radiation is a yellow barrel with something above that looks like lead. She doesn't know anything about it, to be more precise, she didn't know at the time it happened. She didn't have a clue how dangerous it might be for her health. Now I see that the virus has a leaden tone.*

P: *Where could it happen?*

300

L: Caroline served in the military for two years, it must have been there.

P: I think, Igor, we got a clear picture of the past. Let's look at the future now. Hair loss, teeth falling out; spinal column, tendons, joints deteriorate, and the bone marrow is affected.

A: Let's remove that.

(All the tree specialists of the Center work energetically, exchanging a few words now and then, making sure they see the results of their impact the same way).

A: From the liver to the heart. We should adjust. Sergei, look carefully if there's anything else.

S: The hexahedron is vibrating, the vibration gets stronger, I think, it split.

A: We remove the virus in the blood and in the neuron tracks.

P: Where did the sticks go?

S: They assembled into groups. The center is inactive.

A: Everything has to be removed.

P: Is there any information left on the sticks?

S: Yes.

P: It has to go. We need to bring the past and the new future together.

A: I'm simply removing it. Information is now erased. Red and white blood cells begin to interact. They are sending signals: "friend" – "enemy".

S: The hexahedrons are removed from the blood and from the head.

P: How can lead be neutralized? We have to get out the residues on the shells of the virus. The lead's in the blood.

L: Iodine can do it, but it works slowly, milk works faster.

A: The destroyed cells of the virus are like flakes. They settle. When running blood tests, the remains of their bodies might be found. The actual virus is gone.

L: Protein in the milk sticks to the lead, discharging it effectively from the body.

P: So we should generate milk protein right now. Information is confirmed. It is possible to get the lead out at a distance. Let's enter the information on milk protein.

A: Direction – liver and kidneys. The process has begun. The excretion can take place within 24 hours. She has to take diuretics. Her urine will have color spots, like spilled diesel oil. Well, enough for the day.

P: Alright, contact Caroline. We will reconvene at noon on Tuesday.

L: Thank you all.

Time: 6.30 p.m., *signatures of participants, general discussion.*

Soon after, we asked Lyudmila Mikhailovna to get a written response from Caroline Bonzraye about the changes she was experiencing. We received her response. It was sent to the address of Lyudmila Mikhailovna's son. Here it is.

Dear Sergei,

These are some details on my recent hair loss.

I went for a haircut on Saturday 10.02.01, and my stylist told me that I am losing hair. At that time, the entire hair loss was 0.2 inches on the right side of my head. Within just one week the situation deteriorated and the bold spot was already 0.8-1.2 inches in size. Then it began spreading downwards.

Over the course of the following two weeks, the hair loss spread all the way to my neck and the area began having distinct edges.

The size of the bold spot was already 4.3 inches long and 2 inches wide. At that point I contacted my physician. A blood test was taken, and

302

I was informed that I had alopecia areata. When the full blood test results returned, the doctor explained to me that this was an autoimmune disorder. It appears that my white blood cells attacked my red blood cells without any apparent reason.

I went to a private physician, had him examine me thoroughly and took an AIDS test. All the tests came back negative (normal), with the exception of the blood test. Again, I was informed about my excessive number of white blood cells. Besides, I went to the Begravia hospital (a private clinic dealing specifically with hair loss). They weren't of much help, they just wanted my money.

During the past three weeks my hair began to grow back. It continues to fall out but not as intensely as before.

Litovchenko Lyudmila Mikhailovna:

By the end of May the improvement was so dramatic that Caroline was able to go back to work. As a result, we received another patient from Gildford. Mr. Les Allen Verko suffered from severe joint disease. He had difficulty moving even around his apartment. In his young years, Mr. Les was an athlete. It was then that he injured both knees. He underwent several surgeries, but the pain in his legs continued to get progressively worse. My son Litovchenko Sergei Mikhailovich asked the Center for help. The specialists of the Center started working from the gentleman's photos. On that specific day and during the moment when we were working on Mr. Les' illness from his picture, he suddenly felt his joints crack. The snapping sound was very distinct and he was in great pain. After this episode, the pain disappeared and Mr. Les never again experienced any painful sensations associated with his disease."

* * *

It now seemed that the mysteries surrounding the Queen of the Earth and Kali were manifesting themselves in the earthly world around us. Our Center, for instance, received a new visitor – Irina Karysheva. A beautiful young woman, she worked as director of advertising for the "Biomedical", a joint-stock company with a limited number of share-holders. But working in an institution directly involved with medicine could not protect her own health. She sought treatment, went to doctors, followed all of their instructions, but nothing helped. Her condition continued to worsen. And she was not the only one. Irina's father had been bedridden for months. He was clearly fading away, but his daughter did not know how to help him.

The two illnesses were somehow strange, mysterious. The doctors who examined Ms. Karysheva kept changing her diagnosis and contradicting one another. There was only one point on which all agreed: their treatment was not having any practical effect.

With time, as she continued to sink into her illness and began to dig more deeply for its roots, Irina became convinced that the malady was somehow connected with her second job. The thing is that Irina had studied to become a translator, and that was where her heart and interests always lay. Indeed, she specialized in a rare and exotic field: ancient Hindu texts. Her translation from Sanskrit of the great Kalidasa's poem "The Pageant of the Seasons" ("Ritusamhara") earned her admiration and acclaim among experts in the field.

I have the utmost respect for people like Ms. Karysheva, who seek to restore the link between different time periods, to bridge the distance between the cultures of various eras, and to find the common human element in the private lives of different peoples and civilizations. Now I understand that translators of languages long forgotten by most are fulfilling in their own way the very difficult mission of creating the Future by way of the Past. This is an esoteric calling, and it demands not only professional skills, a thorough knowledge of past customs and manners, but also the necessary rectitude of the soul.

These days everyone knows how much harm has been wrought by the unthinking translation of the Latin phrase "Menssana in corporesano." "A healthy mind in a healthy body" suggests that the mind or the spirit will come on its own if you just pump up the muscles and work on your digestion. But, in reality, the saying hails from Juvenal's poem: "It is to be prayed that the mind be sound in a sound body." In other words, the Romans were concerned with the harmonious combination of three elements: the body, the mind, and prayer.

Let's take another example and compare two translations of a single excerpt from Sophocles' tragedy, "Antigone". Here is the first:

> There are many strange and wonderful things,
> but nothing more strangely wonderful than man.
> He moves across the white-capped ocean seas
> blasted by winter storms, carving his way
> under the surging waves engulfing him.
> With his teams of horses he wears down
> the unwearied and immortal earth,
> the oldest of the gods, harassing her,
> as year by year his ploughs move back and forth.*

And here is the second:

* This passage was taken from a translation of Sophocles' "Antigone" by Ian Johnston.

305

Many things cause terror and wonder, yet nothing
is more terrifying and wonderful than man.
This thing goes across the grey sea
on the blasts of winter storms,
passing beneath waters towering ,round him.
The Earth, eldest of the gods,
unwithering and untiring,
this thing wears down
as his plows go back and forth year after year
furrowing her with the issue of horses.*

What a striking difference in the appraisal of mankind! The first text sounds an optimistic note, true to the spirit of the 19th century, the times of Jules Verne and von Krusenstern, of Darwin and Karl Marx, of Nobel and Eiffel. The second, by contrast, is a pessimistic meditation on the duality of the "king of nature".

Preferring one of these versions or the other imperceptibly moves the needle on the compass of one's soul. And to think that there are millions of such deviations; they determine the destiny of individuals, and the fates and paths of nations. But let us return to Irina Karysheva.

"The Pageant of the Seasons" – these are the stages of the ripening, blooming, and withering of a woman's beauty. And it is no accident that the perceptive genius of a poet who lived fifteen hundred years ago so clearly and directly tied the life cycles of human beings to the seasonal changes in Nature:

---

*A passage from Sophocles' "Antigone" translated by Wm. Blake Tyrrell and Larry J. Bennett.

Women's faces with the patterns of leaves,
Tender as the golden lotus,
Covered with drops of perspiration in the spring,
As though with spilled round pearls.
Wives who are tempted in springtime by Kama,
Sit next to their husbands and untie
Every knot of their heavy garb
And become aroused with love.**

The more Irina immersed herself in the spiritual quest for the cause of her personal misfortunes, the more certain she was that the sources of her illness and her father's were to be found far from Russia – in India, in the depths of millennia. Even the name of the poet she had translated means "servant of Kali"– it was believed that the goddess had given him his wisdom. But how does one penetrate the past? And who will help find the answer?

It was then that Irina began to seek out healers and clairvoyants. The reaction that every known psychic had after just barely starting to work with her only further convinced Irina that her current situation hinged upon hidden reasons in the subtle matter world. As soon as the psychics immersed themselves in an alternate state of consciousness, they were horrified, and they refused to work with Ms. Karysheva any further. What they sensed and saw was truly horrific: they saw death.

Someone recommended to Irina that she approach us. What she wanted to hear from us was what she already, by and large, knew herself. That's no surprise – it's a typical move to try to use the eyes of others to

**This is an original translation.

get a closer look at something you already know.

When Igor and I started working with her, we were instantaneously transported into the unusual and mysterious world of another country, another culture.

In the depths of a dark space, we saw a round platform covered in fine yellow sand. In its center we saw a giant stone. It was unusual: a book was hidden inside it. This was a stone book, with stone pages, guarding a secret thousands of years old that had hardened with the end of time.

All around, at the edge where the light sand of time intersected with the dark space of oblivion, twelve columns were arrayed, each with a chalice at the top.

Irina, who was sitting on a chair in our office, facing us, was at that same moment, in that other dimension, kneeling before the massive stone, and the stone pages of the stone book were turning before her. But she was not alone. A little off to the side, slightly elevated amidst the sand was a beautiful and simultaneously terrible goddess, whom I recognized. It was Kali, or her stone likeness, to be more exact. Except that in addition to her other severe attributes, a belt was slung over her shoulder, and on that belt hung a saber. The goddess was armed and preparing for some dangerous ordeal. The stone in which she had been interred evidently could not withstand the strength of her desire to escape it.

There was no one else on the platform. But that was true only of the platform, because higher up in the darkness, in the background, another character in this drama was visible, the mighty Shiva with a golden trident in his hand. His hair was arranged in a pyramid, and a king cobra coiled itself around his neck. Unlike Kali, Shiva was not imprisoned in stone. He was alive. He was looking to see, understanding, and he was not reacting to Igor's appearance on the scene and mine with any warlike gestures. But then again, we did not know in what form he saw us.

That the situation we were in was unusual was further underscored by the fact that as soon as we got a little closer to Shiva, the Creator appeared nearby, just off to the side of us, and began to observe the scene with tense, undivided attention.

The appearance of the Father calmed us. We understood that the events before us were not happenstance, and that they were controlled by the Almighty Himself. And so we began to examine the situation.

Our attention once again turned to the stone, and to the woman kneeling before it. The pages of the stone book were turning on their own: it was the love story of Kali and Shiva. The story is beautiful and tragic, filled with the cruel trials, betrayal, and jealousy through which these Hindu gods nevertheless preserved their love. Kali even had to endure death in the process. And all of these tribulations led to Kali's transformation. After Shiva collected parts of her body, which had been defiled by jealous enemies, and resurrected her using the technology of reincarnation, Kali gained in addition to her former hypostasis, the hypostasis of death in the energy plane. She became the life-giving mother and the destroyer who takes life away. But it seems that with time, the goddess' second hypostasis began to burden her, and she decided to reject her terrible responsibilities. With her divine gifts, she foresaw a time when such a thing would be possible, and in advance created certain future events. This stone, this book, and this story of divine love, called "Kumarasambhava", were the key to the new incarnation of the goddess Kali, to her new mission as the goddess of motherhood.

The story of the two gods' love has been popularized in two classical renditions. Kalidasa wrote the poem "Kumarasambhava" ("The Birth of

309

Kumara," Kumara being the god of war). Then, about six hundred years later, Nannechoda repeated the same plot under the same name. To be fair, this later version deals with Parvati, not Kali, but Kali is one of the hypostases of the wife of the great ascetic and god. And even specialists can be thrown off track in the pantheon of Hindu mythology. As for us, at that moment, we were most interested in knowing what version our patient had read. Perhaps, it was some third one? In the meanwhile, events took an unexpected turn.

A fire burst forth in the chalices on the columns around us, lighting up the platform. Concentric reflections of the flames appeared in the sand. The circles had a way of intersecting with one another that formed a complex energy pattern. But this is what seemed bizarre: not a single spark of light trespassed outside the boundary of the circle defined by the sand. The darkness surrounded it like a wall, containing something that Igor and I could not see.

The stone statue of Kali shivered, and in that same instant, we were transported to another time, into a great nation's distant past. It was there that we saw Ira once again.

Now, she was a very young girl – fourteen years old at the most. She was wearing a beautiful sari and rich ornaments. She was the daughter of a powerful rajah.

We see the rajah himself, lying on his right side in a great hall. Servants with large fans waft cool air over the ruler's body.

There are many people in the hall. Dancers use their wondrous art to tell of the secret of love and passion. The jingle bells they wear on their hands and feet accompany their wild spinning with the harmonious crescendos and diminutions of sound.

Ira (the rajah's daughter) watches the dancing, but then, an idea having

310

sparked within her, furtively slips out of the hall. She takes a small chalice full of sweet from the table and runs from the palace's terrace down a wide staircase. Five stone steps and she encounters a platform, five more, and another platform.

The staircase is long, and there are many platforms on it, all framed by the greenery of a garden with fountains, flowers, guards. But then it comes to an end, culminating in a path, and alongside the path a little stream is quietly humming some tune.

The princess runs along the stream, descended towards a mighty river. For an instant, she stops at the water's edge to throw a flower in. The river's current is so powerful that the flower is immediately carried away.

The young woman joyfully watches her gift to the river disappear and then runs again along the shore towards a temple built on a small mound. The delicate red fabric of her sari billows in the wind behind her, her ornaments jingle, the upturned tips of her elegant slippers glint in the sunshine.

The temple gets closer and closer. And now she ascends its steps to come under a stone overhang supported by columns. She takes off her slippers and enters. This is the temple of Kali. Burning candles and platters with offerings adorn the entry on the left and the right, but the temple is empty.

The princess kneels in front of the goddess' statue and places the sweets she had brought at her feet. She thanks her for some important event in her life, one in which she had previously asked Kali to intercede. The young woman's face is shining with happiness.

At some point, the statue of Kali shivered and came to life for an instant. But the young woman, engrossed in her prayer, did not notice the change. A light sleep had overtaken her consciousness and enveloped her in a dreamlike slumber. In the meanwhile, the goddess, in her moment of

311

coming to life, had pronounced a prophecy: a thousand years hence, at the end of times, the princess will help the goddess return to life.

The momentary slumber releasing its grip, the princess stood from her kneeling position. She remembered something, forgot something else. In her bright oblivion, she stood next to the goddess' statue. Then, as she left the temple, she kept turning to look back.

As soon as the princess left the temple, the prophecy was already having its effect. The young woman suddenly saw what was supposed to happen in the future. It was as though she was running along the path once again, spinning in her dance, rejoicing that she will be able to help gods and people. She was truly happy.

In the meantime, Igor and I were frozen on the platform with the stone that continues to this day to be a holy site for the Indian people. Ira is still on her knees before the stone book, and in keeping with that long ago agreement with Kali, she is trying to read the song of love. But she no longer has the mastery of the ancient language she once did, and she still needs a key that has locked the true meaning of the words. Ira is desperate. She does not know how to fulfill the promise she has made.

Kali looks at Igor and me. Her face is quite decisive and warlike, but now it bespeaks rather a plea for help, an entreaty that we give Ira a hint as to how to find the key to the words' secret. Without these words of love, she cannot reunite with Shiva, cannot leave her hypostasis of death, and cannot become solely a mother.

We look through the text in the stone. The stone pages turn one after the other. Their rustling blends into the murmur of the stream, along which the princess Ira once ran down to the mighty river on the banks of which a temple stood thousands of years ago.

– You must remember the voice of the stream, – Igor hints.

312

No sooner had Igor uttered these words, than something roared and started moving in the darkness that surrounded the platform. Something dangerous and powerful had emerged onto the border between light and darkness, preparing itself to cross the timeless boundary between worlds. Then Kali jumped off her stone and began to run around that dark boundary of pitch blackness. With lightning-fast circular movements, she raised her saber and brought it down. Moans and shrieks of pain and terror accompanied her fighting gestures, as the heads of demons landed in the circle of light and their headless bodies fell away into the darkness. As the goddess circumscribed the platform, tens of heads defined the new boundary of her stay.

Ira continued to kneel by the stone, frightened and amazed. But she already knew the voice of the song, its spirit and its soul. She could begin her work both there on the informational energy plane and here, on the physical one.

– You gave Kali your word that you would help her, – Igor reminded. – She always protected you here, and now, when you fulfill your promise, Kali will bestow upon you the talent to be the best among those who translate the ancient texts of India. You will be able to see, compare, and understand. This song will make you famous. He who will read your song will understand what it means to love and to be loved, and together with that love he will attain an understanding of the higher realms of knowledge.

When Igor finished his admonition, a giant snake appeared at the entrance to the platform, or perhaps a serpent. He crawled around us clockwise, but looked only at me and said something only for me. But I could not hear or understand what he was trying to tell me, and neither Igor nor Kali could help. The voice of the serpent was as inaccessible to them as it was for me. But there was a difference. It seemed that they were

313

not meant to hear him because the serpent was addressing only me. He wanted only for me to absorb the rustling of his thought. But as it turned out, I did not understand it either. Perhaps, this was for the best?

It is strange after all that recently we have been living both here and there. But truth be told, I had never before lived as interestingly as I have over the last year.

* * *

I already recounted at the beginning of the book that we were not particularly successful in the process of treating a woman who was diagnosed with cancer and radiation sickness simultaneously. Although we began working with her when her treating physicians openly acknowledged their helplessness and predicted that she did not have more than ten days to live, we were able to postpone by several months this sad result. More than that, Marina Nikolayevna began to get up from her bed, to read books, and to dream of visiting her summer house in the spring, to putter in the garden. If only it were not for the ill-fated conversation with one of her loved ones... Someone mercilessly and cruelly killed her hopes and ripped the fragile thread that connected her to life.

Some time went by, and Marina Nikolayevna's husband came to visit us. He had become gaunt, his face had darkened. It was apparent how hard it was for him to bear his loss.

We too, as they say, were out of our element. This was the first death of a person we had been trying to help.

He told us about her last days and confirmed that in reality everything was pointing towards her getting better if it weren't for that unfortunate conversation about the summer house... He understood that this conversation broke his wife's will, her commitment to battling her illness. He thanked us for the fact that instead of the several days that the doctors predicted, she had lived several months.

I think to myself that even Jesus was not always able to persuade the people around him. I remember the gospel: "And he did not do many mighty works there, because of their unbelief."

* * *

I saw her and remembered that Abyss of Nothingness that once stirred and flowed with darkness. I remembered how it all began when the voice of the Primordial One appeared in the darkness, which was tired of the illusions of Nothingness. At first, it was not movement that ripened but only the desire for movement. The darkness stirred, and from the center of this disquiet the resonances of energy waves ran in every direction. And darkness began to collide with darkness.

In those places where the waves of darkness struck with particular force against the wall of pitch blackness, tiny sparks of light lit up and went out, pricking with pleasurable warmth the space that was still cold but was destined shortly to become the Universe.

What had happened was good. And the need for movement replaced the desire for movement. The Primordial One opened, and from it burst forth a mighty current of quanta. Their icy breath pierced everything around them, and the flesh of the Universe shuddered, together with the space that it inhabited – pathetically small on the outside and infinitely large within. But the opposites had already come into conflict: everything around flared up and was extinguished in the games of photon currents, red-hot plasma, and cold pitch blackness meeting one

315

another.

Time flowed into new coils of past, present and future, into regulated temporal structures. This was a stage of coordinating the Foundations of Primordial Nothingness with the illusions that had ripened in it, with the vectors and vortexes of ideas, by means of the resonances in the all-encompassing vacuum, the appearance of elementary particles, the orientations and processions of their angular moments of rotation in accordance with their reflections in the Being of the emerging Cosmos. The closed-off nature of the Primordial Singularity was disrupted, and having launched a cascade of vector processes, the eternally unmanifested and indescribable Primordial One began to form yet another "reality".

I see this Abyss. It is in the informational space between Heaven and Earth, and it looks like a cylinder. There is a platform on top with an opening in its center through which the current of the energies of the Cosmos flows down to the Earth. The energy currents of the Earth flow in the opposite direction, rising up alongside the walls of the cylinder. Between the outer rim of the cylinder and the platform in the center, there is a small gap through which the energies of the Earth escape under pressure from below. And now these rising currents are for some reason reoriented towards the center of the Abyss. In other words, they are locked into the cosmic current flowing downward. They escape along the walls of the tunnel, circumscribe an arc out of inertia and then are sucked anew into the primordial roar of the Abyss' central opening.

And there is one more new detail. On the platform near the central opening sits a person on an office chair, wearing a black robe with a hood on his head. He has a book on his lap that resembles the one that opened before Igor and me in the Cosmos – the Book of Knowledge. At times, this person gets up, takes the book under his arm and walks around the central opening of the Abyss. He is clearly waiting for something.

– Who is that? – I ask Igor.

– With the book under his arm? – he clarifies.

– Yes, of course.

– Get closer and you will see yourself, – my partner answers enigmatically.

I move closer to the mysterious personage by the Abyss, and in so doing I pass through the energy current. I want to see his face, but the hood and the shadow falling from it are in the way. I turn this way and that, but the person by the Abyss does not raise his downcast head; it is as though he is playing the children's game of "guess who" with me.

Finally, I cannot bear it any longer, and I simply touch his shoulder with my palm. I do not know why I did this, or indeed why I had this unstoppable desire to find out his identity. To this "why" I received an answer immediately. The person by the Abyss raised his head, and I saw my own smiling face. I unexpectedly met myself there.

Igor was by my side at this point and was carefully observing as my face took on an expression of bewilderment.

– Perhaps you should embrace one another, – he counsels. – It's not every day, after all, that one gets to meet oneself.

I heed the advice of my friend, and hug the person by the Abyss. The past and the present have met and have united. Two "Egos" have become one whole, all while retaining their hypostases.

The Father appears next to us quietly. He stands by us in silence. We bow before Him.

He is dressed for a very special occasion – his whole attire is shimmering with different colors, even the staff in his hand. His face is beautiful and stern. And when He looks at us, it seems that he can see through us. His gaze immediately reaches the very essence of whatever he is looking at.

– The information of the past lives, and the information of the future also lives, – the Father pronounces as though trying to hint at something.

He turns his head, and a piercingly powerful ray beams from his soul onto Igor's.

Igor sees the space into which his soul had been transported on the ray. In addition to the soul, he sees the consciousness, but he does not see the energy or the protein body. Then, he observes the movement of the soul to the earthly layer. It is precisely on the earthly layer that the soul begins to build first the skeleton or the contour, and then the modules of the future body. It does not take much to divine that the Father is showing us the technology of incarnating the soul in the body.

After the modular building is over, information begins to flow from the archival point of the individual. It fills layer by layer all the modular structures of the body, only then passing into the cells and organs. As the final step, a silver ray is directed towards the person's head, filling the body and bringing him to life or manifesting him on the earthly layer. It is in every way identical to the ray that now emanates from the Father to Igor.

– Let us go look at what is happening in My Kingdom, – the Father invites us, and we are instantaneously transported after Him to the boundary that divides the dark and white planes. Paradise and Hell fall on opposite sides of this razor-thin line. In addition to this line of absolute truth, a Chasm divides them. We walk in the Creator's steps on the emptiness above the Abyss, and we can see through the walls that surround these two antagonistic structures of existence. There is disarray on both sides, but for different reasons.

In Paradise, they know about the era of immortality that is beginning and about the impending resurrection. The souls are anxious. Many of them have not been on the earthly plane for hundreds of years, and they worry about how their descendants will respond to them.

Hell is also in a state of anxiety. These souls know that it will all end for them soon. Some of them consider how they might be able to escape to the Father's Kingdom through the Abyss. In the past, some had succeeded at this. They pressed themselves to the edges of the Chasm, where the energies created small zones of stability, and climbed upward by grabbing onto the uneven surfaces. They were scouts who would look out and try to get their bearings without being noticed, and then return with reports of what they had seen. There wasn't much to be gained from such expeditions, but still these missions cemented the belief that someday it will be possible shamelessly to break into the Heavenly Kingdom in this way. They did not know that the situation had radically changed since then, and that by the exit from the Abyss, there was now a guard – the man with the book under his arm.

The Father read my thoughts and smiled.

– You did everything right. Now, your global objective is to resurrect people. But discuss everything in realistic terms, and do not drive others mad with tales of what is happening in the subtle matter world. As for the resurrection of that woman, I will speed up the process and help you. When it comes to the man and Igor's grandfather, the opposite is true. I will go a little slower. The speed is simply too great, and they are not able to catch up quickly enough in capturing the knowledge of events that have happened on earth.

– And the decision about the Abyss is absolutely correct, – He addresses me with a smile, and thin rays of barely contained laughter appear around His eyes. Then He looks down and is silent. Suddenly, He sighs and says:

– Yes-yes, the Earth will be beautiful. And people will live on it with love and enjoyment. Your work will be successful. Never fear. Your worries and emotions will settle down. Everything will be fine.

He turns around and walks away, keeping an even, unhurried pace that allows us to watch Him for a long time as He recedes into the distance.

We look around, and we see in Paradise the garden where Adam lived. We see some implements used to make pottery. One of them is broken, but the information remains that can be input into one's consciousness and read.

The Creator worked here. He liked to work with his hands. He planted flowers in these pots. He experimented before launching the process on Earth. We see the tree by which the serpent explained to Eve that she was naked and turned her attention to those ill-fated apples.

Eve had knowledge and even cognition, but she had not yet attained the absolute truth. Truth and falsehood – these are only the mirror surface of reflection. But she found that she liked looking at herself. She admired her reflection in the water and thought: "Oh, how beautiful I am." And she did not think about the Father Who created her. She thought only about herself, about her outer image. She wanted to live in it. She herself wanted to distance herself from God, and she drew her husband with her.

Events unfolded in accordance with her wish. Nature created the body in the image of man, but the light of the Father grew weaker within him. That is why when Christ was asked about something related to the world, he answered: "Ask your mother, and she will give you of the things which are another's." Did anyone understand what He answered? Yet He is from Nazareth (and "Nazara" means absolute truth), He Who is of absolute truth. Everyone repeats something different: "Protect Mother Nature!" But where is the Father in all this? Who remembers the Cosmos? An understanding of the cause has morphed into the consequence.

Eve tempted Adam to leave the Garden of Eden. They thought that they already knew everything, but the Earth was not yet ready, and the first people were still too weak. The Dark forces turned out to be closer to them and were able to influence them more effectively. Who came up with the words "death" and "fate"? Who used these to govern the world? This is the sad essence of the interrelationships between children and parents – before even knowing why and what for to remake the world to one's own liking. And how did it turn out?

Suddenly a new character appeared between Paradise and Hell: a woman with a braid. Coming out of Hell, she wandered along its walls.

She looks very confused. Her face changes constantly. She has many images – now she's young, now old, now she's beautiful, now she's ugly.

She sees us, but does not come near, keeping her distance.

It seems that she knows that she has lost and will soon be left without work. She is nervous. She wants to speak, but does not speak. She wishes to approach, but does not do so.

She is probably also hampered by the boundary on which we so recently stood with the Creator. Suddenly, her nerves cannot take it anymore, and she shouts:

– Why resurrect? There are those who live for more than a thousand years. Why resurrect everyone?

Igor, seeing how anxious Death has become, immediately begins to tell her why it would be a good thing if people became immortal. Creation, he explains, is endless and comes in many forms. No one will tire of immortality because this is creativity. People get tired of doing nothing, and under such circumstances even a lifespan may seem a very long time. But if a person follows his dreams, even an immortal life seems too short.

321

Death listens to him, and her face changes. Now, she is like a raging fury.

– He, who will soon come, there is no need to resurrect him. He already has all this personally! What are you planning to do about him? He has very great powers, – she cries.

– If this is the absolute truth, – Igor answers, – stand on the boundary line and repeat what you have just said.

– There is no need for me to stand on this boundary line, – Death snaps. – Regardless, everyone knows that I speak the truth. But what's the point of even talking to you. They will no longer accept me where I came from. Nor will you ever take me with you. No one needs me now even though I have strength and power.

Death turned around and trudged back to the gates of Hell. But here is what is surprising: when she got to them, the gates turned out to be locked. Her old friends and allies quickly figured out that if Death were deprived of the opportunity to fulfill her duties in her prior field of work, so to say, then she would immediately find a new one. And no matter how hard the old woman knocked on the gates, no matter how much she cursed, she was not able to enter her prior home. Helpless, she sat next to the wall, leaning on her braid. What a pitiful sight she presented at this moment, considering how recently she made the entire world under the moon tremble before her.

* * *

Igor and I are now living our lives according to the creed of that well-known leader of the world's proletariat: "Learn, learn, and learn!" Of course, we are learning to create rather than to destroy, and that difference is decisive. We are studying the Universe, and we are studying Man, who provides the foundation for everything in our world. We would barely finish one area of study, and immediately move to working through the next one.

I have written before that there is a triangular subtle matter structure above every person's head, in which the secret work of the interactions between the macro and micro-levels is constantly taking place. An energy canal leads to this structure. Bio-energy experts see this precisely in the form of energy, and they are right. But if you are operating at the level of information, then inside the light currents you will discern a structure, consisting of pathways and spheres. Every part of one's DNA, every chromosome, radiates its own impulse or signal into this structure, which Igor and I call THE SOUL'S PATH.

The soul is the repository of all current data about one's body; it correlates that information with the gigantic reserves of original knowledge contained within it and projects it in the form of a row of coordinated spheres into the channel of THE SOUL'S PATH. As the spheres approach the energy pipe, they compress and concentrate into archival points until the flows of the Spirit carries them up the seven lanes of which the Path consists. Above, in the triangle of consciousness, they expand once again. And depending on the specific decision that the consciousness reaches, after analyzing the various scenarios and alternatives the soul suggests, new information control spheres begin to emerge. The interaction happens through the reverse setting of all the lanes to pass information through the soul and into the nucleus of each cell, the consciousness of each cell, found in the chain of DNA.

In the governing triangle of consciousness, the apex is the head and the pituitary gland, the command-administrative structure.

But here is something interesting: if a virus of some dangerous illness

323

infiltrates the organism, it attempts to plant its own informational structure along THE SOUL'S PATH and to capture the functions of control in at least one lane.

Today, we are analyzing cancer, and what do we see? It looks as if a wedge has been driven into one of the lanes. We magnify its structure, and we see that it is also a triangle, whose apex contains information about the cancer. The lower left-hand corner looks like an imitation of the pituitary gland, but in a position subordinate to the triangle's apex. The lower right-hand corner is a hologram of the organ, whose cells and structure of their DNA are intended to receive information about becoming insubordinate. This is a new program, but not of development; instead, it is a program of uncontrollable multiplication, leading to the death of the cell, the organ, and finally, the entire organism. Even the period over which the illness will develop has been determined; its chronometer is contained in the first cell – in the chromosome of the DNA that submits to the false governing system implanted in THE SOUL'S PATH.

Information about AIDS and any other serious disease implants itself in the body in precisely the same way.

How do you battle cancer by using informational technologies?

It is a mistake to treat cancer only on the physical plane. You must work, first and foremost, with information. Thus, you must first find that chromosome or chromosomes, in which the information about cancer was implanted and which is the source of its initial effects.

Then, it is as though you unwind the lane or the tape (this second term also reflects the essence of the process fairly accurately). By the tape, I mean the chronological tape of recorded events, which sequentially registers all the things that happen to a person in his or her life. You must unwind it to the moment when there was no disease, when it had not yet begun.

For example, we erase the information about the illness from a particular patch on the sixth chromosome in the chromosomal chain. In other words, whatever it contains about the cancer, the development of the illness, and the unmanageable division of cells, we get rid of it all. We erase it, and instead record information about the norm, good health, and a life of creation.

Next, we inform the pituitary gland of the fact that it had been deceived by a foreign informational structure (in essence, by a mind foreign to us), and we give it the symptoms that enable it to recognize those cells that have been affected by the cancer. From this moment, the immune system's limitations in recognizing the problem in the body are lifted; the cells are once again under control. The future informational recording about the absence of any illness is combined with the past. And because the future is always more powerful, the eradication of the illness can begin on the physical plane. Two-three months, and the person is healthy.

More generally, this system works in the treatment of all other illnesses, and it is very effective.

But there are even greater things ahead. We confront the question of how to develop the technology to resurrect the dead by analogy to the one developed by Grigori Petrovich Grabovoi. The issue is all the more urgent since we have recently been approached by people asking us about the possibility of resurrecting their loved ones. We are not in a rush, although we have received the technology, and we have launched several exploratory processes to resurrect our loved ones and friends.

We study how this happens, tracing the procedure by which the soul is incarnated in the physical body, the nuances of the reentry from the "other world," where there is no dynamic of external events, where chronological sequences are built through the alternation of discrete holograms of events, like slides in a projector. Those returning to our world spend much time precisely in getting readjusted to the uninterrupted passage of time, which had become foreign to them.

We try to help them by giving repeated impulses to their consciousness that contain a perception of events they need to catch up on. We see how they all want to return to the physical world, which offers a full existence.

Igor and I decided to describe in detail one of these resurrections, so that the reader will know that this is possible in principle. Moreover, all living things in the world strive precisely for resurrection and, as the next step, towards immortal existence, in accordance with Christ's gospel.

The era foretold two thousand years ago has come. The era of immortality has arrived.

We chose just one out of many cases in order methodically to explain all the vicissitudes of resurrection. We provide in this case, as in other similar instances, the true first and last names of our protagonists.

And so: Kuznetsova, Galina Borisovna (passport series II-VG #727239) asked us to resurrect her daughter Kuznetsova, Alexandra Gennadyevna, whose drunken father killed her under terrible circumstances on October 10, 1994. We asked Galina Borisovna to record carefully and in detail everything that will transpire at this time. Let us read together what the voice of Galina Borisovna's soul tells us. Who can recount all this better than a mother's soul:

"On October 10, 1994, a tragedy occurred in our family. Our youngest daughter, Alexandra, whom I called Sasha, passed away. All these years, I have been haunted by one question: why?

The most important thing is that I never sensed the death of my daugh-

326

ter. And I was not the only one. When I used to go to the village, where Tatiana, who was my girlfriend and Sasha's too, lived, she always knew when I would arrive. I arrived at night, and in the morning the phone would ring:

– Hello Galina!

– How do you know I'm here?

– We have already known for three days that you were supposed to arrive today. Sasha came by, plopped down on the couch and said: "I am so tired of these trips. So glad we are finally home..." That's how we knew.

More broadly, over the course of three years, Tanya and I had a constant connection through Sasha: Sasha helped her study, pass her exams, provided information about herself, said who in the village would pass away in the near future (and this came true), and helped to find a person who had disappeared, said what had happened to him and where he was, and explained how to behave in this situation or the other.

In fact, at first (over the course of a year and a half), Sasha visited many people in the village. Even now, everyone remembers her (and indeed, her image is very vivid for people even today). Usually, a person is gone, and people empathize for a little while, then forget. But that's not what happened here. Three years after the tragedy, a girl in the first grade surprised me by asking: "Auntie, it is hard for you without Sasha, right? ..." and broke into tears. I didn't even know this girl. Sometimes, other villagers dreamed about her. Sasha warned of important events to come. Many dreamed about her often.

Then, I went to study at the Center and studied with Igor Arepyev. For my part, I kept thinking about Sasha. One day, he asked me: "So, what are we going to do?"

I showed him the photographs, and he said: "They are waiting, they

327

are asking for something." I was not fully following him; I didn't under-
stand what he was talking about.

But then it came to me. The word "resurrection" resounded in my
consciousness. It was in my subconscious for a long time already, but
somehow lay dormant until Igor's involvement. I had so many questions,
probably because life had fallen out that way. Everything has to be organ-
ized just so and right before your eyes, extend a hand at the right moment,
and you will get what you need. I waited for an opportune moment with
Igor and said:

– They want, they ask to appear? To materialize?

– Finally, – he answered.

This is how our work of resurrecting my youngest daughter began."

In fact, the process of resurrection has several typical technical stages.
The first of these is to obtain the soul's agreement to return to the physical
world. This is very important because it is precisely the structure of the
soul that builds the physical body of the person. We had this agreement, so
we could get to work. Let us read Kuznetsova's notes.

"Something unusual happens at night. I saw an impulse: at first white
(not for long), then platinum and dark blue, a little pink. What do these
colors mean?

I see a space with cells resembling a bee-hive (golden black). What
is this?

I also see a clear pattern (ornament) of snowflakes. They quickly
appear and disappear, and their colors too. How do I stop them and take
a closer look?

The space seems heterogeneous (pink-lavender) with a grey shimmer.

And there is something alive, transparent inside it.

...I dreamed of Sasha. I spoke with her, told her about the period of time that she had missed, about the current events in my life, people, relatives, friends. How life had changed over six years. I dreamt of Sasha. I spoke with her, told her about The space looks heterogeneous (pink-lavender), and I see a grey rippling. There is somethhad

...Igor and Arkady Naumovich ran an experiment in recovering teeth. Once again, I acted as a volunteer. They started the process of growing the teeth – the third and sixth on the upper right. As soon as my thoughts return to the teeth, I feel a pulsation in my gums.

I imagine my teeth as "pearls:" even, white, shining, like a white shell.

...I went to bed around midnight. I had the sensation that someone is walking on top of my blanket (like a cat). I turned on the light, but there was no one there. I addressed Sasha's picture. Everything got quiet, and I immediately "fell" into a deep sleep.

In the morning, I went to the cemetery. The face on the photograph was smiling. It looked somehow enlightened. The mound of the grave under the gravestone was about two inches and three quarters lower than it had been, even though it is reinforced.

...As I recall the teeth, I feel something like a twitch of the nerves. There is some kind of vibration in the place where the gum and the cheek intersect. My cheek tickles.

The sensations are the same in the morning. I decided to take a look. The gum-line by the cheek and on top has gotten red. In the area of the third and sixth tooth, little bumps have appeared – the kind that small children have when they are teething. I have no painful sensations.

...In the evening Tanya (Sasha's friend) called. She was very excited and asked me to explain what was going on. She had had a dream (all

her dreams related to Sasha were like waking dreams, and this had been true in the past as well. The dreams usually predicted the future): Sasha is back in the village. The bell rings, and she opens the door. Sasha is on the doorstep with a girlfriend (that is how she introduced the girl who was with her). They were holding hands. The girl was shorter and a little younger. Sasha had grown older – she looked about 20. She was laughing and full of life.

Tanya said to her: "It has been so long since I dreamed of you or since you came. Where are you coming from? You had, well, sort of died."

Sasha: "What are you talking about?! I am alive as can be! You don't believe me? Soon enough, you will be able to see for yourself. For now, go on and tell me what has happened here while I was away.

Tanya told her about herself, her sister, her mother, about me and about Olga and her husband.

Sasha rejoiced at Tanya's news, played with her daughter, praised the little girl and said: "Until soon, I am alive."

I told Tanya about my work on the resurrection and how to handle herself if faced with some unusual phenomena."

* * *

I feel drawn more and more powerfully to my counterpart by the Abyss. Something ancient is triggered in my memory when I think about him. It is something very ancient, something related to Adam and Eve. When they were leaving the Kingdom of God, they wanted to descend precisely here, through the Abyss. This was a dangerous way for them to go. The Father was angry, but He did not want them to lose their lives. That is why He put a guard in place by the Abyss – the man with the book.

Adam and Eve did not leave the garden of the Father right away. They hid in it for several days. They peeked out from behind the fence trying to see if they could dive into the Abyss? But the man with the book was always there, precisely where his Creator had put him. Thus, the disobedient ones had to descend to Earth in a roundabout way. Later on, Noah's Ark moored in the same place where Adam and Eve had come down to Earth.

I was very concerned at the time with this biblical plot. I wanted to gather more material for my book. That is why at one point, I convinced Igor to visit the Abyss in the center of the Sephiroth with me once again. In reality, he does not particularly like to go there. The place is far from simple, it is insidious. But how does one say no? It was important for our mission, and so we went together.

And there by the Abyss, the serpent is waiting for us, the very same one that once tempted Eve to taste of the apple. He is a healthy reptile, well-groomed. His scales shimmer with gold, and he is not at all hostile. Quite the opposite: he looks to be a domesticated snake. You can do whatever you want with him – wrap him around your neck at the circus or pet his scaly back with your hand.

He opens his mouth and says something, but I can't hear him and don't particularly feel like listening. At the same time, I'm curious.

– What is he trying to say? – I ask Igor.

– How would I know? He is only talking for you. – And he looks away. Either he really cannot hear, or else he doesn't want to meddle in someone else's business.

– I can't hear you, get out of here! – I tsked the serpent sternly, in a business-like way. Since when did I start feeling like such a serpent-slayer and become so arrogant as a result?

The serpent is flabbergasted at this kind of attitude. He does not want to crawl away, but he does not get closer either. He slithers this way and that, waiting for me to change my mind. But his ingratiating gaze and his scandalous reputation seem at odds with one another. Or do they? And what does he want with me anyway?

Go ahead, crawl away, I don't hear you, – I insist again on severing the relationship. What kind of relationship could I have with this reptile? I don't like his eyes – dark, bottomless, like Lapshin's. You cannot mistake this gaze for anything else – he can shave himself bald or grow hair all over, but the gaze will give him away every time. This is the call of the Abyss, of which I am now the guard.

Finally, the duplicitous one crawls away, insulted.

– Well, look at you, – Igor exclaimed either with admiration or, the opposite, in judging the emotional plane of what had transpired.

– Is anything the matter? – I asked, alerted.

– That was the serpent of wisdom... He is power itself... He is trying to transmit something to you, but you don't want to listen. Then, you go even further: he is acting pretty democratically towards you, and you tell him to scram.

– So what, I don't like him, – I say, deploying my foolproof excuse.

– Ah, well, – Igor responds understandingly. – That's a stand.

My second hypostasis by the Abyss observes everything that happens carefully. And he is not just observing. Something is happening to him and to the book that he is holding in his hands. Energy rings are emanating from the book, taking the shape of spheres, then compressing again and disappearing into a white cloud of consciousness over his head.

– What is going on over there? – I ask my friend.

– You are becoming one with the book, – he answers with a sigh of relief. – This is long past due, everyone has been waiting. Technologically, this is like breathing life into someone through the element of the soul. After this, a person starts to remember what had happened to him before, from the Beginning of Beginnings.

And it's true that suddenly something begins to rise up from within the depths of my memory like an awakening. And I see how the Creator tells Igor, Grigori Petrovich and me what is going to transpire many thousands of years later. He is speaking of the very time in which we are living.

And we are not at all as we are now; we are only children. Igor is the smallest of all, standing in the center. And the Father is not as large as we have seen Him become in recent times – He is of quite normal stature, grey-haired, with kind, wise eyes. He is speaking of things that have not yet happened, but are supposed to happen, provided that we are able to do what is predestined for us. He speaks of our challenge, and we listen to Him, but we do not see that there is a huge, athletic looking man hiding behind the wall and listening to our conversation.

He is so huge and powerful, but he is forced to bend down and hide in an uncomfortable and humiliating position. Who is he? How did he trespass over the Abyss that divides Hell from the Father's garden? Pride and ambition are etched on his beautiful face. He is without question one of the ancient gods. But at the same time, he has ears, tense like a dog's, and a face that is stretched, even pointed with attention – and he is spying and eavesdropping to boot. And I have already divined the name: the wings on the arms, legs, shoulders and helmet are too conspicuous a business card. He is Hermes, the herald of the gods. And earlier still – he was the thrice greatest Thoth.

But back then, thousands of years ago, I did not know that we've been

333

eavesdropped on. We were standing with our backs to the wall of the garden. For three days, the Father spoke to us about events to come – about the first, second and third coming of Christ, about the End of Times. And during all three days – that crafty god remained hunched over, cowering, afraid of being discovered and anxious not to miss a single word, spying on the Creator, who gave life to everything – including him.

Moreover, now I also knew that the Creator had seen him then.

I remember what a significant role Hermes or Thoth, as he was known in Atlantis and in Egypt, played in the history of the Earth and of mankind. His role is recorded in books and lauded in the temples. But who guided the hands of the scribes and inspired them? Who governed on Earth, and always had the opportunity to say definitively: "This is how it all happened!" But did what happened actually happen that way? We already know that the people of Atlantis were punished by the Creator for their attempt to start a war with the Heavens, which means that all is not so simple in the history of the creation's relationship with the Creator. And it was not at all the lofty virtues of the kings of Atlantis – Thoth among them – that caused the Great Flood to descend upon the Earth.

Eleven thousand years ago, Thoth replaced Horus on the throne of Egypt and became the keeper of the secrets in the pyramids of Giza.

The information that passes in circles and spheres from the book of my counterpart, the guard of the Abyss, and into him, gradually comes to life in my consciousness as well.

We must immediately go to the Valley of Kings, – I say peremptorily to Igor.

– What for?

– The iput is there.

–The iput is the secret chamber of Thoth. That is where he hid the

334

ancient prophecy he learned about while eavesdropping on the Creator. By doing this he sought to make matters more complicated, to introduce into the action an event no one knows about and that could help challenge the primary narrative.

– Where should we look for it? – Igor involuntarily narrowed his eyes. I know this is one of his professional quirks, left over from his prior work for the police department.

– There are supposed to be three X's there, or three letters "X".*A real Emerald Tablet is concealed between them.

– I understand, – Igor says.

– We hold hands and are transported first onto the earthly layers and then into the Valley of Kings.

–There "x's", three "x's", three "x's", – Igor sings to himself. – I see two – the pyramids are the biggest here. This means that the prophecy was hidden between two pyramids. Although it is not buried deep, finding it will not be easy. Thousands of years ago, every effort was made to prevent this from happening, including a defense against contemporary computer means of discovery and scanners.

A small room in the underground dungeon had been smeared with a special resin and covered in several rows of leaves. This technology is tougher than the contemporary one used for American Stealth fighter jets.

Igor and I are searching for the underground room. We are guided by intuition and the secret knowledge, hidden in the book that my counterpart is holding in his hands. We find it between two pyramids – those of Heops (the word is spelled in Russian as "Хеопс" with a capital X) and Hefren

* The author hints at two uses of "x": it is the twenty-fourth letter in the
modern Latin alphabet but in math it is used to represent an unknown variable.

(the Russian spelling, "Хефрен", also starts with the letter "X"). These are two of the letters X, but we know that there must be a third. Sure enough, it appears at two o'clock in the afternoon. The shadow of the sun, as it hugged the triangular shape of the pyramid, sketched out a third letter X – with the top part dark and the lower part light. The object of our search is at the intersection. This is the tomb, and at the same time, it is the door to immortality. It all depends on the perspective.

When we find the secret room, the information concealed within us awakens and becomes active again. Now we know whose room this is, and we know what Death was hinting at in her last conversation with us, when she said: "He, who will arrive." That "he" – which is the same word in Russian as the name for Thoth – was not used as a pronoun but actually meant here the name of the powerful Hermes Trismegistus (thrice greatest). And it is hardly appropriate for us to introduce him, especially considering that he introduced himself quite well on the Emerald Tablet, hidden in this secret room under the three letters X. I am not speaking of the Emerald Tablet that he purposefully sent into the world to distract the attention of those who seek the absolute truth, but the authentic item that he hid in the secret, protected room in the Valley of Kings.

The Emerald Tablet is suspended in the air, in the center of iput. It is made of stones that look similar to glass from bottles. Thoth made it himself, with his own hands, so that no one could know what was imprinted within it. The stones – green, dark blue, light blue – cast their shadow on the surrounding space. The shadow is a cursed and lethal illness. It is in the back. In front is the promise of greatness, of tremendous power from Hermes. This is the bribe, the promise of a union. The true text is in the center. It reads:

"I am the greatest among the greats! I have accomplished much

upon the earth! Half of the Earth, both land and water, will be my dominion, but it all depends on the one who goes in front and who is higher still than me. It's the one who is three in one or one in three. These will be the sons of man. The one who will open the tomb will suffer inevitable death, but also horrors and incurable diseases. But the one who, while still on the Earth, will descend from the Heavens, the one who is one in three visages and three in one – my destiny will depend on him. This triune will possess real power."

Once again, we ask ourselves, where the greatest of the greats learned about the prophecy? And once again the information trace that remains in the underground room of the thrice greatest immediately shows us the picture of Hermes, who was once also called crafty (do you follow the analogy?), eavesdropping on the conversation between the Creator and the sons. It was after this that he created his Emerald Tablet.

We knew Hermes Trismegistus as one of the teachers of mankind. Hymns were written in his honor, and temples and books were dedicated to him. But was this image of his authentic? The room stored information about a different image of Thoth, who had declared himself an earthly god, an image that practically no one knew about. Thoth was inextricably connected with the fact that man, albeit immortal and possessing power over everything, nonetheless also underwent what mortal beings are forced to endure. He was the one who came up with an intermediary – fate – in order to explain death. He was the one who stimulated the very progress that in the end was supposed to lead to our surrendering the benefits of our intellect to the machine, an effort that almost succeeded, all in order to stop the spiritual development of mankind. The very point of progress is to tempt man, to bend and break him, to throw him off the path of development onto the shoulder of the road, or to drive him off in the wrong direction. The television exists, and this is wonderful. But there is something else that is much better – and that is internal vision. In the first case, we are passive and being controlled. In the second, we are active and engaged in creation. Man retains his will. You can choose whatever you prefer, but then don't whine later about ill will and fate. You choose everything yourselves.

When the Son of the Creator came to the Earth intending to awaken and to aid, those who decided to kill Him, acted through none other than human beings. They were afraid of doing it themselves, but people turned out to be conscientious helpers. The Father taught them the words: LOVE! CREATION! GOODNESS! And they yelled about His Son: "Death to him, crucify him!" Not a single illness is foisted on a person for no reason. Perhaps, many of those, who come to us today for help also yelled on the square in front of the prosecutor's palace: "Kill!" "Crucify!" But illness is redemption. If a person understands everything correctly and grasps the meaning, any malady can disappear in an instant. The Father is merciful. He will forgive even those who would not have forgiven themselves. He has given everyone the opportunity to be redeemed and to make amends.

Many people have seen the Father. They were very gifted. The fire of genius burned in their eyes. Indeed, they were recognized by their eyes. Such people were killed in every era so that they would be unable to pronounce the word of absolute truth.

Those who persecuted God's people had power, title, authority. But they were the ones who elevated themselves and their helpers on these pedestals. All of them but one was able to create. Plotting, conspiring, uniting to make sure that the fruits of other people's labor were directed into their own pockets – all of these things they were more than capable of doing, as well as frightening others with the word "death". But now Death is sitting by Hell's gates and looks to be afraid of something herself.

We have read the prophecy of Thoth. We know of whom it speaks. Everyone awaits justice. And justice must be restored. People must get back the immortality that was stolen from them. The Father must see His children returned.

* * *

Events are unfolding more quickly on the subtle matter plane. Millions of devils, demons, and people climb upward out of Hell along the walls of the Abyss. At the very last moment, when they reach the exit, an energy current picks them up and redirects them back into the Abyss. My counterpart with the book stands at the edge of the energy opening in the center. If anyone succeeds in grasping onto the edge of Abyss, he hits them lightly on the head with the book, and the demons once again catapult downward. The book itself contains tremendous power, and so it is unnecessary to strain one's muscles in order to obtain this result. The Kingdom of God is no place for those who only know how to spoil and to ruin. First, they must undergo a purging. That is why the Abyss is called Purgatory. Blood-curdling shrieks resound within its depths for purging is a painful and slow process. What can you do? These people spend a long time doing whatever they wanted to, and now they must suffer in patience.

Nor is everything the same as before next to Hell. Death is walking around the walls, searching for a way to crawl back through. In the past, this would not have taken her much time. But now she is weakened, powerless. While she has been limping around the walls, those who remained in Hell covered up and concealed the gates as though they had never been there. Then they erected an entire barricade on the other side. It's like they were not demons at all, but some kind of insurgents. They do not want to let their own deadly force back inside the house.

Death is walking around irritated; she can't understand why her very own would not let her back in. She has not figured out that her former allies understood long ago that even if she is left without work in the world, this does not necessarily mean that she will sit around doing nothing in Hell. Her little program, after all, is serious. It's hard to believe that exhortations alone will wean her off swinging her scythe left and right. It is better to heap boulders in front of the entrance just in case. And on the informational bulletin (they also have one of those), an announcement is hanging to the effect that the population of hell has for a long time and with great hope been awaiting a herald from God to determine their further fate. And the letters that signify all this waiting are somehow old, as though they were not written today. It feels like they have been waiting for this herald for a thousand years. They are waiting for the herald, but have sealed up the gate in the meantime. The demons are clever.

And it's not only the gates of hell that are closed, but the gates of the Kingdom of Heaven as well. Someone is standing next to them. We see a mighty half-naked figure, a mask of some bird with a long beak on its head. This is Thoth, whom Death so eagerly awaited. She is still watching from a distance, to see how this standing by the gates of the Kingdom of the Father will end. She does not come any closer – there is such brightness there that her eyes accustomed to darkness cannot tolerate it. On top of that, a lion and eagle are inspecting the guests from their respective side of the gates, just looking for an excuse to pounce on someone.

Igor and I transport ourselves so as to end up between Thoth and the gates. We are, after all, the defenders. He sees us and turns his beak in our direction. He looks at us carefully through the slits of his mask. Unexpectedly, Grigori

Petrovich appears next to us. He is calm, which leads us to conclude that there is no real danger here. Now, all three of us are guarding the gates.

Thoth is the first to speak:

– Children of the Earth and children of Heaven, which is synonymous, I know that the Father gave rights to the three in one and the one in three in accordance with the decree of God's Judgment. Now that you have read the prophecy, I must stand before those who have read it so that my further fate may be determined. A multitude of gods of different peoples and times are likewise awaiting their destiny. Many of them are now gathered at Mount Olympus awaiting my return.

He is silent for a time, waiting for our reaction to his pronouncement. We do not speak, and he is forced to continue.

I know about the Creator's plan, since all of us were informed, the gods first and foremost. We knew that those the Creator would send would be the sons of mankind. They alone will be given the power to resurrect and to continue the new era. I, Thoth, am the only one of my kind to achieve such greatness and such heights in matters of the soul, and thus I was sent to bring news to the gods from the sons of mankind.

He wanted to say something more, but the Creator appeared before him.

– It is too early for you to speak of those events that have not yet occurred. I have warned you that the people will possess knowledge and cognition, so that things will not turn out as they have before, when one or a few lorded over the majority.

The voice of the Father was strict, incriminating.

– Do not look this way at my children. You will achieve nothing. You, gods, possess charms, but I have bestowed on them higher powers. Go on, leave!

Thoth is clearly at a loss, but he obeys and leaves. Death, who had been observing all of this from afar, suddenly took on the likeness of a beautiful young woman. She wants to command sympathy and pity. But the Father turns away, and Death once again becomes an old woman.

– When I sent My Son onto the Earth, in order to pass on knowledge to the people, the gods did not support him.

In pronouncing these few words, the Father gave voice to that which he carried within Himself for two thousand years, without transgressing the cosmic laws that He Himself had established. All the gods had been promised immortality until the End of Times. In fulfilling this promise, the Creator humbled His pain, made it subservient to the law, which he believed to be above a personal grievance. But the gods did not understand. They considered him weak and began to make fun of him on the sly, thinking less and less about their own destiny. They behaved themselves on Olympus and in other closed-off systems of gods the way that tenants in communal apartments act in their shared kitchen. But their quarrels and discords on the subtle matter plane immediately manifested themselves as wars, misfortunes, and natural disasters on Earth. Which of them even considered this? They all knew that until the End of Times, they were immortal. So it was written on the gold bullions of the Creator. It's just that no one explained to them when the End of Times would arrive.

Even in eternity, there are end points, and the End of Times has come. So here is the ambassador of the Gods, Hermes Trismegistus, formerly known as Thoth, who came to ask for an extension of their powers, for a confirmation of the rights of immortality, and he heard the Creator's response: "Go on, leave!"

– What happened is their own fault, – the Father begins to speak again, as though reading our thoughts. – It was convenient for them to keep people ignorant, and what they achieved is a world in which no one believes in any-

342

thing. That is why no one can progress any further, not they, not the people. They live and live, they do something. They try one thing and then another. They decided just to be present for life. All has been achieved – what more is there to desire? It was supposed to be completely different. They even made up honors, prizes, and titles for themselves. Thrice greatest, bah!

Where are the three "T's" in his name? There she is – his friend, – the Creator nodded his head towards the old woman sapped of strength. – Even Hell won't take her now. Look at her all sad. They kept confusing everything and confusing everything, and finally they got confused themselves. Who is their god? They even mixed up all the names. They should have gone to their own god for eternal life; what did they come here for? Now, they are left with that which they wished on others.

The Father grew silent, and looked over the three of us with his long, studying gaze, which immediately sees the essence of the depths and heights.

– I bestow upon you, My children, love and justice. Always be together – three in one and one in three. Watch out for feelings. Feelings let man down. To be courageous in your desires is one thing, but to be courageous in reality is a totally different story. Beware of indifference – indifferent people quickly lose their strength. Do not let evil into your heart – evil pushes you towards the wrong actions and thoughts. Do not fall prey to the illusions of your wishes, since you are among the very few who can always obtain what they wish for. This means that with time, you could stop perceiving life in a real way. Run from the vanity of power. Why? You understand full well yourselves. Do not strive for riches – they are worth nothing. And most importantly beware of falsehood. It is precisely through falsehood that man convinces himself to give in to all the temptations I just recited.

Again, the Father grew silent, reliving past and present days.

343

– Not all those who call themselves people are people. They created my image, that of the Creator, through Nature, through a reflection. And everything became distorted. They changed the shape and created a shell – a body and bones. Let them take these back, and live in them. But they will not have the soul, the consciousness, or the energy of the Cosmos.

How do you think they worked? Nature was able to create animals, but they did not have complete reason – so they run and run around the Earth, having taken a look at how it is above in My Kingdom.

The animals were connected with man, or, rather, man was turned backward in the direction of the animals. Why connect man with an earthly animal that has not passed along the path of evolution? In order to attain superiority over man and to gain power through him. Nature became great. But it is Man, the Creator, who created her. She is good, I don't deny it. But why love oneself with such unearthly love?

When the Creator pronounced these last words, the renowned Russian poet Fyodor Ivanovich Tyutchev's famous verse suddenly resounded clearly and eloquently within me:

Nature – of our past she's clearly unaware,
For our spectral lives she does not care,
Wary of her grandeur, austere and supreme,
We vaguely feel we're nothing but a dream.
In nature's eyes we're all like little kids
Who pride themselves in vain for their heroic deeds.
She treats us equally – to her we're all the same,
Her abyss kindly swallows us in glory and in shame.*

I recalled how unhappy the multiple uses in these verses of the pro-

* This represents an original translation.

344

nouns "our", "we" and "us" made me. The author's poetic genius would clearly have no problem using these pronounces less generously, if there was no other, much more profound, reason for their use. I now understood what it was when I correlated it with the following words: "He in His turn beholding the Form like to Himself, existing in her, in her Water, loved it and willed to live in it; and with the will came actuality, and so Man vivified the Form devoid of reason." ** Original sin is the child born without the involvement of the Father.

The Ego is man's shadow, created by Nature on analogy with the heavenly prototype but without thought and foresight. And an old woman is sitting on the sidelines, who has helped to deprive man of the true meaning of his existence through the mechanism of fear: Death. She so easily took life away from those who had lived only a few decades, but as soon as there was some threat to her own existence, she suddenly lost her calm and her good spirits. Without any discussion, having just traded glances, the three of us approach Death.

She did not turn, but only shuddered in the shoulders as though shivering painfully.

– Go away. I can't tolerate your light. I have no power to command you, but go away. I don't want warmth. I am used to the cold. I owned it all not very long ago, – she pitifully beseeched us, without even turning in our direction.

There was so much we wanted to tell her. But what is there to say to one who is so pathetic and powerless? She is so weak, she feels unwell, and she has no future. We didn't gloat but stepped away as she had asked. Before our very eyes, Death was falling asleep, although she had not pre-

** "Thrice-Greatest Hermes", Vol. 2, from "Corpus Hermeticum: Poemandres, the Shepherd of Men", translated by G.R.S. Mead, a prolific esoteric scholar.

viously been susceptible to sleep. Something was happening to the Dark ones, and it was something they themselves had not expected.

We felt the urge to do a little traveling, and decided to look for ourselves at Olympus, which Thoth had told us about. In an instant, we were already there. It was a gigantic mountain, enclosed in an energy sphere. A powerful wall, the gates ajar, and on those gates we could see the signs of the zodiac, six on each leaf.

The gods who enter through these gates put their hands on the signs of the zodiac. They are convex and made out of gold. The leaves themselves are gold as well.

Igor says that we must simultaneously push on the leaves of the gates, by putting our hands on our signs of the zodiac. We do as he says, and the leaves fly open. There are steps behind them, rising up through the clouds to the summit. A throne stands at the top, with the words "thrice greatest" on its back. So this is who truly ruled Olympus over the preceding millennia. The throne is empty. Hermes did not have the courage to return here with the answer he received from the Creator.

From the peak, we have a good view of everything below. At the foot of the mountain, there is a beautiful valley with groves, gardens, lakes, and castles. In a big clearing, there are thrones, chairs, benches, pillow strewn about. Thousands of gods gathered here to wait for their emissary, who had recently decided to combine his previous duties with sovereignty over the gods. They do not yet know about the most recent events. The atmosphere among them is normal – they are resting, talking to one another. Their servants are bringing them anything they may wish for. It's true, why fill one's head with the problems of people. Everything is already good – in fact, it couldn't be better. The weather is always clear, the food is always delicious, and Hermes had freed them of earthly concerns and obligations. It is some kind of health spa resort. What else could gods and goddesses dream of? Of course, they could set the Greeks upon the Trojans for their own amusement, or stir up some other turmoil. This would be something on the order of a theater in one's own home. Where could such gods lead people? Only to universal atheism. We return from the summit to the gates of Olympus. Now we can clearly see that there is no road that leads here, not even a path. By contrast, throngs of people go to Jesus Christ.

The gods created Death and used her as an instrument to consolidate their sovereignty. "What are you going to do when Thoth, who must arrive, arrives?" – Death asked Igor and me. It seems then that she believed him to be stronger than she was? But as it turns out, even the gods, if they are not protected by immortality, are afraid of their own creation – Death. The people knew in dying that they were going to the Father. But if the gods die – where will they end up? It would clearly have to be before the Creator, because their reincarnation depends on Him and only on Him. That is what Thoth came to ask about – first for himself, then for the other gods. But what could he say, how could he explain it?

* * *

I was suddenly summoned to the ministry, for the first time in a year and a half. Our results are better than ever. Each quarter, despite the general negative outlook in our industry, our profits grow and substantially so. The books now come out looking smart, beautifully adorned. Finally, there is money enough to spend on the decorative elements. If the publishing house received even a little aid from the Federal program for book publishing, our progress could be rapid.

I comforted myself with these illusions for nothing. The bureaucrats

347

had their own views on "KhudLit". The head of the central administration, Nina Sergeyevna Litvinetz – concurrently the head of the publishing house "Raduga", which was privatized for a song just at the right time – laid out the essence of the problem without beating around the bush. She didn't even bother to ask us how things were going or what we were planning to release? She just said, simply and clearly:

– We now have an opportunity to direct some substantial federal resources into publishing, under a serious program.

– That's wonderful, – I responded jubilantly.

– But there must be a different person in the position of director for "KhudLit" under this program, – she tempered my untimely show of enthusiasm.

– I understand. By the pail where the milk is flowing, you always need one of your own.

– Well, you are not planning to fight with the state, are you? – she asked calmly, puffing on a thin cigarette.

Her face – severe, powerful – represented the face of the state, or so it appeared to her in the moment.

So the Moor has done his duty? The Moor can go…* I helped pull the publishing house out of debt. Now you want to kick me out?

– Why would you put it that way? – Litvinetz responded mercifully. – You can name your conditions. We will discuss them.

– For starters, give us a chance to discuss it, – I asked.

– A week, not more, – the "state" agreed.

– What was it that my buddy Volodya Noskov (coincidentally, the editor of this book) said?

Made toast of and tested, alas,

* Reference to a line from Schiller's "Fiesco", which is used idiomatically to imply someone who has completed what was expected of him and can now be discarded as useless.

And yet the day will come,
When the sovereign's hoof
Will kick you, lummox, in the ass,

Under the rusty look you'll cower,
Crying into the red tape void:
"The state – that's us, my friends,
Did you forget it, power!"

Ignoring your pitiful appeal,
The mysterious creature escapes.
Fortunately perhaps, one might say.
Just for whom is this "fortune" real?

Pain killers you will buy galore
To quell your heart's sores in silence...
Where are you bound, Bronze Horseman,*
To the twenty-first century shore?**

Truth be told, recent events have come together in such a way for me
that I needed to concentrate all my efforts on what was most important in
life, and that was controlled clairvoyance. In my heart of hearts, I had long
ago determined that in a few months, I would need to leave my job at the
publishing house. "KhudLit" had become quite successful, and was very
different from where it was five years ago. But what irked me was that

*An equestrian statue of Peter the Great in
St. Petersburg; also the name of a narrative poem by A. Pushkin.
**This represents an original translation.

349

events unfolded according to the scenario that Boris Orlov once predicted so perceptively. He warned that if the publishing house ever recovered, I should then expect unpleasant developments. And here they are. I needed to consult with my friends on how to proceed. And who could be better advisors on such an issue concerning my destiny than Igor and Grigori Petrovich? We got together in the evening, and considered the situation as a whole.

– Yes, it really is the dark kingdom over there. There's not one ray of light. They just steal and lie, – Grigori Petrovich extrapolated from what we saw in the ministry. – You must leave, of course, but only on your own terms. When did you plan to give notice?

– In the middle of April. – Very good, – Grigori Petrovich concurred.

– That's spring. The snow will melt soon, the streams will flow, and once it gets a little warmer, the water will start to wash them away little by little. As for us, we will try to establish a new academy. I trust you have no objections? In any event, their leadership will fall apart no matter what.

– Still, but why are they exerting such powerful pressure, and seemingly out of nowhere? – I inquisitively dig for the root causes of what had transpired.

– There is an information and energy reconfiguration of space, – Grigori Petrovich explains. – They physical plane is their last pillar of support. This is a big source of strength. They have been working their selection here for centuries. Still, without being able to rely on the subtle matter plane, they will have a harder time working. But, first, far from all their people are aware of the global events that have taken place. If they were, you would have been surrounded on all sides by deserters by now. But how could you even work in their midst? They don't know how to create anything.

All they know is how to conspire and inform on others. And second, what else can they do if not that which they are so used to doing always? A habit is second nature. And it's not like everything is going so well with their first. You have to be patient. For the Dark ones, this is the last year when they can still seriously throw their weight around. What, you think they haven't put pressure on me?

But the bad pressure was not directed only at me. Irina Karysheva came to see us. The translation of the "song of the stone book" was going more or less well. She had translated the chapter on the birth of the goddess. Now she is translating the Samadhi –the code of conduct. Some very interesting parallels present themselves in these different divine stories. Kali's mother was born of the thoughts of seven fathers.

The proto Archon also created the prototype of man for Earth, the mother, with the help of seven Archon monarchs. But then, out of ignorance, he breathed the soul, or the force of life into man.

As a parallel to the Hindu epic, the theme of a battle between gods and man pervades the Apocrypha of Ancient Christians as well: "And they brought him (Adam) into the shadow of death, in order that they might form (him) again from earth and water and fire and the spirit which originates in matter, which is the ignorance of darkness and desire, and their counterfeit spirit. This is the tomb of the newly-formed body with which the robbers had clothed the man, the bond of forgetfulness; and he became a mortal man. This is the first one who came down and the first separation" (from the "Apocryphon of John", translated by Frederik Wisse).

In one form or another, the story of humanity's enslavement to the gods exists in every major world religion. And this is no coincidence. Our ever growing capacity to heal people, to foresee events that take place on the information plane, and even to influence them, is a testament precisely to this.

If humanity's potential will truly be fully realized, then no one will need technical progress in that dangerous form in which we see it developing now. Of course, no one will surrender his or her privileges without a fight. But it is unlikely that such a fight will lead to any positive outcomes for those who instigate it. Even Kali, who personifies death on the energy plane, has decided to reject her own terrifying hypostasis, has remembered her maternal functions, and is now dancing her dance of abdication, which is gradually morphing into a dance of love. There are changes afoot on the platform where she dances as well. People have appeared there who want to help the goddess. There are pregnant women and musicians playing a new rhythm for the divine dance, the rhythm of life, on their drums. Shiva, who awaits the changes along with his beloved, has approached the platform with the stone, but still cannot enter the circle of light.

Irina listens to the roar of the drums, takes note of the splashes of light illuminating the circle, commits to memory the jingling of the bracelets Kali wears on her wrists and feet. All of these rhythms assist her in her translation, and she is ready to spend every free minute on her beloved craft. But here is the problem: notwithstanding the fact that Irina is a world-class expert in her field and is not at all prone to conflicts, her boss has started to pick on her at work. She has no reason to be angry, but that is exactly what she is, and she takes her anger out on Irina for no reason at all. She is a strong, heavyset woman, and she yells, screams, and insults Irina over any trifling matter or just because. It did not use to be this way. Perhaps, she is doing someone else's bidding?

Someone is standing by the gates to the Heavenly Kingdom once again. Igor and I transport ourselves there immediately. Perhaps, our help will come in handy. We see the familiar figure of Thoth. But now he is wearing a different mask, that of the jackal. But why did he decide to switch masks? Does he think that this one will be more pleasing to the Creator? He came out of the dark plane, but a dark mantle is dragging behind him. This is Death. She somehow managed to get into Hell; having gathered her strength and taken stock of the situation, she passed directly through the wall. Afterward, she lowered herself onto the level of the Earth in the spot where the gods gathered by Olympus. Then she dragged herself again in the form of Thoth's mantle to the gates of the Kingdom of Heaven.

Back there, by Olympus, they did not tell the gods anything. After all, what was there to say? "Everything will be fine." Or something else of that sort?

We stand face to face, but Thoth is looking past us, at the gates. His patience is rewarded. The gates open, the Creator comes out, and stands opposite us.

– You see how everything turned out. It is the people who have described the true reality that exists. They have become closer to me, and I will bestow upon them My love. They now stand between Me and all of you. What do you expect from me? Now you must address your plea to them, since, as a matter of right, they have taken your place. Why make it harder on yourself and come directly to Me, when I have been so far from you for so long. I understand that you are so important, so great. Indeed, thrice greatest? One source of greatness is in goodness, another in evil, but where is the third? Is it in the absolute truth? You were not thrice greatest.

353

Thoth froze in painful concentration. He was in an absolutely hopeless situation. Everything is in keeping with the rules – both the battles and these changes. But how are you to accept change if for thousands of years you have been a god and suddenly you are no one?

– Go away. I have nothing to add, – the Creator says, and something fearsome pools within His pupils.

Thoth wishes to answer, but the dark mantle in which Death is hiding pulls him back. He attempts to struggle against it, his powerful muscles flexing with tension. His efforts are in vain. Death is dragging him away.

The Creator turns to us:

– Please record with extra care what I am saying and what is happening here.

He gestures with his hand towards Thoth, being dragged down by Death.

– He is Alpha and Omega? For whom? Who can approach both Beginning and End?

He tosses his staff from his right hand to his left and strikes the ground with it. Thunder and lightning immediately respond to the staff's call.

– What is the logical conclusion to the whole matter? It is building and creation. Arranging and imposing a structure on information provide great strength to aid in creation, strength that people have.

– Come with me, – the Father commands.

And we follow over the black velvet of the Cosmos.

– As for the main events, you can see eternity before you. I have permitted you to enter it. – We walked and walked. On the left and the right, we could take information, but we keep walking further, and there is less and less information. And what if we look back? We need something to push ourselves off of. There are events there, history, evolution, civiliza-

354

tion – so many things. Everything that has existed has a beginning and an end. But the future has no end. In the future, one can create and strengthen for eternity, to get closer faster to the real future. If, for example, the present positively connects with those events that are desirable, then, depending on the people and circumstances, the future comes closer. As it turns out, it is not that we are approaching the future, but that the future that is getting closer to us because we create with our will power elements of the world in this information space. And it opens for us any field of activity. We speak of controlling, which is indeed what we are doing now. We must control, and space will unfurl to come meet us. The more we create, the more we receive, and the more information we can connect between ourselves. Or, to be more precise, the more information we can receive. The more information you receive, the more you realize your desires and the greater volume of information you control. It turns out this way because, when you orient yourself away from Earth and into infinity, and you array events from the present forward, you end up controlling events.

You can build events in any situation when its future causes you some concern. You can move even closer to space and attain even greater powers because you are creating and getting rid of negative information. Space gives you harmony and freedom.

As to the second question – reading the book – you should look at this from the point (although it is not a point) where information spreads out onto all of space. You must understand that the information derived from this point is positive for the whole world, and for all people. I archive this information and give of it to all.

Why do I draw your attention to this? So that you can understand the meaning of the text, how this is given, and why it affects everyone without exception. The most important point is that it will be active for a

355

great period of time, which is to say for eternity. You must understand all these principles of the world in order to create more profoundly and more thoroughly.

For the duration of time that I was not opening the book, you must see, I created a particular archival point. It is very capacious, and that is clear from looking at it. Any person who has read the text of the book, who can put it next to him or herself will be cured of all diseases.

What does this stem from? It stems from the fact that you must create an archival point for the second book? How do you create it? In what point? How do you find the right point in space? How do you create it so that it is for everyone, for the whole world, for all the elements of the world, for all people? For people to know what they are pushing off of, what fundamental parameters they should use to build all this. And regardless of where you are and what you are doing, help must be provided. Such points in space do, of course, exist.

All is clear – where to get it, how to go? You can create a different space and a different world. You can create everything. You can also develop our Earth. It is better to encompass all this fully, from above.

The archival points of information have many layers. But how does one work with them? How do you access the information that is archived within then? It is easy to find the point. Moreover, we can create it ourselves. Indeed, we can do this closer in space to the events at issue than we could previously do. But again: focus on the principles of the work. Why does the plant grow? Quite simply because someone waters it. This is also a way of controlling events.

The archival point can be brought closer, can be created. But this is an element of the world. That's why the principle exists that if we do not understand something, we do not interfere with it. The same is true in

creation: if we do not know it, we do not do it. To create information a͟
to archive it is already an attainable goal. But it must be made manifest
in the unmanifested space. This, we have not yet observed. It is not being
manifested. Today, we can work here to create something there, and vice-
versa, work there to create something here. We have already reached this
stage. But why does it not manifest 100%? You have been given these
principles, but where are they?

You can't develop only in one direction, for example, by specializ-
ing in resurrection. You must treat, diagnose, and materialize as well. In
space, there are very many points of information, and space creates, but
we have moved forward and several points have appeared there. Imagine,
for instance, that there are eight, and they contain global information that
creates and gives direction to the entire universe, to all space.

Rays and channels must extend from the points into this space. But
how does this line go? You must know the principles. If we know the principles of how a cell is built, then we can successfully examine it now. But
what if you do not know the principles?

The cell is the most complicated part. It follows then that the cell
is correlated in complexity with these points in space. Focusing on the
nucleus of the cell, there too we can observe the plasticity of information.
Nucleus and space. I would put it this way: space is like the cell since there
are many points of information in it as well.

If we know how to work with the cell, we must work with space in an
analogous manner.

Here are the elements of the world. We have moved forward, forward,
forward, and here we have arrived at the most interesting part – controlling. But this must be in the phase of creation for the whole world, for all
people. Now, we must create that which we have studied.

357

We have already examined how the Sephiroth are connected with the levels. That linkage is clear. Now, the archival points have come into the picture. They too must necessarily be connected to the Sephiroth.

The levels of planetary consciousness are built on account of the Sephiroth. The Sephiroth were built because of the information on controlling the world and space. Space is built because of the elements of understanding the world. Everything is interdependent – one to one.

These points contain all the potential of the world. At any moment, the Sephiroth can call up the information within them and transfer it to the levels. Humanity has never gone further than the Sephiroth. Man does not know that this too is only a structure.

But every cell in the body is marked with the figure eight – the mark of infinity. How do we understand this eight? A cell can potentially multiply for an unspecified period of time – it contains the potential for thousands of years. That seems to be the case, but is it everything? There is another possibility: the information in the nucleus of the cell is archived in such a way that it connects two world planes – the manifested and the unmanifested ones. It is not for nothing that out of a single cell we can build a body, then bodies, then bodies enough to fill the entire planet, etc. But there can be a third point: the microscopic cell is the equivalent of the whole universe because the image of the Creator is imprinted on it. Ponder this subject for yourselves. The potential for infinity exists, and so it is better not to die. Those who have been resurrected and those with an expanded consciousness have been marked with the infinity sign.

The soul is also a principle of the endlessness of space.

An armchair appears next to Him, an armchair not a throne. The Father sits down.

– Come closer, – He commands sternly. – I will show you how to cre-

358

ate properly. It all begins with a single cell. Look. Here is just one cell. With the power of my thought I will create a flower from it. There is soil too, but the flower dies. Why? It's because it needs energy. I can provide that directly from my hand. I can take a pitcher and pour water onto the soil. Do you see how each cell of this plant comes to life?

Isn't treating people the same thing? Giving energy, watering, helping? If you look at where I will now place this flower, you will see an entire garden. I am like the gardener who likes flowers and who loves to tend to then. When there are many flowers, the result is a beautiful garden.

What am I telling you about? Is helping people not like this work in the garden? There are flowers with broken stems. I bandage up the flower, nurture it, and water it like all the others. What's not to understand about this? Consider it and you will understand everything quickly. I did not tell you anything complicated. I just wanted to show you my garden. It is so simple, and it is a miracle! But it is a miracle with an explanation.

There is no miracle for Me in this. Nor is there one for you because all of this can be explained. And there is nothing that you wouldn't be able to master. But what do we have? At times in life, you were moving very quickly and in some places you didn't notice someone or something. There are so many flowers, and you must be very sensitive to perceive which flower asks for help. If you have heard a voice calling you, you must stop and listen, then take the pitcher and water the flowers.

We take the pitcher and water those that have asked us for help. Now all the ailing flowers are indistinguishable from the healthy ones. And they express their gratitude to us. But who is thanking us? All the flowers ripple and thank us. We helped a few, but all are grateful. With this, our lesson ends. Go with God.

We express our thanks. The Creator stands up, and the armchair immediately disappears. He walks away, leaning on His staff.

* * *

The Ministry grew tired of waiting. I've been getting calls from them practically every day, with the staff of the Managing agency being the most persistent. This agency was created precisely to look for anything that isn't nailed down and to redistribute what they find to the benefit of the team that has arrived to take charge of printing, television, and book publishing. Since the staff of the Managing agency was purposefully comprised of people well-versed in pressure, blackmail, and all sorts of shady dealings, they – as specialists – were the ones tasked with cultivating at atmosphere of anxiety, instability, and hopelessness at "KhudLit". At first, they decided to limit themselves to small, preventive measures. The deputy for Shubin, general director of the Managing agency, called nearly every day on behalf of his boss with issues concerning rental space. The conversation always unfolded in roughly the same way:

– We need a space on the first floor of your building for a firm we are on friendly terms with, two hundred to three hundred square meters.

If any objections were voiced, the man's tone immediately changed. It filled with notes of indignation and barely concealed threats.

– This is not your building. The minister charged the Managing agency, and none other, with disposing of space for the industry's concerns. It seems that you don't understand who you are talking to, and what the consequences for you will be if you stand in the way of our plans. This request comes directly from Shubin. If you do not succeed at finding a common language with us, we will come over and sort the situation out ourselves.

– The first floor of our building houses a store, a cafeteria, and the distribution department. Where will all these things go?

– Move them to some other floor. And if you can't do it yourselves, we will come over for a visit and help you develop a reorganization plan.

From there, the agency's interest in the publishing house only expanded. They were interested in our vacation retreat in the Odintsovo district called the "Green town" – almost two and a half acres of land worth no less than a million dollars. It is an immutable law of nature that if you take something valuable from one person and sell it cheaply to someone else, you always have the opportunity to earn enough in the transaction for a villa and a Mercedes. What's more, there will be no traces of any crime. You don't need to break into a safe. The interested parties will bring everything to you in a case and will keep quiet. What would they talk for? So that they, in turn, could be questioned about where they found what they so carefully stashed in the case?

Even in the most difficult years, no one from the publishing house's administration gave in to the temptations that arose again and again around the "Green town". They all thought that the tough times could last for a long time, perhaps a very long time, but not forever. And at some point, the organization will once again have enough energy to develop the retreat and to put into effect the longtime plans for its reconstruction. We wanted to return to the literary Olympus with everything that had for many decades already been the history of "KhudLit". We had regularly hosted great writers and famous artists at this retreat. It was part of our fame and our history. How could we turn our backs on this? How could we sell it off?

Faxes began to arrive from the Ministry, describing in great detail how we were to effect the transfer of the "Green town" to the Managing agency, and to whose name we should address the letters requesting that our fame and our past be expropriated from us.

– What do you even care? – Shubin's staff members yelled on the phone. – You are practically not even the director anymore.

I did care, and the pressure mounted.

How strange are our bureaucrats, or should I say the public servants we have hired for the benefit of the Motherland – the servants of the people, to put it in Soviet terms.

Unwittingly, I remember the textbook aphorisms of Po Chü-i, a Chinese satirical poet from the 9th century:

"In the old days, they killed a man and were angry; today they kill a man and laugh.

In the old days, they appointed bureaucrats to disperse the thieves; today they appoint bureaucrats to steal.

In the old days, he who ruled over people took upon his own shoulders the whole world, and the people mourned for him; today, those who rule over people are perched on top of the whole world, and the people mourn for it."

Persecution, persecution, persecution... What can I say? These are also life lessons, albeit unpleasant ones. Patience, patience, patience... We can't begin to act like these people or to learn from them how to solve our problems with lies, aggression, and force. At times, Igor and I lost it, wanted to get back at them without reservation, using our newfound capabilities: an eye for an eye, a tooth for a tooth! But at the very last second, we always stopped. That was precisely what they were expecting from us. In time, we remembered the Father's words: "How do you get into the Heavenly Kingdom? Only by means of the soul. And so they are fighting for human souls. They wanted to get into heaven in the protective guise of a human being. But you didn't let them through. And now they are raging out of fear. They want eternal life, but how do you get it? Their days on

362

Earth will be over before they know it, and no one has promised them any other days."

* * *

For the third time, Thoth has appeared by the gates leading to the Father's Kingdom. Igor and I immediately reentered the subtle matter plane and stood facing him, blocking the path. Thoth did not ever stir. It seemed he had more important things to deal with and other problems to tend to. He was once again in the mast of the jackal. But Death was no longer with him. She remained by Olympus, also waiting. Even from a distance, we could read her thoughts. They were much like a person's thoughts: how do we live and what do we do?

Death has undergone new transformations, and they are not for the better. She has now lost the outer shell of her skin, and only her skeleton remains. To cover up this shame, she has thrown the black cape with the hood over herself. The scythe is missing for some reason – either she is so weak that she does not want to carry around any extra weight, or someone has taken it from her for their own needs. She is one of the gods and even has a seat on their supreme council. There are only two women on the council, and Death is one of them.

The gods await the decision of the Creator. Death waits next to them. For the first time, she is not within their control, and they glance at her askance, fearfully. For one thing, her ugly skinless skull is unpleasant to behold. But they also understand that this skeleton-like machine of destruction could turn against them too, for gods deprived of their immortality have become like people.

Many of the gods, those with more foresight, divined even sooner how everything could end up and left Olympus. They went by way of birth, like regular people, so that at the end of their days, they could meet with the Creator, and depending on their deeds, earn either forgiveness or oblivion.

Everyone had traded places – the gods became like people, and the people like gods. Well, this is not only a gift but also a lesson that the situation can at any second reverse by 180 degrees, if we, human beings, turn out to be unworthy of the great gift of the Creator.

When the Creator was talking about flowers yesterday, this was not just an allegory. It was technology that He was imparting to us. He was showing us how it is possible, by transporting a large of objects onto the subtle matter plane, to replace the procedures of the physical process with consciousness, the soul, and the spirit. It is easy to hear the slightest vibration of an ailing plant on the subtle matter plane. This allowed us to address the situation with all the flowers right away and to find out precisely what was happening to them, and, significantly, not just to some of their separate parts – stems, leaves, buds – but to each cell of the entire organism. In essence, we were shown the system according to which all connections were organized – the physical space, the space of perception, the space of cognition – and how it was possible, in working with any objects in the world, to change them with the local phenomenon of a human being.

The Father spoke of the system, and he watered the flowers not just in any way, but systematically. After this the flowers of the subtle matter world came back and blended into the other flowers. And how can we now distinguish them from one another?

In this one picture, there are so many motifs – diagnostics, synthesis, decision, controlling the information of an event and the instrument of control. In other words, the consciousness, the soul, and the spirit of a person are capable of instantaneously harmonizing an object in need. Moreover, this is the practice of controlling reality, and not just some experiments with unknown endings – maybe it will work, maybe it won't, how will it turn out for us?

When the Creator waters the flowers, He shows us how He creates the sphere of information, then the matter, then from the matter the cell with which He reenergizes the area that is in need. He can create an entire organism from the cell – a flower that has the ability constantly to develop and divide, in other words, the capacity for self-realization and self-development. A flower has the capacity for processes of exchange both within itself and with the outside world; it has the ability to adjust to different weather conditions – wind and rain. It is supposed to live peacefully for a certain period of time, and it will live out that time peacefully. But if something happens to it again, this time we too – Igor, Grigori Petrovich, and I – can help. We can reenergize the injured organ or even resurrect it to new life and make the flower immortal. The Creator gave us the necessary technology, gave us the right, and marked it by striking the ground with His staff, which immediately led to a change in spatial information correlating to His decision.

There are times when the consciousness of the flower is afraid of what is happening. In those instances, the Creator takes it in His hand, calmly listens and explains things in a way that will not shock the easily frightened flower, so that it too can calmly grasp the situation and not fear new life changes.

As for Thoth, he continues to stand there; he does not leave. He has turned his side to us, and a shadow has fallen over his face. This is a very significant circumstance, related to the prophecy from the tomb. The third inscription of the prophecy falls like the shadow of the first, a shadow on the stone. Half of the god's face has now been obscured in darkness. Or, to

365

be more precise, it isn't his face but his mask. His mask, by the way, has also changed. It is once again the head of an ibis with a long and curving back, just like the first time.

We sense his mood and his thoughts. He did not want to switch masks. He can remain forever in this mask. It was in this mask that he once began his path of ascent. Now he has the same face in two planes – the Dark and the Light. He no longer has two faces, two bodies, two options: to be simultaneously both here and there. Instead of the second mask, there is a shadow – the premonition of death. Behind it is the night. Night equals darkness. Neither people nor things are visible in darkness. Secret things happen in the dark – something can be born, something can die. The boundary that divides birth from life hides within it. Who can remain on it without help, without support? Who will extend the hand of assistance? Death saw what was happening by Olympus. She gathered her remaining strength and ascended to the top. She wants to give her hand to the one she followed for thousands of years in a row. She loves Thoth and trusts him. But will Thoth rely on Death's hand? And where will she lead him?

The boundary is thin, colorless, transparent, and it leads to Olympus. But will he be able to complete the journey, without having asked the Father for forgiveness?

The boundary falls to the earth from Olympus and divides it into parts – the one where Death can still remain for some time, and the one in which her rights have been extinguished, where the time of continuing life and resurrection is arriving.

What hand does Hermes, twice greatest – in good and evil – extend to his loyal partner: the right or the left? Much will depend on which hand he gives her and from which side she will lead him along the boundary. He can give his hand from the side of the Dark forces, or he can do the opposite. But Olympus, to which Hermes is after all connected by some feelings and ties, is, despite its betrayal of people, on the side of the Light forces. And he, after some hesitation, still gives Death his hand from the side of the dark plane. And Death leads him along the thin razor of the absolute truth. She leads the one who once came from Atlantis to Egypt and became its king, who then seized the reigns of Olympus, and who did both bad and good and always sought to maintain harmony between his two hypostases of good and evil. But now he is standing on the boundary of the absolute truth, and he cannot find another, named Life, to support him on this dangerous line. The scales of life on which he so often dispassionately weighed the good and bad deeds of people are this time weighing him. And the dark side turned out to be the weightier.

But even in parting, Hermes remembered something from his great past. When the boundary had led him to Olympus, he took several steps downward to bring Death to the lower levels where she did not want to go. Death resisted, and as he practically dragged her by force, he lost his balance, and the boundary consumed him. From these levels, there is nowhere to go but the Abyss. And what is Death to do there – eat her own? Things turned out very badly for her indeed, and she had no one to complain to. It was empty down below – no Lucifer, whose image had been invoked for so long to frighten people, no Satan, no devil, all of whom were one and the same but with different names. What was she to do now? She had no strength, and no one to eat to improve her health.

Yet in the end, on the boundary of the absolute truth, Thoth did something that redeemed many of his unseemly deeds. If he had given Death his other hand, the magnetic fields of the Earth would have changed. Many people would have perished, and Olympus would have as well, since the gods were no longer protected by immortality. Perhaps that is why the

Creator gave Thoth one more chance. We could see how a grey pigeon, not white, nor black, fluttered up from the boundary that had consumed the god. It is not for nothing that the last of Thoth's masks was the bird mask. But the bird is a celestial creature, which means that there is still some opportunity, after passing through the coils of the evolutionary spiral, to ascend to the apex of life.

Three days later, we heard an announcement on the television in the evening. The commercial ship "Mercury's Memory", which was sailing from Turkey to Eupatoria, suddenly sank. Without any external cause whatsoever, it capsized and nine minutes later sank to the bottom. These events coincided with those that had occurred in the information space. No one had heard any SOS signal.

A raft with several surviving sailors was found completely by accident. None of them could explain what had occurred. Was it a coincidence? But they say that a coincidence is just another name for God. And more than that: Mercury, Hermes, Thoth – these are all names for the very same persona. Also a coincidence? And the nine minutes it took for the vessel to sink, another coincidence? The nine destroyed Mercury, who is also Hermes and Thoth.

* * *

Up above, at the Beginning of Beginnings, all the chief members of the Light powers were assembled. There were thousands of them: archangels, saints, the legion of Jesus Christ, the eagle and the lion. The three of us – Grigori Petrovich, Igor and I. The Father stands with His staff in his right hand. The throne is behind him. We have been placed to His right and closer to Him than anyone, although compared to others in stature, we were still quite small.

The Creator was very pensive. He was waiting for something, some very important moment that only He was aware of. We have been standing like this for a long time, for almost an entire day. The Father said: "Everyone must abandon what they are doing and be here next to me. There is nothing more important than that, which is about to transpire."

Everyone is looking at each other but waiting calmly and patiently. Our closeness to the Creator also does not appear to surprise anyone. From here, the Beginning of Beginnings, I see my second hypostasis by the Abyss. The man with the book under his arm is still standing next to the opening in the center, which is now closed off with a heavy lid. The evil spirits are no longer flying. All have been sent to Purgatory, and no one has broken through to the Beginning of Beginnings. Death has receded into the Abyss. When I was about to strike up a conversation, Igor pulled me back in time.

– Be quiet. You will start talking to her, but here's her way of thinking: "Aha, you are interested in me. That means I can somehow use this to my advantage."

I remained silent and saw her off to the Abyss with my gaze. Where else is she supposed to go if not back to her own?

On Olympus, the scene did not at all correspond to the situation. The gods had gathered in the valley. They were sitting on their thrones, chairs, and benches. Some were walking in pairs; others were relaxing on padded stools or basking in the comfort of pillows. There were waiting for some great happiness.

They should have scaled the mountain and looked – here is the earth, here are people, here is life. They should have thought to themselves: "What are we doing here?" But no, they were lying around and relaxing.

369

Finally, whatever signal the Father was waiting for had arrived, and He began to speak:

– All the chief members of the hierarchy can help people directly. There are no longer any intermediaries. You are permitted to exert a benevolent influence directly on segments of the soul.

For three days, He gave instructions about precisely who should do what. He proclaimed that the information structure of space will be recoded and reoriented only for positive interaction. Later, this recoding will spread to other planes.

Then, he lets everyone go and addresses us.

– The people do not stop to think about the fact that the sequence of events was not built upon the Earth. They do not even know what an event sequence and infinity mean. That is why they live so briefly and in such an unsettled way, and their soul undergoes pain and sorrow. People search for oil. They obtain gas. They are hypnotized with the word "progress". But perhaps one should study the soul and oneself? When the first rocket left the Earth for the Cosmos, everyone rejoiced. But now, they have stopped celebrating, for the ozone layer is disappearing. Your primary goal is to transform the negative into the positive.

We walk next to the Father and listen carefully to what He is saying. His words are so simple. He absolutely does not try to embellish the figures of His speech in any way. But it is as though what He says reveals the very essence of the problem. We approach the garden. The Father glances over the flowers:

– You have treated them correctly, and the results you have achieved are weightier than ever. I permit you to write and speak about this. The time has come. But not everyone will hear what I am telling them through you. Situations can be different, and everything can be interpreted in different ways. You will encounter such people, but pay no heed. Remember, you are helping people move towards the enlightenment of their consciousness. And now that no matter what happens, no matter how events unfold, I always know how they are going. No one will be able interfere. No one will be able stop what has begun.

He smiles. He is content, although the last few days have been full of pressure.

The gods were very afraid of losing power. Thoth used their fear, and invented magic. At times, he so fully lost his dignity that he made his way to the Beginning of Beginnings and eavesdropped on My words. That is how he learned the words of resurrection. And the gods believed that he was the pinnacle of the divine. So that no one would make an attempt on his power, he made Death his ally. After this, he began to select his outward images. He could have selected the image of the lion or the eagle, but he chose the images of the jackal and the ibis. The ibis is like your crow. He pronounced himself the boundary between life and death – he judged, he weighed on the balance human deeds, and he rendered the sentences. But his primary goal was to give birth to god-man. Only if he had succeeded, he would have given birth only to man-god, exactly like himself, and this is the polar opposite of god-man. The first god-man, of course, was My Son, Jesus Christ.

And here, I remembered the boy Kirill, who spoke incessantly about the last-last in his lineage, and that he was prepared to destroy all humanity for his unborn son. But who was hiding beneath the mask of the infant and circling nearby?

– Nature helped them at first, – the Father uttered. – Original sin implies birth without a Father. And since it was without the Father, it means that the newborn did not have a soul. Not everyone who now has the image of a person has a soul. Examine carefully. They have created a likeness, but the qualities and properties of a soul are unbreakable. First and foremost, look to see whether the person has a soul.

He stopped, and so did we. The Father looks at me.

– Arkady wants to get to Olympus faster, to talk to the gods. He needs this for his book, and he probably thinks that he will hear more there than I am telling him now.

The Father is not chiding me. He is telling me this, knowing ahead of time that I will not be very satisfied with my mission.

– Well, well, I also have much to do. Go with God, as I am always with you.

He turned around and left.

We looked at each other. It turned out so awkwardly. Why did I start thinking about Olympus?

–Alright, to Olympus? – Igor asks, but I can hear the accusatory note in his voice.

Grigori Petrovich does not agree. He says he has too much work to do, and he also disappears. How did he ever learn how to do that? In the blink of an eye, he is gone.

Now, it is just the two of us. Igor has assumed a position of neutrality with respect to this poorly timed problem of visiting Olympus, but I am very concerned about the psychological aspect of what is happening. I am tasked with describing events, so that they are no lost in the past. Something from within is leading me into a strange world that we know from myths and legends and that has turned out to be both so similar to and so unlike them. And there is something else that I cannot fully comprehend yet, some feeling from long ago that has hidden itself in the depths of my memory that I was at some point involved in this world disappearing into nothingness.

The feeling was very indefinite, comprised of some shards of reality that my consciousness simply could not assemble into a single whole. Something was surfacing from oblivion – one moment a face, the next a fleeting scene. Then, it all settled down once again in the darkness of ignorance.

For some reason, I could see most clearly three beautiful women in ancient Greek garb and three small children about their own business – puttering, playing with toys, chasing one another. It seemed to me that I was also part of their group. One of these children – chubby, curly-haired, with a small child's bow in his hand was particularly friendly with me. The second one did not like to play for long. He sequestered himself with books and studied. And sometimes he came and tried to give some book to me. (The books were, for some reason, contemporary in style and not the scrolls of antiquity.) But one of the women deftly intercepted his attempts. Each time, she shielded me with her body and said that I was still young and would have time yet to pore over the books. It is now as I am writing that everything has come together into a more or less coherent image. At that time, when Igor and I were preparing to descend to Olympus, it was more like the fragments of recollections than an integrated plot.

When we descended to the second information level of the Earth, where, under the dome, the society of ancient gods had for so long isolated itself from its preordained duties and responsibilities and been shielded from life's turmoil and unwelcome energy influences, the first thing that came into my mind was Tolstoy's famous phrase: "The Oblonsky home was in turmoil."*

Less than half of the gods remained on Olympus, and they no longer looked quite so carefree. The gates were wide open, and one group of gods after another, having made its choice between oblivion and reincarnation passes through them. Those who have decided to "go among the people" enter through the gates (it appears that yet another one of our classics prophesied looking up at the Heavens).** They know that if their last reincarnation is successful and they are able to overcome the tests of karmic programs, their reward will be eternal life and positive creation.

Another group of gods, and a fairly sizeable one at that, is frozen in hesitation over Olympus. They do not want to go to the Earth because they have been the source of much evil there, and are afraid that they will not be able to surmount the karmic programs. Their situation is a terrible one. Events are unfolding rapidly. Uncertainty of the final decision is also a sentence. We see how a quiet but powerful centrifugal current begins to pick up the gods. They feel the heavenly current at work, and a panic sets in. It is strange to see such famous gods, personifying for the most part the functions of war, fear, arbitration, in this condition. They can no longer catch up with the positive information currents. They are being carried in the direction away from Earth, into the open Cosmos, where more likely than not, they will finally dissolve into the fabric of nothingness. This is, in essence, preordained. After all, they do not know how to create anything. Their functions are destruction, betrayal, indulgence in temptations and weaknesses. These are far from the habits you need when you are called upon to create your own world out of nothing.

The remaining gods, seeing what is going on before their very eyes,

* From Lev Tolstoy's "Anna Karenina", used idiomatically to symbolize chaos and confusion.
**Ironic reference to Maxim Gorky's "In the World".

become more entrenched in their decision to descend to Earth. No one is forcing them to do anything, but this is not an easy choice. After all, life on Earth, as it exists, is the one they have created. And it is very far from what they would have wanted for themselves. Now, they needed to try to live like people, but it was clear from everything that they did not feel like it. Of course, things are better in the Valley of the gods. One can engage in pleasant conversation, flirt with nymphs and naiads, lap one's ambrosia and enjoy the sight of people struggling down below.

The insular information system of the ancient gods was crumbling before our very eyes. Another group that has been carried away by the cosmic wind has wholly disappeared from view. Many others left even earlier. The palaces, parks, and temples of the Valley of the gods are emptying out before our eyes. We can read the thoughts of those who are leaving. The god of fertility is making plans to create plenty. He has a lot of thoughts on the topic – he just never got around to business before. But now he wants to fix everything, all at once, in one earthly incarnation. Would he ever be a great minister of agriculture!

The god of arbitration is thinking about how to resolve problems between adversaries. He is in a very constructive mood now, but the Supreme Court has been trying to get him since the days when Gorbachev was in power. One of the Oceanids is very concerned with ecology and the loss of vessels in the ocean. For whatever reason, she is particularly preoccupied with the fate of commercial ships. Military flotillas do not concern her at all, and perhaps that is how it should be.

It looks like everyone who is returning to Earth is in a constructive mood.

Good luck to the new recruits! Just don't trip on the Russian army custom of new boy bullying.

The goddess of astrology stopped, facing us. She is a very beautiful woman with kind eyes.

– I was the one who created the gates to Olympus and the signs of the zodiac on them, – she ventured. – But Hermes erected the wall. I thought that people would come to us, but no one has. Hermes deceived me and the other gods. These gates can be created only by a man. Hermes possesses the secret power to switch the male and female foundations, and so he gave me a male name and a male hypostasis. But I am a woman. Everyone believed that a man had created the gates. They walked up to them, put their hands on the signs of the zodiac, but no one could leave. That is because I had both a male and female foundation within me at the same time. No one guessed that they needed simultaneously to place a male palm on one leaf of the gate and a female palm on the other. Only those gods who fell in love with one another and decided to escape the rule of Hermes succeeded in leaving the Valley of the gods because they pushed the leaves of the gates together. We do not know what happened to those who left us. Hermes told us terrible stories about these escapees, and it is very difficult to discern them in the guise of humans. Our gratitude goes out to you for showing us the true path. Our knowledge will help people.

Igor and I make eye contact. That is precisely how we entered the gates of Olympus during our last expedition, by pushing the two leaves of the gates simultaneously.

And one more similar thought: why do they consider us fomenters of the heavenly revolution? We ourselves, this whole world and all the events in it are possible thanks only to one – the Triune, Who created the Universe and will not allow His creation to be willfully distorted by irresponsible co-creators.

We wish the goddess luck and say goodbye to her.

The Egyptian god who created the secret room between the pyramids of Heops and Hefren where we read the prophecy approaches us.

– It was I who made the room invisible to all the capabilities of the twentieth century, – he said. – Hermes endowed it with two powers and walked out into the world as a man and a woman. His prophecy is a pledge to the Primordial One. Everything in exchange for everything. Thanks to this, he obtained a second power – Night, the hypostasis of Death. This is a great strength and power. Even the Sun has a shadow that Hermes could now dispose of, but only until such time as the three in one and one in three would arrive. He wanted power more than he wanted immortality. He could have won everything, but instead he lost everything. Be careful in your wishes. Now it is within your power to have anything you wish for.

Another god approached us and immediately struck up a conversation:

– I saw that men were given of the female essence, and women of the male essence. This was all changed on Olympus and was fortified with fear and death. Women were weighted down with fear, men – with death. Then, they were united in a single whole with love. But is it necessary for the horror of nothingness to be the fruit of love?

The gods are leaving Olympus. They are descending to the Earth, and now, as you are reading this book, many of them are already among you. You can recognize them by their eyes, knowledge, talents, and abilities. They want to help us and themselves as well.

Now, a large group of gods passes by us. They are carrying an ancient sage, dressed like a Tibetan monk, on a litter. One of them stops next to us, and gesturing towards the procession with his hand, says:

– He is the wisest of them all, and many ask for his advice. What he says is very important, but not everyone can understand it.

One more goddess decided to say something. She looks like a Roman deity. On her head, she wears a high hat. Her earlobes are adorned with earrings bright as the sun. Her sleeves have triangular slits. The goddess appears very emotional and pathetic. She just needs to air out her feelings to someone:

– Before we were capable of reincarnation and often found ourselves among people. But that was not for long, and now we must live in human bodies our whole lives –in ordinary earthly bodies. This is so difficult. But we are descending to the earth to understand man's essence, and we are going to try to be useful to you.

The very ancient god stops next to us. He is patiently waiting for us to finish our rendezvous with the goddess. As she steps away, the sage sighs heavily and begins:

– I was the one who built the first pyramids on earth. They are like an accumulator of energy. With the help of the pyramids, one can obtain predictions of future events, move stone plates and towers, and influence the world around. With the help of the pyramids, people could obtain great knowledge, and this was not to the liking of all the kings and gods. That is why they ensured that no one would be able to use the capabilities of cosmic technologies. Secret knowledge opens up during the solstice. The perspective of the Sun stores a great deal of information, if you look at the Valley of the Kings from above. That is where energy words appear, although they can only be read when the axes of the pyramids coincide with the cosmic text. Only the initiated can find the necessary perspective and sightline to read the solar missive that appears only briefly and quickly dissolves.

You can also use the pyramids to unravel electromagnetic forces and to control their signs. That is how you can create a strong wave and wind on the sea. Jesus Christ had the greatest energy under his control – he could part waters and walk through them, as though through a tunnel. I do not have that kind of power. I can only create waves, whirlwinds, and tornadoes. After all, this is nothing more than a big funnel of air. You can use the tornado to clear sand in the desert, to move soil and water onto the clearing you have prepared, and to create an oasis. This could come in quite handy for people. They do not want chaos. They seek harmony and beauty.

He sighed, and turned to go away, but then turned back towards us once again.

– Ah yes, that sage they carried away on the litter, you could have asked him about something important. It's a shame you didn't.

Igor and I glanced at each other. We grasped that we had missed some opportunity, but perhaps it was not yet too late to fix it? We gave chase, and it did not take long. The sage on the litter, and the gods around him were waiting for us close to the gates.

– I knew that you would want to ask me about something, – the sage began, anticipating our questions, and little rays of wrinkles in the corner his eyes betrayed the internal mirth he could barely conceal.

– I am a sage, and I have mastered the art of wisdom. That is why I do not speak in a way that will allow everyone to understand me. I do not know if you will understand. The sage you were just speaking to is the most ancient. You, however, existed before him.

The first thing that will be is a dream. What can be better than the one who is the closest to Him, and who holds the book that contains the absolute truth? What can be better than the absolute truth? After all, he stands by the chasm, but he did not fear it, on his way to Him.

The second is also a dream. When a little boy was seven years old, there were 24 sages on the upper platform, and the boy was climbing a big mountain. But there are no such mountains on Earth, even on platforms. He lost his grip and fell, but he did not die, and he started climbing again. Again, he saw the summit, and again he lost his grip.

Now, he climbed up a third time and he met the one with whom he is speaking now. He listened, but he did not hear everything. But who can be higher than him? No one. And, you know, the answer to the third question is also very simple: I waited for you and I fulfilled my mission.

We bow before him and say some words of gratitude. His litter is lifted and carried away, but the sage turns and yells to us:

– He, Who is higher than all others and greater than all others, He who taught you everything, – I give myself to Him completely, I trust Him implicitly – this child, who is more ancient than all others.

We think we have solved the riddle, and we glance at each other. I give voice to the opinion we both share.

– We got five answers to three questions. But did we understand everything correctly?

– I remember that dream about the mountain. I have had that dream my whole life, – Igor says suddenly. – I climbed for an entire day and fell off. The second day, I climbed and saw him, but then fell again. The wind was too strong. The third day, I climbed, and did not get spooked. I came up to the Father, and the Father said something. I listened to him carefully, but did not hear everything.

– And I remember about the Abyss, – I echo the words of my friend. – This Abyss is both madness and the absolute truth. I was walking towards the Father along the boundary of madness and absolute truth, and I did not even understand that I could fall from it.

– Where shall we direct our eyes and our quest from now on? – Igor asks. He always cedes to me when it comes to making decisions. It is as though he himself is only agreeing. That is why I have recently started to make sure that he is participating in collaborative decisions.

– Where do you want to go?

– Whatever you say, – my partner tries to evade the circle of responsibility.

– Who knows where I will say to go? Let's decide together.

– I would look at the pyramids, – Igor gives in.

– Let's look, – I agree.

– We are transported to the pyramids, and we figure out the time based on the position of the sun. We search for the spot where the text imparted by the Sun's code is not merely a game of shadows. Above the pyramids, at the intersection of their axes, golden letters come into view. But they go in completely different directions, – left to right and right to left. It is impossible to read them. We are discouraged once again, and we no longer feel nearly as important as we did half an hour ago. And on top of that, the letters are appearing and disappearing very quickly.

The Creator appears next to us, leaning on His staff. He looks at us searchingly.

– You can see, He says. – In this book, there is one space and then another. How do you read it then?

We are silent. Nothing brings enlightenment to our heads.

– You are going in the right direction thinking about heads,– the Father picks up on our thoughts. – There are likewise two spaces in the head – the left hemisphere and the right hemisphere.

He looks at us expectantly once again, hoping that we will finally grasp such a simple concept in the art of decoding.

We do not give up and remain obstinate in our ignorance.

– You do not have time to read the letters? You should try moving the way the sun moves, with the same speed, and even a little faster so that you can get ahead of events. Start together with the sun, but be a little more nimble. This is the first thing.

The Father is waiting again, looking searchingly into our faces.

– The letters are running off in different directions, – I complain.

– Those who wrote the letters in different directions wrote only one letter each and could not know what is written here. No one has yet read this text. You will be the first, not counting Me. There is a heavenly prophecy contained here, and it has more than one meaning. It has several meanings, and you must understand everything. So, where is your decoding device?

– In our heads, – I am trying to guess rather than actually guessing.

Igor immediately picks up the same idea more successfully:

– When we look at the letters, we must transform the energy in the left and right hemispheres and concentrate it in the area of the third eye.

– Yes, – the Father agrees. – If you read our scripts using a certain technology, you will find a completely different meaning and answers like those of the sage. Everything begins with a point. A cell is created out of a point, matter is created out of a point, and the Bible is created out of a point. Read your text.

We find the point and begin to move around the pyramids at a speed somewhat greater than the sun's. Under the control of some internal impulse, the energy of our brains' hemispheres builds from the glowing strands a strange stencil. As the text is caught in its compartments, it gains meaning: "Three in one and one in three will come to the Earth, and the mercy of the Heavenly Father will descend upon the earth. And people will gain the power to build and to create, and the people will grow closer to the Father and will understand the Father. But the people will have many intermediaries who will attempt to close the visage of the Heavenly Father with the hands and to instill fear, so that everything would become

382

afraid of the Father's visage.

Those people who will attain the heavenly prophecy...

We lost the running line once again, having failed to maintain the necessary speed.

You can change the stencils, preloaded in your consciousness, – the Creator hints.

We now understand what He is talking about, and we begin to read anew. These are the prophecies:

Year 2001. A dark spot will darken the north of Russia, and everyone will be sorry that it had happened.

Year 2002. A great flame will appear amongst the people of Europe that they themselves had stoked. This is not a fire, but it will burn everything around it.

Year 2003. Those who are on the left and who take pride in their power will create a technology that will terrify the world. The technology will assume a power of its own, and the isles may be flooded. Those who created weapons scanning the information space and changing the vectors of time will not be able to encompass their creation within their consciousness, and it will began to threaten its own creators.

Year 2004. Two countries with large populations will be so unhappy with one another that only a tiny straw of prudence will buoy them up on the surface of an ocean of troubles.

Year 2005. A people who share one skin color and live on one continent will gather such forces and such an army as no one had previously assembled until that time.

Year 2006. There will be a war between two peoples that will grow into a war among three. And those who will be on the left and the right will march against the one in the middle. But the war will stop to give the people peace. America and Russia will stand up for one small country in the South.

There will be great disturbances among the people as a result of war. The one in the middle will be unable to withstand the people. The one on the left will not know what to do with the people. The one on the right will die.

– Now do you understand how you can read these texts? – the Father asks.

– Yes, we do, – we nod our heads in unison.

Finally, the Father smiles. He is pleased.

– There is one more factor that you need to take into account. Those who read this text and look from Heaven to the Earth can change the course of events. But you must not forget the word responsibility.

* * *

The tabloids, which, between scandals and describing the private lives of "stars" of different calibers, also write about astrologists and other predictors of the future, contain frequent reproaches against these figures as well. They promised something, the critique goes, but it didn't happen. Their science thinks highly of itself, but it is far from perfect!

There is, of course, no shortage of charlatans, but I am speaking about real, genuine predictors. There are not many of them – you can count them on your fingers – and their visions are true. Their problem (if it can be called a problem) is that they do not make any correction for the existence of clairvoyants who are capable of changing the course of events and who frequently prevent disasters. In the book "Save Yourself", I provided facts about the number of accidents that Grabovoi prevented, all of which are documented. It may be that someone predicted these impending accidents and informed of them publicly. But the events did not happen thanks to the intervention of another power that the predictor did not take into account. In other words, it was business as usual.

Some people suggest that nothing would be simpler than having all the experts in the subtle matter world unite. Why not have the masters of extrasensory work and other esotericism consult with one another about impending events, reach a common opinion, and undertake collaborative actions to permit or to change the course of likely events, and then everything will be, as they say, tip-top. That would be great, but it won't happen, at least not in the foreseeable future.

Not all of these magicians represent Light forces. There are still many who are with Lapshin, which means that agreement is impossible.

Imagine that we have segmented off the Dark ones. (Although who would be competent to do so? A more powerful clairvoyant, whatever his stripe will always be able to conceal his true nature from a weaker one.) The remaining ones are so different in their worldviews and paradigms, their technologies, their proclivities, that it is very unlikely that they could find a common terminology and language. They say that two masters will always find common ground in their craft but never in their art. But in this case, it is extraordinarily difficult to find agreement in the craft as well.

And now we come to the so-called "human factor". All of these "chosen ones of fortune" are also people, meaning that they are conceited and vain. In this enclave, too many will hog the covers for themselves, purportedly "in the interest of mankind". Each will consider his opinion and the action he recommends the only correct one. In such cases in civic organizations, the final word belongs to the chairman, the president, etc. It is interesting to think who will elect or appoint this person and according to what criteria? The Lord God? He does not become involved in vain human affairs.

Truth be told, all human organizations, societies, and institutions have a fairly low proportion of useful activity. This is true even of the Church, which calls itself the "daughter of Christ". But we want for the predictions of the future to be one hundred percent accurate. I suspect that the one-off predictions taken in their totality provide more truthful information than we would get out of a "collective mind".

So what is the trusting reader supposed to do? Insofar as possible given whatever limited capacities, he should influence events. Why did the Creator give him freedom? One can wring one's hands and run around the gossip-houses and the smoking rooms, enthusiastically spreading the word about some future misfortune. That is enjoyable, to be sure. As the satirist Ludwig Ashkenazi believed: "Everyone wants for something to happen already and also fears that something might happen." You haven't noticed a certain sweet satisfaction within yourself upon learning of some catastrophe? You thoroughly conceal this petty feeling, but it is there nonetheless, right? Instead, you could resist the impending negative event with all your soul and extinguish it at least on the information plane.

That is how collective consciousness is formed, and whether a given event will occur or not depends on it.

Chapter 6

The process of resurrecting the daughter of Galina Borisovna Kuznetzova, it seems, is gaining momentum. She is carefully noting what is happening to her, her relatives and people close to her, as well as unusual events. When one reads the things she writes it creates a feeling that a ray of magic light has pierced the everyday gray, poverty-stricken, dirty life:

"April 13, 2001. My older daughter Olga and I went to Bogdanovshchina village in Smolensk Region, where we have a house and where Aleksandra is buried, to clean the grave after the winter and to visit our native places.

April 14, 2001. In the morning, we were going to visit the cemetery. I set out a little earlier. Suddenly, I heard my older daughter cry out: "Mom, come here - am I going crazy?!" She showed me an alarm clock on which the hands were moving backwards. She said: "I feel scary, this creepy, maybe something happened to Aleksandra!"

And I felt some sort of excitement, even joy: with all my being I felt - this is our Sashka*! She is feeling mischievous and playful!

I told Olga about resurrection, told her how to behave, how to treat this with understanding. We left the alarm clock alone. We observed over the course of two days: it precisely counted the time backwards.

April 16, 2001. Our departure for Moscow was scheduled for 9:00 a.m.. After waking up, Olga called me into her bedroom and showed me the alarm clock. It was working properly, as if it had not been going backwards for two days.

* Sasha and Sashka are diminutive forms of Aleksandra (or Alexandra).

387

We looked at each other; there was nothing to say.

At night I had a dream. I clearly saw a road leading to the village from the cemetery. The cemetery itself was not there – it had disappeared. The road was empty, it was early morning. It was cool from the dew that was sparkling in multicolored drops in the rays of gently warm sun. The birds are chirping! And Sashka was walking at a flying gait, smiling, turning her face to the sun and squinting her eyes. She was even wishing that there be no one in the street.

Here she is, walking towards the house already through the village; she passed by the kindergarten and the monument, looked at the school, and turned off from the road onto the path leading to the pond, and came out on the road leading to the village. A nurse assistant was watching her from the clinic window. It is Tanya (her godmother). She could not believe her eyes, was bewildered and baffled. She could not understand what was going on. She was standing astounded. Sasha passed by without as much as a glance in her direction. She walked along the street she had known since childhood. Smiling, she greeted a man as he was passing by. I did not recognize him. Another man came up. She greeted him playfully, laughing inside. She turned towards the well. She entered the garden gate and I came down the porch stairs. Flowers were blooming along the sides of the garden path leading to the house, and the grass was wet and very, very green.

There was no feeling of the unexpected. She embraced me. She was slender, tall and young.

"Oh, finally, I have been waiting for you for so long", – I thought. I did not say it out loud, but she understood everything. We sort of dissolved within each other, but I could feel her body.

The state and feeling was as if we simply had not seen each other for a long time. There was an excitement in the chest, no, some kind of stirring, movement – rather the work of Soul and Spirit.

A new scenario came along at once. I see the Alekseyevskaya Metro Station, a square in front of the subway entrance. And suddenly she appeared. I led her along Mir Avenue. She was walking with determination, not distracted by anything, crossed a small park diagonally, and went down Kulakov Lane. She was taking in the freshness of the morning, looking at the larch trees. She crossed the street at the pedestrian crossing, turned into a courtyard, and went into an entrance-way to the building. I, in some state of bewilderment, took her hand and we slowly walked or rather floated into the office of Igor Vitalyevich.

I was extremely glad and embarrassed.

I said: "Igor, meet our Sasha! I don't know what to say, I don't know how to thank you!" The three of us were sitting together, my hands and feet felt like they were made of pudding, I didn't know what to do with them, what to say ...

And Igor said: "So, Okay ... What shall we talk about?"

I came to. I was standing next to the bed. I was dreaming while awake. It was time to get dressed and go to work.

Regarding the teeth. The redness was gone, the gums had become uniformly pink, but where there were no lumps, the gums were pale pink. When the protruding lumps are touched with a finger, it is possible to feel hardness inside. I rarely wear my denture (only sometimes) because it rubs on the outside of the gums. Another thing I noticed: throughout the entire week I had an off-taste in the mouth, as if some liquid was seeping. Sometimes there are springs of saliva. But there is some other liquid that leaves an aftertaste similar to blood. But there is no actual blood.

There is a faint lump on the left that is barely felt. There are more on the right, and they are larger".

* * *

The situation at "Khudlit" is becoming more complicated – they are not letting us do our work, they are trying to set everyone up for an emotional breakdown practically on a daily basis. But I am pretty good, too – I was able to halt the procedure of merging several publishing facilities into a holding company. It is too obvious that those with whom that had been done successfully in the past are now gradually sinking into oblivion. I publicly characterized Grigoryev's efforts in that direction as creating a mass grave for the state-run publishing houses. And, as agreed with our team members – Igor and Grigori Petrovich – I handed in my letter of resignation effective April 18. Otherwise I would not be able to do what's most important, if I get pulled into the struggle. My conscience is clear: the publishing house is in a good position. There are no debts, the trends for profit growth and output of printed matter are good. It is interesting how in this situation they will be able to explain to the press the change of command. On the other hand, does the press really care?

Strange and unbelievable things started happening almost on a daily basis. One day, the doors of my office opened and a skinny gray-haired man walked in. Despite his impressive appearance, he held himself stiffly, even bashfully. When he introduced himself, my surprise had no bounds.

– I am Professor Mark Aleksandrovich Mokulskiy, lead specialist at the Institute of Molecular Genetics, – he said, and added: – Arkady Naumovich, I have come to request that you take me on as an apprentice. Will you turn an old man out?

The request was so unusual and so out of line with my understanding of my knowledge and place in scholarly research that I felt lost. Mokulskiy was not just a lead specialist at the Institute. In the recent past, he had been director of the Institute. His name was well known among scientists in Russia and abroad.

– Mark Aleksandrovich, for the love of God, – I tried to steer the situation back to a relationship more suitable to the status of my guest. – If you were to ask me just two or three questions regarding your specialty, I would hardly be able to qualify not only as your teacher but even as your assistant. I am the one who should be learning from you.

– As for the specialty, possibly. But I would like to learn about other things, things that I am not capable of doing by myself, – Mokulskiy delicately interrupted my self-deprecation. – Professor Pytyev from Moscow State University told me about you, and also I read a few articles about your work, including a number of your own publications. I know that such an unusual phenomenon as clairvoyance really does exist. Many years ago, at the request of then-President of the Academy of Sciences of the USSR, Anatoliy Petrovich Aleksandrov, I studied this phenomenon. I am very well familiar with all of the experiments with Kuleshova, Kulagina, and Juna.* But what you are doing goes beyond the boundaries of extrasensory perception.

– Well, probably, – I agree. – True, we are working already not so much at the energy level, but at the information level. It is the most complex level, but at the same time the most promising one.

– And that is what I would like to learn, – Mark Aleksandrovich at this time indicated the area of his interest.

I am still a little unsettled. For an apprentice the professor is too eminent.

Our relationship with Mark Aleksandrovich at one point led to the development of quite an interesting project. We decided to conduct a series

* Kuleshova, Kulagina, and Juna are all names of famous Russian psychic healers.

of experiments to prove the real effects on biological objects from psycho-physical exposure. Unexpectedly, a well-known scientist joined our group, Andrey Igorevich Poletayev, who headed the group for molecular and cellular technologies at the Engelgardt Institute of Molecular Biology. It was he who became both the script writer and director for the main events of our research work. He had planned a rather extensive set of experiments both with a cellular culture and computer devices whose software we were supposed to influence and control.

The very first orientation experiment yielded an amazing, although expected, result. In the laboratory setting, Igor and I were supposed to influence a cellular culture in such a way as to cause accelerated division of the cells compared to the control samples. Both the control samples and the ones that were part of the experiment contained the same culture. It was simply divided into several Petri dishes, and half of those were brought into our lab. The other half were left in the room where the culture was grown initially.

In order to rule out the subjective influence of human consciousness on the study materials, the results were supposed to be measured by a special automated computerized laser unit, that functioned in autonomous automatic mode.

The experiment process itself went on as a normal everyday work routine. Poletayev brought the Petri dishes, Mokulskiy maintained the registry records.

The setting was to increase the rate of cell nuclei division rate by 50 percent. At this stage, Igor described the external appearance of the cells. He described the shape of the cells and the sequence of the division process. The appearance of the cells under the microscope fully corresponded to the description that Igor had made several minutes prior to the beginning of the programmed accelerated division of the cells. This fact alone seemed so unusual that Andrey Igorevich, without even waiting for the results to be processed by the measuring instruments, started discussing new possible experiments. Later on, this work led us to very promising directions of psychophysical influence in the area of accelerated regeneration of human tissues. But that would happen afterwards. Meanwhile...

As early as after two days, Andrey Igorevich reported the anomalous, from the scientific standpoint, behavior of the exposed samples. The cells were indeed dividing at a much higher rate than that observed in the controls. Specifically – in the control groups the mitosis cycle of the cells occurred over the course of 28 hours, which was normal. In the Petri dishes, where the cells were exposed to psychophysical influence, it took 12 hours. It was decided to start preparation for long-distance influence on the biological materials.

* * *

I am trying to understand the events that occurred at the edge of the Abyss and on Olympus. Why God, who was revered on Earth as the most ancient teacher of humankind, like Prometheus, in reality turned out to be a traitor. His gifts are like the Trojan horse – beautiful on the outside and dangerous within.

There are many official descriptions of the life of the God Thoth, but I chose the version presented in the book "The Ancient Secret of the Flower of Life" by Drunvalo Melchizedek. This individual is a physicist by education; he is considered one of the most powerful clairvoyants. Moreover, Drunvalo did not hide the fact that he received his knowledge to a significant extent due to Thoth. This was one of those rare cases when it was

393

possible to analyze varying versions from the original sources and find the truth. A peculiar psychological investigation of the rise and fall.

The history of Thoth from Egypt, of this Human-God (may Vladimir Solovyov, the author of "Readings on Anthropomorphism", forgive me!), goes back to the distant past, almost to the beginning of Atlantis. Some 52,000 years ago he discovered for himself the way to continuously stay conscious without dying, staying in the same body. Since then Thoth lived in his own body until he transcended to a new way of existence which is far outside the bounds of our understanding. He lived almost throughout the time Atlantis existed, and for 16,000 years he was even a king there. Throughout that time he was called Chiquetet Arlich Vomalites. Actually his name was Arlich Vomalites, and Chiquetet is a title that meant "seeker of wisdom" because he wanted to become wisdom itself. After Atlantis sank, Arlich Vomalites and other highly developed beings had to wait for about 6,000 years, before they could start restoring the lost civilization.

When Egyptian civilization started to appear, Arlich Vomalites made his contribution to its history and called himself Thoth; he kept that name throughout the existence of Egypt. When Egypt succumbed, it was Thoth who became the founder of the next great culture, the culture of Greece. Our history books name Pythagoras as the Father of Greece, and state that on the foundation of the Pythagorean school and due to its existence Greece appeared, and our modern civilization stemmed from it. Pythagoras in his works asserts that Thoth took him by the hand, descended with him under the Great Pyramid and revealed to him the knowledge of geometry and the nature of reality. When Greece arose due to Pythagoras, Thoth entered that culture in the same body as in Atlantis, and named himself Hermes. Thus, Arlich Vomalites, Thoth and Hermes are one and the same person. Is this true? Read the "Emerald Tablet of Thoth-Atlas", written

2,000 years ago by Hermes, and decide for yourself.

Among other things, due to Thoth history began as a science. During the existence of Egypt, where he was also called the Scribe, he wrote down everything that happened then.

Generally, the acquaintance of Drunvalo with Thoth, described by the author himself, leads one to suspect some covetous aims on the part of God. See for yourself: by the time Thoth started communicating with Melchizedek, Drunvalo possessed some secret related to sacral geometry. Moreover, his first and fundamental knowledge Drunvalo received long before his friendship with the cunning God. This is his text:

"While in Vancouver (Canada), my wife and I decided we wanted to know about meditation, so we started studying with a Hindu teacher who lived in the area. We were very serious in wanting to understand what meditation was about. We had made white silk robes with hoods and were very serious about this new endeavor we had begun.

Then, one day, after practicing meditation for about four or five months, two tall angels about ten feet high appeared in our room! They were right there. One was green and one was purple. We could see through their transparent bodies, but they were definitely there. We did not expect this appearance to take place. We were just following the instructions that our Hindu teacher was giving us. I don't believe he fully understood, as he kept asking us many questions, and he didn't seem to understand either. From that moment on, my life was never the same. It wasn't even close.

The first words the angels said were, "We are you." I had no idea what they meant. I said, "You're me?" Then, slowly they began to teach me various things about myself and the world, and about the nature of consciousness ... until finally my heart just completely opened to them. I could feel tremendous love from them which totally changed my life.

Over a period of many years, they led me to about seventy different teachers. They would actually tell me the address and the phone number of the teacher I was to go see. They would tell me either to call first or just show up at his or her house. So I would do this — and it would always be the right person! Then I would be instructed to stay with that person for a certain length of time. Sometimes, right in the middle of a particular teaching, the angels would say, "Okay, you're done. You may leave."

Therefore, Thoth appeared in Drunvalo's fate for a reason. He was extremely interested in something, and it was specifically something that he was not able to take from the new teachings by himself. But let us get back to Drunvalo's story.

"Three or four months after I returned from Egypt, Thoth appeared and said: "I want to see the geometric figures given to you by the angels". Angels gave me information regarding the geometry of ties of the reality with the Spirit and taught me the form of meditation that I am going to pass on to you. This meditation was the first thing that Thoth wanted to learn from me. It was an exchange: I received his memories, and he received the meditation. He needed the meditation, because it was much simpler than the method he had used. His way for continuing to stay alive for 52,000 years was very unreliable – it was the same as hanging by a thread. He needed to spend two hours daily in meditation, otherwise he could die. He had to spend one hour performing a very specialized meditation, lying with his head pointing north and his feet pointing south; and then for another hour to stay in the reversed position performing a different meditation. In addition to that, once every 50 years, to preserve the viability of his body, he had to go to the place called the Halls of Amenti and sit there for 10 years or so in front of the Flower of Life (this is a pure flame of consciousness that remains deep within the Earth)".

From this point everything starts to fall into place. Drunvalo received information concerning subtle matter technologies from the angels. And Thoth wanted to receive the same, but from Melchizedek. Why did he need an intermediary? Simply because Thoth belonged to the opposing camp. The angels would have given him nothing.

Now let's proceed to what Thoth exchanged for the practices of Heaven that were not accessible to him. It was his memories, that is, his past. Not a bad exchange: to exchange the past for the present. And, most importantly, Drunvalo, not suspecting a catch, agreed voluntarily. I am afraid he will still have to face in his life the consequences of this rash promise. Because in the fine plane material world the word is worth a lot. Remember I told you about the lesson in the desert when, grateful that the Teacher held us over the chasm, I promised him "to always offer a hand to help". And received a severe rebuff: "But you do not know what I could demand for that! Let's consider that we just had a simple chat!"

Igor and I are trying to trace in the levels of the Earth, through the planes, at the Beginning of Beginnings, information traces of Hermes starting from the most ancient times. And what we find turns out to be quite different from what has been written about this God. So, history may be falsified not only with respect to the lives of people, but also with respect to descriptions of the lives of gods. And how come the system of gods – those who were supposed to help the Earth and the people, – ended up closed? It is necessary to discover the meaning of what had happened and is happening. Now, seeing events both on the energy and information planes, we still have barely a billionth part of what it is necessary to know. In addition, a lot of things shown to us are allegories. They are similar to the answers of the wise man at Olympus: three questions, five meanings. One has to look from the beginning, from the very beginning. I probably bore Igor with those endless excursions into the past. But he cannot leave me by myself, as there are quite real dangers lying in wait for anyone in the latent Universe. We are always together, as it was before, as in the battles.

We are looking for the beginning – and we see the soul. We try to figure out what is soul, – and we get matter. Matter and soul are the same thing, but they are not identical to each other because they exist in different planes of space. Soul is the ideal reality. And everything we see around us is the materialization of the ideal, that is, of the soul. Therefore, soul is generally everything, the entire Cosmos. And the spirit within the soul creates movement, activation – it is a force within a force.

We see that even though consciousness is a part of the triad of the creation of the world, it is set apart from the soul as a separate structure. This is what defines reality, and at the same time it is a control structure. But it is control through the soul. Soul is like the Sun in the infinity of the Cosmos. Soul and spirit are inseparable, they are two in one. And consciousness is separate, by itself. It is the Kingdom, the Kingdom of the Son; it is like various planets around the Sole One. Like life on those planets.

I again think through the results of our research. The Ideal (Father) with the help of Spirit (the second power of the triad, dividing and uniting) implements itself in our plane of space as matter and form. And form is already control as a function of consciousness. Therefore, consciousness, soul and spirit are the Sons in our world. That's why the ancients always spoke about the single God, Triune in nature. About God with a capital "G". The remainder of the pantheon of the gods are assistants of the Creator, of One, Who is the Father there, and Sons are here.

But some assistants, it seems, decided that they would be better at dealing with the entire Universe, managing it more effectively. Why did that happen? On the face of it – due to a very serious error that occurred in creation. But is it really an error? And can the Creator err at all?

Soul and spirit are two in one. In the latent world there is a single Absolute, which comprises the male and the female unmanifested. In our world there are two: soul and spirit. It is not necessary that the soul in a material reflection of it in the personality of an individual must be female. The human body at the level of macrocosm is just a small element of the gigantic cosmic structure of macrolevel. What happens as a result? The Father had three sons. Remember, almost every fairy tale starts this way. We know one of them: it is Christ. There are three, but we know only one. Why is that? Because there is again the same universal tripartite principle of the macrocosm and world creation – three in one. Three in the Father, three in the Son. Christ, as consciousness, was the first to reveal Himself among the people. So He was noticed first.

The Father was building the temple – the temple of the body of the Son. As you can see, it is quite a different temple than the one people in church cassocks are trying to tell us about. How was He building it? In the apocryphal books of the ancient Christians, which have been lately drawing the attention of many scientists, there is a strange sentence found: "These are the twelve Aeons which stand before the Son, the great Autogeny, Christ, through the will and the gift of the invisible Spirit. And the twelve Aeons belong to the Son of Autogeny. And the All was firmly founded through the will of the holy Spirit, through Autogeny. And from the Foreknowledge of the perfect Mind through the revelation of the will of the invisible Spirit and the will of Autogeny, the invisible Spirit named the perfect Human, the first revelation and the absolute truth ... " ("Apocryphon of John", StPb., 1999, p. 13).

Between the names Autogeny and Christ there is a sign of equality.

What kind of a strange name is that – Autogeny? Some parts of it sound very modern; and not just one, but two at once. "Auto" comes from the Greek word "auto", "self". And "geny" also comes from a Greek word: "qenos", "genus", "origin". Again we have two in one. Plus the internal sign of equality, so there is the familiar construct: 1+2=3. Triad! Isn't that interesting: the word is ancient, but the meaning is quite modern. And there is no need to pay particular mind to the word "apocrypha". It's just that the fathers of the church didn't quite understand something in this holy writing. It happens. They lack understanding of quite a few things. Even reincarnation, which Christ demonstrated by His very presence on Earth, was announced as invalid by the bishops gathered in Constantinople five centuries after the acts of Christ. And the Gospels books were cleaned up in view of this quite a bit, but they could not rub all of this out. So we read there that when Jesus was asked about the fact that Elijah is supposed to precede him, Jesus replied that Elijah had already come, but no one had noticed him. Is that not about reincarnation? For us this is the starting point on the road to the absolute truth.

So, the meaning of the word "Autogeny" – "self genus" or "first in genus", if you find it more convenient.

Gene is a functionally indivisible unit of three-dimensional structure of DNA. Three-dimensional!

Why is it that in the esoteric teachings so much attention is drawn to the building of the temple, and it is specially underscored that it was being built for forty and six years (40 and 6!)? Six is for some reason separated from forty. And in the human cell nucleus the DNA divides into forty six chromosomes. Is this yet another coincidence? And one more observation: when Igor and I worked with AIDS patients, we saw that the virus in the information plane also affected six chromosomes. But did not touch the other forty… Looks like it could not even touch them.

Let us try to sum up the results, using not so much the famous deductive method of Sherlock Holmes (it is only famous until the reader becomes familiar with formal logic), but common clairvoyance and informational traces in the planetary Internet.

Nature was creating, using a reflection, a son without a Father. Actually, she wanted a daughter. But the daughter that she tried to bear without the male origin turned out to be a son, and a very unsightly one at that. The mother disliked him so much that she threw him away from herself and wrapped him in clouds.

The boy was born without a Father, and the Father is intelligence, among other things. Thus, the boy that appeared did not have a mind. But instead he was very strong: his strength was inherited from his mother without fail. So, if one is strong he needn't think. Such a son is a threat to everything. And besides, he was born immediately older than his brothers – because he developed in reverse, turning from a man with a beard into a baby in the cradle. Another unforeseen anomaly. Why did he have a beard? Because he was born already as old as Dolly the sheep (oh, those classics of genetic engineering).

That's when cunning Thoth conceived the idea to use the strong boy with a beard. Thoth himself had no problems in terms of amount of intelligence. So that's how he decided – his brawn, my brains – and we need no one else. So that's how the creative process started that I have already talked about to some extent in this book.

Thoth together with his accomplices decided to replace the Creator in everything, even in creating man. They knew that man had to be "made in his image", and took the image from Nature, via a reflection. But a reflection of a reflection is a distortion. As a result they changed the form. What they created was not the body of a man but a shell and bones. They created those. That's what the Creator left for them. But they could not obtain the soul, consciousness, energy. All that went to the kingdom of heaven.

They pried and spied, and what did they get? People live 40 – 50 years, and have a bunch of diseases besides. Therefore, they needed to cheat everybody as to why they do not live eternally, to hide the original reason. So they made up whatever they could.

Then they created the analog of night down there for themselves: pitch darkness. They invented fate.

Igor and I attempted to communicate with Fate in the levels. She was quite an attractive girl, but sort of obnoxious. Whatever we were starting to create, she would think up some resistance on the sly. And if we were trying to clear it out with her – she would immediately take off somewhere. Her beauty was cold and her energy was cold as well. She does not like Igor and myself, but she is afraid of us.

Fear was also invented by the gods, who started helping Hermes. On top of Olympus they created a secret council made up of twelve gods. They did everything similarly to the Divine Kingdom, but changed the polarity from plus to minus, and the meaning changed accordingly. They included two women there – one was Death, and the other was the lover of Hermes, a high priestess. But there are gods and gods. It is for a reason that in one of his works that survived till our days, Hermes lets it slip: "But I pray you, Asclepius, do not think that actions of the Earthly gods are the result of accidental events. The Heavenly gods reside in the heights of Heaven, each filling the place that fell to its care, and overseeing it, while those our gods (Earthly gods, demons), each in his own manner – by overseeing some things, predicting others via foretelling and prophesizing and

402

helping them to happen in due manner, – act as allies of men, as if they were our relatives and friends " ("The Perfect Sermon or Asclepius". M., "Aleteia", 2000, p. 272). And there is another important admission there: "Man is the creator of the gods".

Why, talking about collaboration with people, with mankind – ostensibly – did Hermes speak in the singular? We looked at this point through clairvoyance – and realized that "thrice-greatest" did not misspeak. He indeed meant just one man, the one that his mother abhorred and threw away from herself having seen his serpentine nature. And another obvious point that is impossible to overlook, – he subdivides the gods into the earthly and heavenly ones. It is not quite as though the heavenly gods would be performing some duties on Earth. No, these are two different camps. The heavens created the Earth, and on Earth some kind of power appeared, separating itself into a different entity. And as relationships developed, the matter in question was not just the autonomy, but the expansion of its power into the Heavenly Realm. The wars started – the armageddons in which at first the victories were won by the Dark Powers of Mugen, headed on Earth by his seven Archons. They were doing the same way as it was on high, only the other way round. They tried to confuse people whose clairvoyance they had already taken away, so that immortal man would stop seeking a way to the absolute truth.

In heaven Life is a man. As a counterbalance they, down below, created Death – a woman. Thoth-Hermes, the slightly cunning God, was working on all the tricks of that nature. The great [Russian poet] Tyutchev, who could hear the voice of the heavens as no other, poetically summarized the quintessence of those two ideologies:

403

"Our unity is bound with blood and steel,"
That's what the modern prophet said.
But we shall tie the bond with love instead
And see which of the two proves a better deal.*

("Two Unities", 1870)

If gods were people, the way the Creator wanted, they would have progressed quickly, would have grasped the essence of the idea, and would have started helping the Father in his creation. But Hermes and Mugen created the enclosed system of Olympus in order to cut people off from interacting with the gods. All the effort was directed to the end so that mankind would not find out about its destiny, nor about its great capabilities. Even the Church served mostly not to the ones whom it undertook to serve.

Why were the inquisition fire stakes blazing throughout Europe? A bloodless method of fighting heresy? When was the Church scared of blood? No, the people were burnt so that the soul would be immediately consumed by the fire and would not be able to tell anything either via prophesies or by prophetic dreams. That is how they banished the word of the Father from the Earth.

And they wanted to transfer Christ specifically with the help of Death into the enclosed system of the gods. Because on Earth Death is an intermediary during the transition. But at the last moment the Creator Himself replaced the Son on the cross. And Death retreated, couldn't make it, this kind of opposition was beyond its strength. That is why Jesus rose, and left – not for Olympus, but to the Father, to the Divine Kingdom.

Behind these external events there are internal depths which were not

* This represents an original translation.

404

noticed before. Jesus was the first human who, in accordance with the idea of the Creator, connected to His Divine Essence. He was bringing people knowledge regarding the resurrection. Because if one person was able to avoid dying, the mercy of the Father and His blessing, then others can do it as well. Even on the cross He addresses the Father and does not acknowledge anyone, neither kings, nor earthly gods. And He was capable of doing the most important thing: took the Holy Spirit from the earthly gods, and after that they were called the Dark Ones.

And a short while prior to that He wrecked everything in the temple that had been turned into a place of trade. People, incited by Mugen and Hermes, created idols for themselves and were trading in the house of the Father. No one sought the absolute truth. And how can it be found in the midst of false values?

Why did Thoth-Hermes know so much? Because he carefully observed the Creator and eavesdropped. He would hide behind a wall, or send his assistant who was quite crafty, who called himself the God of wind, to scout out the situation. So this wind would peek out from the Abyss, look around, and then dive back down again. Because at the edge of the Abyss a man was standing with the book under his arm – the Book of Life. And not only a wind, but Death herself was afraid to look him in the eye. The wind could see noting, but he would lie and make up whatever he could. He tried to look more impressive in the eyes of his master who lied all the time as well. So that way they led each other around the bush. That's why everything for them worked only half-way – for the twice-greatest and twice-the-last-scion.

In the hermetic works Thoth-Hermes pointed out his especial closeness to the Creator, stating that he was His scribe and wrote everything down. However, Igor and I did not find in the information plane any trace of this activity. If he wrote everything down after the Creator, he did that only by being deep in hiding and on the sly. But no matter how he tried to hide – it does not at all mean that the Creator did not see him; no matter how the formerly light-bearing angel tried to deceive – only in his own dreams was he not found out and not unmasked.

The traitor, betraying the One Who created everything – that is the third name of Thoth-Hermes known by [those] two [other names]. Is it still not clear who appointed the gods to rule over men? The Father created Man, and there is no evidence anywhere that He directed anybody to be a boss over man.

But, oh, reader, should we judge Thoth-Hermes, flighty and winged? Even the apostle Peter (Greek for rock!) renounced Christ three times in the span of one night. Man, due to the freedom given him, is deceptive and volatile. Ambivalent. In that, at the higher level, lies the basis for free development. And at the lower one, should the Creator be forgotten, – the basis for various abominations.

There is a parable – I can't recall where I heard or read it. There was an artist who looked for a long time for a model from whom to paint Judas. Finally in the slums, at the bottom of city life among "people without a particular place of residence" or, to put it simply, the homeless, he found just the right type of model. And started painting him, session after session. Meanwhile, the model continuously looked at the artist somewhat oddly, sometimes winking, sometimes smiling ironically. "What's the matter?" – the master asked sternly. "Sir, do you not remember me?" – asked the model. "No, I don't." – "But you are the artist, you must have excellent visual memory. Look at me again". – "I don't remember you." – "Well, you see, five years ago I was your model for Jesus Christ."

We can very quickly lose our external appearance and our internal spiritual support, which is the foundation of this appearance, like the person with the crooked neck from my first dreams. He did not want to betray, but became a traitor and put up with that. In the same way Peter did not want to renounce Christ, but, having renounced Him thrice, maintained his faith in Him in his soul. And later died as a martyr on the cross for his faith; he himself asked his executioners to crucify him upside down, as he considered he was not worthy to meet Death the way Christ did, whom he had rejected three times that fateful night. The face is the mirror of the soul. People who have depth, can even do without that when they determine others' character. "You may keep your mouth closed, and you may conceal your face. But whoever's worth something, will not be able to hide that", – considered Goethe. How quickly, practically overnight the functionaries of the different district party committees turned into democrats! Just yesterday they would shout: "What, are you against Soviet Rule?" And today they are already waving tricolor flags in front of the building of the Government of Russia, which is called "The White House" as a matter of brown-nosing to the West. How easily people rush from side to side it they don't have an internal moral core, the guiding star of Bethlehem!

We, due to our own lack of will, reluctant to accept responsibility for the world, for its development, for the processes of creation, made our superiors who have confidently inserted themselves between the Son and the Father. And the "managers" liked that position on top, the position of supervision, management, being in a position to condemn and pass judgment. Space has psychophysical characteristics and is oriented towards desires of people. Dream carefully, for there is always a danger that your dreams may come true. But what has come true is just one link in the chain of cause and effect. And what happens in real life afterwards? One of the well-known "people in power" was arrested, and the whole country named the Kremlin is worried and bewildered: "What is it that they have against him? Everyone is stealing here – but it doesn't mean that everyone should go to jail. It is important to understand who should be imprisoned, and who shouldn't be". They are working on the basis of understanding, you see. No matter how many Russian people throughout the world are facing troubles – not a word about them. And here, as in the scary children's tale by Korney Chukovskiy – it's as if the crocodile had swallowed the Sun.

About understanding – this word did not appear randomly at all. The thing is that in our country, given the conditions set forth by the laws, as well as current rules and regulations, it is not possible to live normally. It is only possible to survive. And that if you are lucky. Not a single person can go through life without breaking some rule or other. They, those laws, are crafted like that on purpose, so that the law-enforcement authorities could say at any moment and to any individual: the fact that you are still not in prison does not mean that you have not violated something; and, if the directions to correct that were received, we would be happy to correct this error.

That's why the whole country is divided, in the same way as it was during the time of Ivan the Terrible, into those who live within the "law" and those who act based on the concept of oprichnina.*

* * *

In the evening Ira** Karysheva came over. She is a translator. She feels terrible. For three days in a row she has been in unrelenting physical discomfort. Everything is trembling inside. She has stomach pains.

* The oprichnina is the period of terror during the reign of Ivan the Terrible through his henchmen.
** Ira – diminutive form of the Russian female name Irina.

Igor and I activated the internal vision screens. The situation is related to Kali, to the fact that the Goddess gave up that part of its nature which is death. Death has come forth from the Goddess. Igor sees it as a beautiful young woman, the internal essence of whom is horrific. I see her both as a woman and as a huge snake. It is strange to watch this: two Goddesses are dancing on the stage face to face. Death is stepping backwards, hypnotizing the one who used to dominate her. Kali is very much afraid of its former nature, but continues the dance of love. She has already given birth to Ganesha – a boy with a nose like a baby elephant. Cute child, with a round belly, four arms... and his elephant head has just one tusk. He is the God who removes obstacles.

Igor and I teleport to the stage. I stand between Death and Kali. Death is puzzled but not afraid. She even tries to intimidate me. The snake feigns an attack but stops within a millimeter of my face. She does that several times, but I am not afraid. Had I been frightened, then an intermediary would have appeared, which is fear, – and then Death would immediately have found a new persona for herself. This is a direct confrontation of Life and Death.

– Where are we going to put her? – I ask Igor.

– I am thinking.

– We can't put her into the Abyss, for it is sealed.

– I know. And besides, this is not an informational, but the energy-based essence of Death. It is weaker, but it is still pretty nasty.

– What should I do with her? – I push Igor for an answer.

– Let's imprison her in the stone statue of Kali. This is the past anyway. She will stay in it forever.

Kali, who had calmed down due to our appearance, quickened her dance.

Using the energy of the Holy Spirit we start to crowd Death towards the statue on a pedestal. She resists and wriggles but is forced to retreat. That's it, we chase her into the stone. She is in the center of a motionless image. Now she is in the past, there is no need to be wary of her. There is one personification of death remaining on the earthly plane – it is a young woman (about twenty eight); she is beautiful; she has black hair that falls down her shoulders. An Angel of darkness as Kirill warned us. We will be on our guard.

When we were returning home, a very bright star appeared on the left of the road. It had ten distinct rays and was surrounded by a sphere. The star quickly approached Igor and me; it appeared to be a demonstration of some kind.

– What does it want to tell us? – I asked my friend.

– It says that life has won.

– Wonderful, – I agree with a feeling of joyful contentment.

After that the star moved away from us.

So who was it that sent us such a powerful sign of affection and approval?

* * *

The day came that I had set to be my last day at "Khudlit". I came to the Ministry, picked up the directive concerning my dismissal, went around the offices of our Chief Directorate, and said my farewells. I was on good terms with everyone who worked there. Even the head of the directorate, Nina Sergeyevna Litvinets, gave in at the last moment and asked, while shaking my hand:

– Don't hold it against me. As you understand, it wasn't at my initiative.

410

I understood: another person forced into the position of being a stupid mechanism.

I offered her a farewell wish:

– What you need now is not to let "Khudlit" sink. Otherwise no one will be able to understand why you did all that. The press is looking at the situation already.

– No one cares what they write in their rags, – Litvinets responded.

– That is surely true. That makes you remember the Soviet times with their headlines like "Our newspaper took up an issue. So, what has been done to follow up?" No, I am not being overly optimistic; after all, I started working as a journalist about thirty years ago and I know very well who and how rationed critical statements in those years. Mayakovskiy, an idealist and romantic, like all true poets, at the time the one-party system first came into existence, wrote ironically: "Criticism from the grassroots is like a poison; from the top down – that's what the doctor ordered". But this is exactly how it worked in the 1930s, and that's how it continued all the way until perestroika.

And we can still see relapses of this formula to this day. Oh well, the people at the helm are still the same ones, brought up with the communism of the military barracks variety.

And as for the other side of the coin – the attitude towards mass media. Oh what about freedom of the press? What did you, a little man of no account, gain from that freedom? The yellow press, little scandals in the top echelons of power and in the families of nobility? Tons of ads and all the talk about sex – at the edge of what is acceptable? Alas, the common man is generally quite satisfied with that; there are plenty of crossword puzzles and jokes; now he knows what to buy, where, and how much it costs.

411

And what about the government authorities – how do they regard "the fourth estate"? They have a number of publications that are being hand-fed through the Ministry by Mr. Lesin and others who are obedient to the instructions of the management. Meanwhile those who are really free are lumped with the "yellow" press which does not deserve to be given the time of day, since it only exists for the purpose of blowing off steam in the society. And no matter how much an honest journalist writes about corruption among those in power, the authorities couldn't care less about it: those authorities are self-sufficient now and do not report to anyone. On the contrary – everyone reports to them. And if a journalist becomes too persistent – they will just have him killed, and no one will ever find any clues.

So, what about our Ministry? Oh well, it has people fit for the time they live in. It's a pity that they have even forgotten their classics as well. Otherwise they would have remembered the caustic words of Alexey Tolstoy:

All-mighty Lord, what a pity
That Your brilliant plan
Is unknown to the Chairman
Of the Publishing Committee.*

So, they cannot understand why a girl can sing about her lost love, but there was not a single time when a miser would sing about his lost money.

They shape the world after their own fashion, and for this they shall be punished. But I did not tell Nina Sergeyevna about that. She is smart, she has no ideals or illusions, and she knows what life is really like. If she only would not forget about God.

* This represents an original translation.

Then there was a farewell party at the publishing house. Tea and cakes, and everyone saying only the nice things and being afraid of the future. Must have been for a reason. It was already the next day when the arrogant attitude of Ministry officials towards the statements in the press with respect to "Khudlit" was tested for truthfulness. The newspaper "Sovershenno Secretno" published a big article by a journalist Taisiya Belousova, titled "Game with No Rules: Redistribution of Property in the Book Publishing Business".

This killer material (in terms of the facts collected there) opened with a photograph of the building of our publishing house, above which, wearing the smile of a cat that just ate a canary, hovered the Minister of Press – Mikhail Yuryevich Lesin. I will quote a few excerpts from this article:

"In reality, the list of those who had received money from the Ministry is for some reason heavily guarded; that makes one suspect the officials of playing dirty. There are rumors that federal money was paid to private entities (for example, the publishing house "Raduga"); and that not the whole amount allocated to support the publishing houses printing technical literature was used as intended...

Director of "Panorama" V.S. Buyanov, a person of skill and understanding, turned his publishing house into a very successful enterprise. They received practically no money from the government, however, they were not suffering from the lack of it. When the staff decided to attempt to convert the publishing house into a joint stock company, Mr. Grigoryev rejected the attempt by stating: "The Ministry considers that privatization is not feasible". Could it be because the ministry had its own designs for "Panorama"?

The publishing house is located in a beautiful multistory building at

413

Bolshoy Tishinskiy Pereulok; the building was at one point given by the Central Committee of the Communist Party of the USSR. The management of the Ministry of Press decided to place its Executive Directorate in the same building as well. And Buyanov was standing in their way.

According to the President of the Association of Book Publishers of Russia, M.V. Shishigin, the directors of the state-run publishing houses had complained to him that Deputy Minister Grigoryev attempts to intimidate those who resist him by threatening inspections and bringing criminal charges against them. Officials from the Ministry of the Press do not have any qualms about threatening to drag people's names through all the possible mud and throw them into jail for attempting to fight against the team "which brings the presidents into power or replaces them as it sees fit" according to one of the victims.

There was talk that Grigoryev was attempting to scare, among others, the director of "Panorama" – and it went so badly that Mr. Buyanov ended up in the hospital. Despite that, there were eight inspections. There were talks about criminal charges... Buyanov succumbed and left of his own volition.

The editor-in-chief of the newspaper "Knizhnoye Obozreniye" was one of the first to be fired by the Ministry of the Press. It's important to note that Grigoryev and Yatsenko go back a long time. As the director of the private publishing house "Vagrius", Grigoryev constantly placed ads in "Knizhnoye Obozreniye", aggressively demanding significant discounts, to which the editor-in-chief would not agree. When the saga of firing the director of "Panorama" started, Buyanov, who fell into disfavor, was given an opportunity to state his views in the "Knizhnoye Obozreniye". There was criticism against Deputy Minister Grigoryev. And besides, it became known in the Ministry that Yatsenko, who did not like

414

the reorganization of the publishing houses, undertaken surreptitiously, was planning to ask, from the pages of the newspaper, some challenging questions: how are reform projects related to the interests of the economic, scientific and cultural development of the country; have the financial and economic consequences of creating the new structures been evaluated; what are their advantages compared to existing ones; do they offer any guarantees against further reduction of scientific, technical and industry publications; will they not be harmful for development of the different fields of sciences, the demand for which is bound to grow, etc.

It is rumored that the editor-in-chief was fired in great haste. While Yatsenko was on sick leave, two orders signed by Minister M.Yu. Lesin, were sent to the editor's office – regarding dismissal of Yatsenko (stated as "by mutual consent of the parties") and appointment of the new manager, who started immediately.

Yatsenko is battling in court with the Ministry of Press to this day. Despite the threats (anonymous "well-wishers" telephoned his son, threatening that they could arrange for a search during which drugs would be found in his possession) which resulted in the need to apply to FSB [new name of KGB] for protection – he intends to seek justice. Meanwhile, over 20 employees have left "Knizhnoye Obozreniye".

"Detskaya Literatura" was merged with "Malysh". However, this merger is in appearance only. "Malysh" was already "dead" back in 1999: there were just the director and the accountant left in that publishing house, and they sold the manuscripts that had been prepared before to private entities. An employee from a commercial publishing house "Egmond Russia Ltd", who was accustomed to working with Western investments, was appointed to manage the holding. Now, according to the unkind rumors, he is openly on strike: he is not a publisher, nor is he a

printer; he is just a manager; he knows how to manage money, and the money was promised to him, but never provided.

The merger of "Sovremennik" and "Molodaya Gvardiya", who would be housed together with the "Sovremennik" staff at Khoroshevskoe Shosse. "Khudlit" was not included in that holding. We will talk about it separately.

By 1995, "Khudlit" became poorer than a church-mouse. The staff were forced to come to the Goskomizdat [State Committee for Publishing, Printing and Book Sales] and the Writers' Union; after that a tender was announced for filling the vacancy of the director. They say that the current Deputy Minister, Grigoryev, was among the candidates. But for some reason the committee, headed by a well-known writer, Boris Mozhayev, did not like him, and "Khudlit" was entrusted to the care of the director of publishing house "Culture", A. N. Petrov.

"Khudlit" is located in a five-story building (38,750 square feet) in the Baumanskiy District of Moscow. The first two stories are an architectural landmark of the 19th century; the upper storeys were built in the 1950s using the funds of the publishing house. The building is in need of repairs. But the Ministry of the Press likes it. At first the officials were going to attempt a restoration (having first removed the actual owners) which would have taken about three years. Then the rumor appeared that the building was about to be sold urgently because... the country needed foreign currency to repay debts to the Paris Club. When the sale did not work out, the officials suggested that the premises on the first floor be rented out to a company that was friendly with them. However, since there was no location to which the warehouse and bookstore of the publishing house could be relocated, the tenants did not make it in.

In January 2001, the Ministry of the Press decided to take over (using

416

its Executive Directorate for the task) the summer vacation retreat of "Khudlit" in the area called "Forest Settlement"; employees had spent their vacations there since the 1930s. The building of the retreat itself was nothing worthwhile, but the land was worth USD 1.5 – 2 million (it's in Odintsovo Region, just under 20 miles from Moscow, all the utilities and communications are in place, it's a beautiful area with a forest, fields and river, surrounded by summer houses of "new Russians"). The "expropriation" was explained by a plausible excuse: we will sell the retreat and improve publishing capacity using the money.

The Executive Directorate spent a long time attempting to force A.N. Petrov to transfer the retreat to its balance sheet. From a legal standpoint the director has no right to do that. The Executive Directorate is the same type of state unitary enterprise as "Khudlit". Neither the Directorate, nor the publishing house, nor even the Ministry of the Press have any right of disposal of the retreat, because it belongs to the Ministry of Government Property and the latter is the only entity who as the owner is in a position to transfer it from one balance sheet to another.

According to rumors, the negotiations devolved to threats: if you do not sign the transfer documents, we will start an inspection, followed by the arrival of "our" criminal investigators. Apparently, it turned out to be impossible to break the resistance of the director, since on March 5, 2001, Minister of the Press M.Yu. Lesin signed a directive to initiate an inspection of the financial and economic activities of the state unitary enterprise "Khudlit"…"

This is what happens when people who live, not according to the law, but to an unwritten criminal code of honor, come to power. Once this article was printed, "Khudlit", on the heels of the director who had already left, was beset by a mighty swarm of inspectors.

Earlier they had said that they were not bothered by possible articles in the press. They must have been joking… Judging from the level of nervousness with which about a score of inspectors were turning "Khudlit" inside out for two months, they were in fact offended by the criticism. At least it is a good thing that literally within a month from the intradepartmental inspection, another one took place, less influenced by the Lesin's team. There were differences in the results. Oh well, that happens…

But what is going to happen to "Khudlit" now? God knows… Their old game plan became too widely known, and they have not yet been able to make up a new one. Will they be able to do it before time runs out?

* * *

In our Pushkin branch, we had two new interesting students. A postgraduate student from Moscow State University – Alexei, and a 10th grade school student from Ivanteyevka – Natasha. Already during the initial classes they amazed their instructors – their clairvoyance manifested practically at the drop of a hat. And it did not just manifest itself, but started operating at such a high level that the instructors requested an immediate consultation with Igor and myself regarding this phenomenon. We scheduled the day and had a meeting.

At first we decided to work with the girl.

Natasha was very beautiful and effeminate. She had some kind of magical, hypnotizing gaze. As a subject for diagnostics we called in another girl from a group studying in the adjacent room, and asked Natasha to scan her and make a conclusion regarding the girl's health problems.

Over two or three minutes Natasha listed a whole set of illnesses. And, most importantly, did not make any mistakes in listing the reasons that caused them. Her abilities were truly phenomenal.

– So how about treatment? – I reminded her.

– In general that would not be difficult, –Natasha responded, – but should it be done? All illnesses are sent upon people for their transgressions. She must feel that through first; let her stay as she is for a while.

– Did you explain to her what needs to be corrected and what areas require special attention?

– Let her think for herself.

– Why are you so harsh? There are no serious crimes there. Just everyday life errors. – I tried to defend the subject of our diagnostics.

– In any case – illnesses are not given to people without reason.

– There it is – the arrogance of the gods, – Igor suddenly states. – And the one here is actually the best of them.

I was bewildered – what gods was he talking about. And then suddenly I saw the shore of an ocean – forbidding and rocky. A girl with long light hair falling freely comes up from the water. She is wearing a light blue dress. The waves next to her body are behaving oddly – they seem to be petting her. The girl comes out onto the shore, walks up the stones onto the rock that juts out towards the sea and lies down on the wet dark stone. Her face looks very similar to the face of the girl sitting now next to us, in a completely different place and on the brink of a different millennium.

Igor, who was following the scenario appearing on my screen, briefly confirms:

– That's right, that's exactly that very character.

– Natasha, you really like the sea, don't you? – I ask our student. The girl's face lights up with a happy smile.

– I really love it.

– And does the word "Oceanid" tell you anything?

419

– It has to do with water, – she answers uncertainly.

– And what about the God Poseidon? Who is he to you? – I continue questioning her.

– I don't know, –Natasha is at a loss. – But that name calls to me in a strange way. I feel that it is pleasant, there is something dear to me about it.

– There is an earthly body and a heavenly one, – I explain. – And for each of these bodies there is its own family history – its own father, its own mother, sisters and brothers.

– I remember something vaguely. My dreams are kind of strange, – Natasha says suddenly. – In the dreams it seems to me for some reason that I have a lot of sisters and we are very close. I saw in my dream my sisters and myself running around on the beach sand at some island and then we heard a lovely voice singing a song. We ran towards the voice and saw a beautiful young man wearing rather strange clothes.

– It is called a chiton, – I suggest to her.

– Yes, wearing a chiton, – the girl agrees. – He had a lyre in his hands. And he sang a song about love. About some love of his whom he lost because he looked back. We listened to his song, and tears were running from our eyes. He sang about his loss in such a way as if he had lost part of his soul. Neither I, nor my sisters knew how to help him. And when I woke up my pillow was all wet. I really did cry in my sleep. What a strange vision.

– This is not a vision, this is the memory of the soul, – I explain to the former Goddess. We have two types of memory: memory of the body, which is the dominant one, and memory of the soul, which, until a certain time, hides its treasures. Until the earthly "I" and the heavenly one combine into one. It is like two persons within one. There is one body but two internal essences. One is here and the other one there. They are separated

420

not only by time, but also by space, to be precise – by a number of planes of space. Let's try to do one thing. Natasha, you will imagine the Valley of the Kings in Egypt. Just imagine it, and that's all, and then tell us whatever you see.

I am acting on the basis of intuition, not trying to achieve a particular goal. But what is happening surprises others, not only me. There are about ten of us in the room where Natasha is attempting to awaken the memory of her soul. There are Igor and I and a few other students who are attending out of curiosity rather than need. And in front of all of this audience of people, who gathered there, basically, at random, a girl who seems on the face of it quite an ordinary girl, a high school student, suddenly starts her completely unbelievable narrative:

– It's the Valley of the Kings, the pyramids. I can see them very clearly, even more clearly than I would with my ordinary vision. The sensation is as if I am there in Egypt myself. But I understand that I am here at the same time, in the room where we are all sitting together. I am both here and there at the same time. However, these are different countries and, it seems, different points in time.

– Look around and listen to your intuition. Where are you drawn, to which pyramid? – I try to orient the girl while at the same time writing down in a hurry everything she tells us.

– I am drawn to the mountains. There is a secret library there that houses tremendous knowledge. It was build at the command of the gods.

– How do you know? – I try to get clarification on the unexpected statement of our student.

– I took part in it myself, – the girl replies in a somewhat surprised voice. – At the entrance of the library there is a curse, but it does not affect me, I can enter. Also there is a spirit guarding that cave. But it is not going to oppose me.

421

– Why do you think so?

– I know that this is the case. The spirit obeys my command. I can walk around and do as I please here.

Suddenly the post-graduate student from Moscow State University, Alexei, who had been silent until then joined our research process.

– I am in the clairvoyant mode and I am near the library in the cave, but I cannot enter it. The spell at the entrance is dangerous for me. I am watching the events through a small window near the entrance. I can see Natasha. There is a painting on the wall in there. It shows a pharaoh, and a young woman next to him; she is wearing a circle diadem with a snake. The girl in the painting and Natasha are the same person.

– What else can you see? – I am starting to develop this new lead.

– The room contains a lot of bookshelves and there is also a table that looks like a writing desk. It is convenient for reading those huge tomes.

– So let's read, – Igor suggests. – Natasha, can you see a very old book at the bottom shelf right in front of you?

– Yes, and I feel drawn towards it.

– Are you not surprised that these are books, and not papyrus scrolls?

– No. It is shown to us this way for convenience.

– Take it, place it on the stand, and let it open on a page where it refers to two people known to you.

– The book opens in the middle. And when I look at it, I do not feel like I am reading a text, it's rather that I know it and watch it as if it were a movie, – Natasha informed us.

– So what do you see?

– I see Arkady Naumovich and you dressed in the robes of priests. This book is about you! – the girl exclaims in surprise. – You are priests of Amon Ra and are very famous for your actions. You are trying to bring your faith to the people. But there is a menace of danger for you. It was reported to the young pharaoh, who destroyed the faith of his father, that you have ostensible stated that there are no gods other than the one who created everything, and – the most horrific accusation – you have been telling people that the pharaohs are mortal as well.

You are caught by the pharaoh's guards. The pharaoh is young – he is just eighteen. He has a very beautiful wife, whose name everybody knows. He is unable to restrain his feelings and be wise. He wants you dead.

And then a third one appears. He is closely connected to you by some unbreakable bond: you are always together, yet independent at the same time. This third one is very wise. He has nothing – neither wealth, nor power – but his word is a form of power as well. It is so unusual that people succumb to the mysterious newcomer. He is allowed into the presence of the pharaoh even though those deciding on whether to let him in or not don't understand themselves why they parted their ranks and let him approach the throne.

This new man speaks very highly of you. And he asks them to let you go and not to persecute you any more.

Pharaoh gets angry, starts screaming and threatening.

And then that man says to him: "What are those two to you, if you are great? And what do you have against those two if you have the glory? They say that God is one, and you say – a multitude. But have you thought, pharaoh, – from where does a multitude appear? And in Egypt there are many people, but they are ruled by one. So how did the multitude turn into oneness?"

Pharaoh is thinking. He is calm, he is in contemplation. Then he orders the release of the priests.

– And what happened to the third one? – I ask.

423

– He went off into the desert. He is going towards Israel. He walks from village to village and tells people about a single God. He says that a word can bring life or extinguish life. Life is given to the word by sincerity, kindness, love. And it is taken away by envy, betrayal, lack of faith.

People listen to him, but it seems they don't understand. He will keep saying this for hundreds of years. Then those two will appear next to him. They will enter cities, and people will gather around them. But there is a strange thing: when they come out of the city gates, at first they walk along the road. But then they vanish and reappear somewhere far away from the place where they were. They could appear in China, India, Tibet – anywhere they want.

* * *

A few days later we gather again in the same room and practically the same people are there. Natasha is full of enthusiasm. What she had seen has not overwhelmed, but rather inspired her. She is ready to travel through the library storage rooms as far as needed. Alexei has not been wasting time either: he has worked on sorting out his past. He already knows who he is. And we know as well. We had never thought that we were going to meet the closest companion of our enemy face to face like this. But whatever happened in past incarnations should not be automatically extended to relationships in the new incarnations. That's what the Father taught: "It may be that a person has gone through many lives badly, and through the last one – well. Or the other way round. How can you judge?"

We do not judge. We just sit in the same room, look at each other, answer questions, speak about clairvoyance, and work.

This time Natasha was drawn into even earlier times. As soon as she appeared in the secret library, the book that was set on the special stand in anticipation of her return opened by itself at a page determined by someone in advance, and the young clairvoyant appeared on Olympus, but back at a time when it had not yet been surrounded by a wall and covered with an energy dome. She was standing on the very top of the mountain and looking at the gardens, fountains and palaces. Not for a moment was she doubting that she was seeing things that were familiar to her and that she had known for a long time.

– This is Olympus. I used to live here, but my relationship to those who are in power is rather complicated, – this tenth-grader from the secondary school of Ivanteyevka village tells us. – I walk down. At the bottom of the mountain in a cave there is a blacksmith's shop. There is the anvil and next to it a sturdy man with a black beard; he is dressed in a tunic. He has seen me and has stopped working; he is looking me in the eye. He is surprised and, it seems, scared. He lowers his head and sets the hammer aside. I ask him whether he remembers me. He does not answer and responds with another question: "Why have you returned?"

I tell him that now I have come from the future. Suddenly he laughs ruefully and lifts his head: "So, a disaster happened to the gods?"

Far away behind the trees a beautiful slender woman appears; she has a very stern, commanding expression on her face. Hephaestus becomes nervous (for the first time Natasha states the name of the God, with whom she was conversing – without hesitation, as if she had known him for an eternity). Hephaestus is afraid of that woman. He asks the girl: "Hide behind the stones. Hera should not see you". I hide. Hera comes up to Hephaestus and tells him something. A boy with dark hair runs up. Hera looks at him with hidden irritation, but restrains herself when the child interrupts her conversation. Then she tells him something – in other words, sends him away politely. The boy runs off. He runs into a very beautiful palace surrounded with lots of lush plants and flowers. Hera continues to speak with Hephaestus. She wants him to make something to order. He promises to do it, and she leaves.

Another young woman appears, dressed in short clothing (a top and a skirt, as Natasha describes the dress of the new character). On her shoulder she carries a bow, and on her back there is a quiver full of arrows. This is Diana.

("Why Diana, and not Artemis? Why are Greek, Roman and other gods living together on Olympus?" – I think to myself, but don't interrupt our storyteller.)

She saw me and was very glad of that. We embraced each other. Diana is also surprised by my presence there. "Watch out that Hera would not see you", – she warns.

We walk along the path among the trees. We approach the house into which the boy had run. I tell her that I want to go inside. She asks: "To see Demeter?" Then says her farewells and leaves.

I stop Natasha and suggest to her:

– Create a mirror sphere around yourself to become unnoticeable. It will not protect you for a long time: after all, a Goddess is not an ordinary human. But for some time, till you get your bearings, you will be invisible.

It feels as if suddenly an invisibility hat covers Natasha. Now it is possible to continue the investigation without attracting undue attention.

– I enter the palace. Everything here is vast and beautiful. There are two women, or actually Goddesses, inside, and the boy, who is telling a funny story to Demeter. Then he speaks about how he met Hera in the afternoon and she could not get rid of him.

426

The women laugh. Demeter lightly, affectionately slaps the boy on the forehead with her palm.

– Today for Hera even ambrosia will taste like bile because of you.

Another boy appears. He was running around the palace and now rushes to his mother. She is the second woman, the one who had been talking to Demeter. The boy is mischievous, his hair is curly and he is carrying a small bow. This is Eros. His mother is the Goddess Aphrodite. She embraces him, turns him around so that she is standing behind his back, takes his small bow and shows the right way to nock it and put the arrow in place. Some other boy appears. He is very serious and holds a book in his hands. He wants to give it to his friend, the son of Demeter. For some reason it is very important, but the Goddess apparently does not want her son to have the book. The book is associated with a lot of responsibility, and she is trying to shield her child from the work and duties that come, in her opinion, too early. She considers that he is not grown yet, that he is too young, that he ought to play and run around rather than sit over books. Especially since this is an uncommon book. The one who owns it will have a lot of powers but also a lot of responsibilities.

– I have been discovered, – Natasha suddenly becomes agitated. – Demeter suspects that I am there. What should I do?

– Leave the palace, – I order her.

Natasha complies. She is walking within her invisibility sphere along the alleys set about with evergreen trees, passing by the fountains and sculptures. She sees another beautiful palace and enters it.

– In the center of the hall there is a large pool, – she starts telling us. – It is square, and the water in it is not ordinary water. If you wade into the water and stand in the middle, a thick white ray will beam from above. It grants a connection to all the levels of the planetary management structures. Behind the pool there is a throne on a pedestal, and Hera is sitting on the throne. She is looking in my direction, then puts her finger to her temple and waggles it, showing that I am crazy. She can see me; what should I do?!

– Leave! Leave at once! – I order.

Natasha immediately leaves Olympus; a second later she is among us, in our physical space and not in any other. She wipes her face with her hand and seems to be overwhelmed by her discoveries.

– Those boys are quite extraordinary. Something very important for the Earth is associated with them. There is some kind of mystery about them. There is a feeling that their presence on Olympus is quite different from others. I don't know how to convey that. They are, well, in some kind of a different situation. And the gods, perhaps with the exception of Demeter and Aphrodite, do not know that these children are different from all the other children of the gods.

Igor and I exchange glances. We know what Natasha is trying to say and we are amazed at her perceptiveness.

– Do you know what will happen to one of those children? – Igor asks.

Unexpectedly, Natasha starts seeing the informational level again and starts talking.

– I see a man with curly hair. He is young. He is about thirty. He has wings behind his back. I think this is the one who was the boy called Eros. He is standing on a cloud. He is wearing a red cloak with a brooch on the shoulder. He is looking down. There is the main city of the country of the Jewish people: Jerusalem.

Another man is walking through the city; a crowd of people is following him. He has a staff with three rings on it: a black one, a white one and a silvery one; however, no one can see the rings. They can just see a plain

428

stick. I am next to him, and the man with wings is above us and observes what we do. He is sort of guarding [us]. A door opens in one of the houses. A gray-haired man appears in the open door. He invites the man with the staff to enter his house. This is a city resident who is writing a book of great importance for the people; however, everyone around says that he is just crazy.

The man with the staff nods to him as if he were an old friend and enters the door.

The master of the house bows and offers to his guest, whom he addresses as Teacher, a seat at the table. The Teacher agrees, but then suddenly turns to me and says: "Natasha, come here!" I kiss the edge of his robe, and he stretches his hand above me and asks: "Will you share a meal with me?" I decline mildly. He smiles: "Running to the library?"

– How does he know about the library? – Natasha asks us.

– You are talking to Christ, – I explain to the girl.

The man with gray beard approaches, also smiling: "It is not difficult to set out a feast, but it is hard to make it so that everyone likes the food". They sit down at the table – Christ and several other people with Him. He asks Natasha to tell them about her travels and whether she liked the city.

Natasha responds with some sort of generic platitudes to the effect that she really liked it and is amazed. Then her story sort of fizzles out.

– What, is it hard for you to tell what you saw? – I am slightly angry.

– No, but he feels even the slightest lie. And besides, I don't have to tell Him: – He can see everything right away. Now He raises the goblet, and everyone follows suit. He tells a parable, teaches the people. Then he raises the goblet again and says that soon it will be time to leave. Everyone becomes worried. He touches my forehead. He knows where I am from, He sees all of us and smiles.

Natasha comes back from the past. She is overwhelmed by that meeting. Her eyes are shining with delight.

– This really was the real Christ, – she says in astonishment.

Alexei, another God from Olympus – and in the modern world a post-graduate student from Moscow State University, – looks at Igor and myself silently in concentration and suddenly says:

– And all the while they thought you were a false target, just a distracting maneuver. They looked everywhere, except close to themselves.

– I hope you won't let them know where to look? – Igor asks with a stern expectant expression on his face.

– What would be the point? What is done is done. And who am I now, anyway? – with bitter regret notes Alexei.

– You have also met Natasha previously, – I prompt him. – And your relationship was far from perfect, to put it mildly.

– I know – Alexei confirms – I have already looked through my past lives by tracing my soul.

– You were a very pugnacious man, remember that? – Igor reminds him. – You had a short red cloak. In one hand you carried a torch with which you lit a space all around you looking for enemies. It was not just a simple torch, but one that contained the wrath of the gods within it. And in the other hand you carried a sword. Once we met in the sephira of Saturn. Do you remember that? It was after Armageddon. You wanted to attack us, but wise Saturn said something to you, and you chilled out.

The people in the same room with us are listening to this conversation in bewilderment. But Alexei himself is not surprised at all.

– What's the use talking about it now? I am now a person, just an ordinary human.

430

– Leaving Olympus, you promised to teach people stern self-control – not wars and battles.

Natasha, who has closely followed the nuances of this dialogue, suddenly goes into the clairvoyant mode again.

– I see the ocean, sand, a large rock in the distance and near the shore there is a man wearing a black tunic; in his hand he is carrying a lance. This is Alexei, but at the same time it is Ares, the God of War. He calls out, calling Poseidon, and threatening him. The ocean surges. Poseidon comes forth from the waves. At first he is not very tall, but then he starts growing. He is holding a trident. Behind his back some sea monsters are appearing and a lot of girl warriors in armor, riding dolphins.

Ares grows larger as well. He becomes very tall. He threatens Poseidon. The waves behind Poseidon start to look like people. A huge dragon emerges from the water. Poseidon asks in a thundering voice:

– What do you need, silly boy? Come to your senses or you will perish!

Ares laughs and looks back. Behind him a black whirlwind rises from the ground. This is Death, this is darkness.

The whirlwind forms, solidifies and starts towards the ocean. The battle is about to begin.

From behind Poseidon a girl in armor appears. She is wearing a helmet and carries a shield in her hand. This is an oceanid, Poseidon's daughter.

– This is I – Natasha states in a suddenly flat voice. – I yell at him to stop. Ares is looking on. He is thinking. He has some kind of strange thoughts regarding me. He is hesitating. Another man appears. This is the God Hermes. He is urging his ally to start the battle. Ares stops hesitating. He is ready for action.

All of a sudden, from above, from Olympus, another woman carrying a spear rushes in on a chariot – Pallas Athena. She stands in the middle demanding that the battle about to start be called off.

I approach the shore and call out to Ares: "I, Oceanid Electra, challenge you to a duel. If I win the battle you will leave and take Death with you ".

Ares is silent. He does not want to fight me. It is not that he is afraid; it is just that he has strange ideas about me. He imagines me to be his woman. I egg him on: "Fight me! You will become known as the one who wins fights with girls".

Ares turns around. He leaves. He leads Hermes and Death away with him. That's how it ends.

Natasha is with us again and looks questioningly at Alexei.

– I believe that now you have another chance to make each other's acquaintance again, – I smile. – Good thing you are not carrying weapons or wearing armor today.

Chapter 7

The hardest audience for reaching understanding is medical professionals. Even if the results of our work are monitored and documented and irrefutably demonstrate the recovery of some incurable patient, they are inclined to ascribe this to the self-activation of mysterious reserve powers of the body. Recently we entered into a contract on joint activities with a regional association – the "Medical Treatment and Health Enhancement League" associated with the clinic of the scientific research, development and experimental manufacturing facility "Quantum", which specializes in aerospace research. The clinic had excellent diagnostic equipment and advanced laboratories. It was convenient to perform diagnostics and record the results at this prestigious institution. I decided to start with myself.

I have already described in the first book the way Igor and I restored my gallbladder, which had been removed thirteen years ago in Pushkino Municipal Hospital by the then head of the surgical department Lev Moiseyevich Ginsburg. I had with me the x-rays and medical statements regarding cholecystectomy due to gallstones. In addition, there were x-rays of the kidneys where over ten stones were observed up to one centimeter in diameter. In addition to those problems there were a stomach ulcer, pancreatitis, immunologic thyroiditis, two slipped discs and fatty hepatitis of the liver. And so with this fine collection of well-documented illnesses I came to the head physician of the clinic, Vladimir Anatolyevich Kushnir.

We had met before. I told him a little about our technology. He listened politely, and the expression on his face indicated: "Oh well, there are all sorts of patients out there".

Now I requested that he perform examination using diagnostic equipment, having given him the folder with the copies of my diagnoses and x-rays.

– Where shall we start? – Vladimir Anatolyevich asks in a business-like way. And again behind his question one could hear rather clearly: "It's one thing to mess with people's minds, but instruments is another matter. They cannot be cheated".

I suggest that we start with the gallbladder. He looks in doubt at the long scar – a memory of the surgical work of Lev Moiseyevich – and inquires somewhat skeptically:

– You think you already have grown one?

I don't respond even though I know that the gallbladder is two-thirds restored. The gallbladder matrix is in place, and its energy scaffolding. Moreover, the cells have also finished regeneration. But now, when one looks at them with clairvoyance, they look transparent as if made of glass. What can one see in this case with an ultrasound examination? – I don't know myself.

So I try to be careful in my assumptions.

– Let's take a look and document it.

I lie down on the couch. Vladimir Anatolyevich turns on the equipment, smears my stomach with some sticky disgusting stuff and starts the examination.

He turns me this way and that way, makes me puff up my stomach, tells me to breathe, then to hold my breath. Finally, he pronounces his verdict:

– There are no miracles. If they cut it out – it stays cut out.

I do not argue. I only request that it all be documented. That a medical statement be written, signed and verified with the clinic's seal.

434

Two days later I come again to see Vladimir Anatolyevich. He asks with doubt in his eyes:

– Are you really hoping that you will grow a new organ?

– I am, – I answer briefly: lengthy comments would not be appropriate now.

– Fine, – agrees Vladimir Anatolyevich, and we proceed to the ultrasound lab.

But this time something seems to have changed, after all. Vladimir Anatolyevich is somewhat puzzled.

– Stay on the couch for a little while, – he asks. – I am going to call in another specialist.

A few minutes later already two physicians are peering at the screen, exchanging short phrases:

– What is this shadow?

– It's not clear.

– And it is right in the area of the gallbladder. And the shape is similar.

The other physician huffs and puffs as he is thinking.

– Maybe something is wrong with the instrument?

I request again that everything be recorded the way it is. If there is a shadow – let there be a shadow. I'd rather come back again in a couple of days.

When I return for re-examination several days later, Vladimir Anatolyevich warns me at once:

– There are going to be two of us performing the diagnostic procedure today. I invited a very competent specialist so that we could figure out this incomprehensible shadow.

There is the couch again – it feels like my own furniture by now. Two physicians are looking at the screen and I hear their brief, but very expressive statements.

– The size is almost normal.

– The wall thickness is 3-4 millimeters.

– Why are the edges vague on the top?

– It's really sharp at the bottom. Here is the gallbladder wall, and here is the duct.

The consultant soon left. I sat up on the couch.

Vladimir Anatolievich was sitting barely a meter away from me, but he was looking through me into the wall. His gaze was strangely absent.

I touched his hand.

– Are you all right?

He startled and came out of the stunned state into which he had obviously drifted prior to that.

– But I know that it is not there, – he said, sounding lost.

It was impossible to look at him without pain. It left a feeling that he had suddenly lost his grounding in life.

– And is it there now? – I asked.

– Now it is, – he confirmed. – Only at the top the edges are fuzzy.

– Let's look again in two or three days, – I suggest. – Maybe it will fully materialize?

– Are you sure this is regeneration?

– What else would it be?

– I don't know.

– But this is not the first time you have encountered that, – I pull my biggest ace from my sleeve.

The chief physician is looking at me with mute surprise.

– Let me pull out a few papers from my briefcase.

He moves away, letting me stand up.

– Two weeks ago a woman came to your clinic with a request for an examination of her thyroid gland. She also happens to be a doctor – a general practitioner.

– Yes, I vaguely recall that, – Kushnir confirms.

– Here is the medical statement you wrote. You note the absence of the left lobe of the thyroid gland that, in fact, had been surgically removed.

– Yes – I remember.

– And several days later you examined that woman again; naturally, she was not trying to remind you about herself. And what was the result?

– What was it? – he asks back.

– Here is your conclusion where you describe the left lobe as being in place.

He looks through his statements, comparing the records.

– This is impossible.

– Why? You have documented in my case, besides regeneration of the gallbladder, completely healthy liver, kidneys that do not have stones in them any more, a normal pancreas. But you did not treat them, did you? Why would they have become such normal ones, while we have documents that state exactly the opposite. And can there be anything normal about this at my age? Just think about it.

Vladimir Anatolyevich is very puzzled. Questions are running around in his head. He is trying to remember at least a single case of clearly documented organ regeneration. He is thinking about mechanisms that could activate these processes.

He is not an ordinary physician. He is involved in scientific research, and he set a goal for himself: to defend his doctoral thesis. He asks at what level we activate the rehabilitation processes – at the cellular, molecular or even at a deeper level – at the level of elementary particles?

The answer is obvious. Neither at the cellular nor at the molecular level would it be possible to work with the DNA, cell nuclei and genes. For that much finer methods of vision and influence have to be used: those can be only sub-elementary particles and bioenergy, which can precisely record both damaged and normal areas of atoms and molecules. Even at the molecular level it is impossible to create the laser effect of targeted point influence on the tissues and pathological concrements (for example stones in the kidneys and liver), and destroy them.

A week later we met again. Vladimir Anatolyevich again conducted the examination. This time several specialists from our Center participated as well. My regenerated gallbladder showed up on the display screen with even, clear lines. It grew darker and larger, accumulated bile within and generally looked very convincing.

– That's what can come from a common shadow, – I stated, not without a slight dig in my voice. – The process of regenerating a vital organ occurs like common event, without broad coverage by the mass media and television.

– Oh well, – Igor gained his footing right in time. – They are not interested in that. They are busy talking about how, for millions of dollars, machines have been purchased abroad that would be able to cut up your body into highly decorative pieces. TV does not advertise miracles. There is no money in them. By the way, doctor, he suddenly addressed Vladimir Anatolyevich. – It would be high time for you to think about your own stomach and something else besides. About a kidney, for example.

Kushnir was embarrassed and lowered his eyes. A week later he admitted that Igor, without any kind of ultrasound, had precisely pointed to the doctor's personal health problems.

Soon the clinic of the scientific research, development and experimental manufacturing facility "Quantum" saw a new stream of clients. Physicians could observe with their own eyes how the absent organs had been restored and cancerous tumors disappeared literally within two or three weeks.

Sometimes Vladimir Anatolyevich became unbalanced and sent our patients away. That's what happened to one of the women who had extensive benign growths in her chest.

– I cannot document this, – he was trying to convince himself rather than the woman we sent to him for examination. – Two days ago I personally examined you. You had growths, knots in your chest, cysts and something else. And now there is nothing. I need to call a conference. We will invite breast specialists, do additional blood tests and then we shall decide. If I sign all this now – my colleagues will decide that I have gone mad.

A day later the conference, called by the chief physician, after a heated discussion, was still forced to document the fact of a miraculous recovery.

* * *

Even among people close to Grigori Petrovich Grabovoi, few know that he writes poetry. The poetic form conceals some kind of cipher – behind the common meanings there is the technology of resurrection, immortality, non-dying. Here is one of those poems:

> Oh Man!
> You are the world. You are eternity.
> There are unmeasured forces in you.
> You capacities are boundless.
> You are the embodiment of the Creator.
> In you there is His will,

By His intended purpose you transform the world.

In you there is His love,

Love everything alive, as He does,

Who created you.

Do not harden your heart.

Contemplate good,

Do good deeds.

The good will return as longevity.

Love will grant immortality,

Faith and hope are wisdom.

With faith and hope

Your unknown forces will come forth,

And you will obtain what you are dreaming about.

Immortality is the face of life.

The same way life is

A trace of Eternity.

Create in order to live in Eternity.

Live in order to create an Eternity.*

I will take it upon myself to bring look at those poetic lines as being close to some statements by Grigori Petrovich:

1. Each object in the Universe is balanced by ties of development with respect to all other objects.

2. After the word there is an eternity of existence.

3. Eternity is the longing of the spirit of Freedom.

4. The difference between perception and deviation from perception forms the object of perception.

* This represents an original translation.

5. The mind is the process of transformation of space.

6. The matter of the Universe is oriented in accordance with the mind.

7. By changing consciousness it is possible to change the world.

8. Each myth possesses the absolute truth of a postscript.

What I have quoted is born from the holographic consciousness. I am not going to explain this term to the reader – it is evident from the contents of this book. These are not just images – this is precise knowledge clothed in the flesh of words. Here are the mathematics, physics and philosophy of immortality. In centuries past they preferred to talk about this subject differently. In one of the ancient alchemists' manuscripts there is a recipe for the elixir of eternal life: "You needed to take a toad that had lived for 10,000 years (I hope, you have one of those?) and a bat that had lived for a thousand years (it must be simpler with bats, it seems), dry them in the shade, them to powder and take that".

It's a simple recipe – just two components. If it had been really capable of helping, then, despite the unsavory components, there would be hordes of those willing to partake of eternity. But it's unlikely that those who made up this manual for magic seriously counted on direct positive results. There are some other tricky circumstances at play here. It is either quackery or a secret code. For example, ten thousand years for the toad is a chain of incarnations and accumulation of experience. A thousand years for the bat is also an accumulation of experience, but this time in the fine plane. Drying in the shade means comprehension in silence. "Reducing to powder" is to extract the essence. To take is to apply. We will not go into that in depth. What is important for us is different – resurrection and immortality are really possible. People have thought about them both in the past and at present. People have never wanted to nor could they give up their right to immortal existence. Even science cannot refute that right of man.

Here is a witty statement by an American physicist, Nobel laureate Richard Feynman: "If man were to create a *perpetuum* mobile, he would find it impossible due to the first law of thermodynamics. But if he were to take on the problem of extending the life of an individual to an indefinitely long time, there would be no law of the theory of biology that would prevent him from being successful". And Feynman concluded that the only question was how long it would take to solve this task.

A completely different approach to the problem of immortality was developed by a Russian thinker N.F. Fedorov. "God, – he proclaimed – did not create death". And therefore man can and must find a way to get rid of it, using scientific methods as the foundation.

Fedorov sees ways to resolve the problem: "science of infinitely small molecular movements", light and chemical rays which preserve the images of people past, "construction activity of the rays". "But the business of resurrection, – Fedorov writes, – is not just the business of external forces, directed by the collective mind of all, but is also the personal business of everyone, as a son, as a relative ".

The viewpoint of our great compatriot is close to us. Both in the fact that God did not create death, and that the solution must be based on scientific methods.

It is exactly the combination of the Divine and the scientific that is, in our view, the true guiding indicator towards not-dying, immortality, resurrection.

We have already activated the processes for returning many people who were close to us. Those processes are underway, moreover, hundreds of people who come in contact with these procedures in one way or another, confirm, both verbally and in writing, the stages of resurrection. Igor and I have never met many of those witnesses in person. They send their written testimonies to us. Galina Borisovna Kuznetsova brought one of them from a friend of her daughter Sasha, who died several years ago:

"This started long ago, almost immediately after Sasha passed away. From the very beginning I frequently saw her in my dreams: we talked, went for walks together, she gave me advice. I constantly felt her presence... Then the dreams stopped. Several years passed.

In May of this year (some time around the twentieth) I saw Sasha in a dream again. I dreamt that I was in my village, at home. Suddenly the doorbell rang. I opened the door and Sasha was standing at the door and said, laughing:

– Hi!

– Hi, Sasha! – I responded, pleasantly surprised. I also noted that she was not alone. There was a girl standing next to her, short, dark-haired, 12-13 years old. Sasha followed my eyes and said:

– This is a friend of mine...

– Sasha, you were away for so long! Where had you disappeared to? – I asked.

– Oh, just so, – she vaguely waved off the question. – Better if you tell me what is new here.

– I live in Moscow now. I am married, and I have a daughter, – I told her and relayed another pile of news. And then I asked: – But how is this possible? Because you... don't exist...

Sasha laughed:

– But why? I am very much alive! And soon you will see that for yourself! We'll still go out dancing together!

443

After that she became hurried and started leaving. At the end she said I should not forget that she is alive now!

In the morning I recalled my dream and in the evening called Borisovna. And that's when I was extremely surprised when I heard about the resurrection program. Borisovna gave me some advice on how to behave. I became more attentive. At that time my husband left on a trip and strange things started happening in the apartment: steps, rustles. And once I clearly heard the click of a switch... I looked out into the hallway and discovered that lights were on in the bathroom even though I had not turned them on.

Some time later – I was about to leave and was styling my hair in front of the mirror – while a transparent silhouette flicked by behind me. I turned around, but did not see anything. Two days later I dreamt about a road divided by a green strip of grass. I was walking along one side, and then heard steps along the other side, but could not see anything.

– Sasha! Is it you?

– Yes, it is.

– But why can't I see you?

– There are two reasons: the first one is that someone does not fully believe that I have returned; because of that I cannot materialize; and the second reason...

– And was that you at the mirror?

Quiet laughter:

– Yes, it was. Did I scare you?

– No.

I wonder who it is among the people close to her that does not believe in her return.? The night of June 11 (before the visit to the cemetery) I had a dream that I came to her grave with Borisovna. I was looking as if through the ground and saw an absolutely empty space there. I exclaimed in bewilderment: "But there is no one there!"

(Of course, we will add on our own behalf: there had not been anyone there even before, just some dead flesh; the soul was long since in a different dimension. And the fact that a normal ordinary woman, of whom there are millions all around, felt a completely non-physical connection with the state of the grave, and realized that something had departed from there – is worth a lot. It's unlikely that any of those visiting the graves of those dear to them have gone through this state. – A.P.)

"Since I started communicating with Sasha again through dreams, I again feel her help. Now I have been presented with an opportunity for free training, a good and interesting job, and even career growth. She is with me again. I know that!"

Here is an independent testimony by Galina Borisovna concerning the ongoing process of resurrection of her daughter. Moreover, similar observations are recorded by relatives of other people being resurrected. A comparison of these observations presents very serious material to researchers in order to discover so-called standard procedures and technical stages. But it seems more important to me at this time to not distract the attention of readers by presenting dozens of concurrent processes, but to study them thoroughly and in more detail using one example. We shall continue quoting from the diary of Galina Borisovna:

"May 28, 2001.

Apparently nothing happens by accident in the universe. I was walking towards the subway, and remembered how recently I had gone to the theater with a friend. The play was "The Last Don Juan". During the intermission, going down the stairs with Natasha Sotnikova, we saw two girls right in front of us. One of them was extremely graceful. Natasha and I admired her, if I can put it that way. And I immediately thought about my daughter. I told Natasha about it, only Sasha's hips were shaped differently, and I thought (the thought of resurrection lives within me every second, one can say that, it is in my every breath like air): "May Sasha have the perfect shape (so that she would be shaped like that girl) based on the principle of the "golden ratio", the way Nature, the Creator had intended". And the suit that girl was wearing was really swell. And another thought: "It's Sasha's style and color". I could practically see her wearing it.

Once I was in the metro I continued reading a book by Grabovoi, "Resurrection" (this is the only time I have for reading, even though it would be really nice to read sitting at my own desk in silence, with my desk lamp lit).

I am reading page 86, item 9. "Body control during resurrection". I have already seen several times that it is not accidental. I read the book without haste (I would like to do it fast), as it happens. It seems that some-one leads my thoughts on, and then the book confirms that and convinces me that the thoughts have been right and imposes on me an obligation to work on the details seriously and not just in passing.

May 29, 2001.

I did not feel like getting up. My thoughts were in disarray. I have come back again to the village, to that morning. In my subconscious there was a number 12, (this is a play on words: three (the sum of numbers), one in three, three in one, twelve). I see again the green woods, pasture and the field. Already clearly I can see Sasha in a trouser suit of heavy silk, wearing black sandals; she is carrying the long jacket over her hand. But

446

the blouse that I see under her vest shows sometimes white and sometimes purple. The trousers are really flowing along her legs.

In Grabovoi's work I read on p. 17. "Shaping the image of the resurrected one from the standpoint of your consciousness". Straight to the point again!!! (Yes, Galina Borisovna! You must be more serious about this, and not just go with the flow. – A. P.)

I am already thinking about the future of my child, and this is good! A lot depends on the thoughts of the mother – she has to wish passionately and see the child's future. But without pressure: it is, naturally, the choice of the child.

My girl was a "tough" manager (I used to say: "Sasha, I do not envy your future subordinates"). Even though the great advantage was that she was kind and forgiving. I dream and want to see her near men like those in the Center, as their assistant, colleague, student...

Regarding teeth: I had an appointment at the clinic with our dentists – Yaroshevich and Kolesnikova. They, together with Andrey Igorevich Poletayev from the Institute of Molecular Biology are performing an experiment for the regeneration of teeth. It seemed as though they did not believe their eyes: they kept looking and touching...

Lena Yaroshevich said: I will believe my eyes when I can touch them with a spoon. Marina's eyes showed admiration and surprise.

On the gum deep in the back (on the right), another hard spot developed. On the left there is a tooth under a crown – something is oozing from the gum. It had been suggested that this tooth be removed 3 years ago. Pulp was growing on the root. But my physician provided treatment twice over 2.5 years by injecting medication in the root area.

Now the tooth is not aching, but I constantly have this thought that there is something happening to it, some processes are occurring.

447

The resulting medical conclusion stated:

"During the examination of the patient Kuznetsova B. the following was found: Partial secondary anodontia of the upper jaw. Alveolar ridges are pale pink, without pain during examination, smooth, without bony prominences.

Re-examination.

The upper jaw shows increased bone prominences in the areas of tooth six and three respectively, type: osseous exostosis. During examination the bone prominences are slightly sensitive, sharp edges can be felt. In the jaw the bone tissue is without abnormalities, the mucous lining is pale pink; at the edge of alveolar ridge the edge of the bone ridge is thickened observably.

Kolesnikova, Dentist"

Let's leave aside for the moment the odyssey of the dental treatments of Galina Borisovna and look via clairvoyance at the body structure of those who at some point pass away from life, and now due to new capabilities of development of human society, have a chance to return from that world back into this one.

Let's look at it backwards. What happens when a person dies?

When a person dies – first the soul leaves, and it leaves not alone but together with the spirit – penetrating and permeating. This duality is always together. After them consciousness leaves. And so that's it! There is no soul, no spirit, no consciousness. What is left is what our scientist are so fond of studying – the physical body. There are still some chemical and physical reactions going on. There are still some programs that were created specifically for this level, controlling something, regulating something. But the person is no longer, because the soul left together with

448

spirit. And the spirit is the energy of life that gives growth and limits it.

With the help of the spirit cells can divide, and in its absence – only decay. Soul is life. And the spirit is the energy of life. Everything has a life: a blade of grass, Dolly the sheep, Spot the dog. Spirit is everywhere, in everything. And it is not some sort of cloud, as people commonly imagine. It is energy which has organization and structure. If you plug a TV set into an electrical outlet, the screen will light up. If we use this analogy to describe a person, then the TV set is the body, energy is the spirit, the image on the screen is consciousness; and the diagram of the TV set, its operating principle, is the soul. But this is permissible only as an analogy, because consciousness is by hundreds of orders of magnitude higher and more complicated; this is the principle of the infinity of space. And, unlike a television receiver, consciousness is very complex: it has thousands of screens, thousands of channels, and each channel shows its own films.

After what was revealed to us, Igor Arepyev and I proceed in our perception of the world from the premise that none of the commonly used neurolinguistic constructs are random, and even more so ones like God, soul, spirit and consciousness. These words are the key and original ones; they are the very ones that form the foundation and formation of the world, religion, philosophy, exact sciences and language as the consolidating structure.

The knowledge that we use, and by the help of which we achieve results that are impossible from the standpoint of orthodox science, demonstrates that it is the spiritual structures of the universe that are the original cause of everything existing on earth, and that they are the transforming factor of reality.

Our practice proves that fully physical results correspond to certain mental operations performed by man in his consciousness. In other words, there are real manifestations of instances when mental reactions of the internal world start influencing objects of the external world. For example, there is the full recovery of people affected by diseases which are incurable from the standpoint of modern medicine; regeneration of organs and tissues previously removed from the person's body.

The triad structure – soul, spirit, consciousnesse – is the complete structure comprising both the levels of material and spiritual organization. Therefore, there is a need to provide definitions for this concept and a number of others directly related to it, from the position of our research and our practice. More so that this tri-unity is capable of reproducing its own field of dynamic reality, in which the spirit is not opposed to matter. And here more than anywhere else fits the saying of Plato that the scientists do not invent absolute truth – they discover it.

The glossary that we are about to offer you includes not only our work (of Arkady Petrov and Igor Arepyev) but also, first and foremost, the work of the Academician Grigori Petrovich Grabovoi.

So…

God – True Man, Creator and Creator of eternity and infinity. As the origin of the Cosmos and Universe, He is reflected in any world and in his spiritual manifestation is equal to everything created by Him in the past, present and future. By taking on the image of Man, God has the material, personified manifestation in the World of His existence of which He is the center. Re-creation of the World occurs on the basis of the law that the image of man leads to creation of each element of the World in accordance with the principle of self-creation.

God is eternal, He has never died and therefore represents the basis which re-creates all the elements and structures of the Universe. In the

Divine reality the concept of time does not exist.

In the World of Creation God is manifested by the triad of the soul, the spirit and consciousness, which are the single essence structures of His personality and personify their activities in physical space as the Sons of the Creator, that is, the Creators.

Soul – is the substance of the Beginning of Beginnings, which is partially outside of the capacity of perception of man, because it is what forms that perception, which is consciousness. It is the highest form of development of information. The principle which realizes itself through the structure.

Soul is eternal, sacrosanct and exists as the organizing structure of the World. It is that which performs the process of manifestation of the physical in physical, the material in material. It is possible to say about it that it is the World of worlds, the Life of life, the Temple of temples, the Word of words, the Absolute Truth of absolute truths, the Good of all good, the Measure of measures, the Depth of depths, Light and reflection, United in the whole. It is everything. It is in the soul that information, space and time develop.

The first thing that was created by the Creator in the process of re-creating Himself was the soul, and He placed it into a special absolutized space.

In order to understand the design of the World it is necessary to know that the Creator is the cause, the soul is the principle, the spirit is the action of the soul, and the consciousness is structure.

Spirit is a vector structure which implements impulses from the soul or consciousness during the transition from the external to the internal and

451

from the internal to the external, and also from the manifest into the latent and back again.

Spirit shows, directs and builds, while at the same time acting as a system of informational control. Spirit is all-pervading, resolving and delivering. It is the spirit that transfers information from the soul to the consciousness and back, as the carrier of light. In physical space it is manifested as energy. That's why they say: "Where a thought goes, energy goes; where energy goes – blood flows".

Consciousness – projection of the soul in the area of transformation into the material, which makes it possible in the process of evolutionary development to adequately reflect the reality of the World in infinite time and space. This is the area of reverse reaction to the event, that is, the process of self-awareness, and of the reflection of the events of the world by the local factor of the person, animal, plant and any other physical object. It is through the structure of consciousness that the soul interacts with physical reality. In the broad sense, consciousness is a structure which unites spiritual and physical matter. The entire external world is built on the basis of consciousness that is mediated by the brain, not born within it.

The source of consciousness is separated by the matter from the area of perception. The source of consciousness and the area of perception must be regarded as one of the structures of the World. By changing consciousness and perception it is possible to change the World.

In our science the principles of time are viewed as single-type elements of consciousness, and space as a structure of time. Therefore, space is secondary with respect to the consciousness of man, in case of a certain level of its concentration and development, space will start obeying the will impulses of man.

Each element of consciousness has within it everything that is connected to the entire external world, including the elements consciousness of other beings.

Consciousness can be: mundane, expanded and true.

Mundane consciousness perceives as reality the averaged results of concepts about the world by those who inhabit it. In the mundane state of consciousness at the informational level no object in principle can intersect with another external object or with itself, since the area of consciousness is separated from the area of perception of consciousness, and the reaction interval corresponds to separate areas at the time of understanding.

Expanded consciousnesse is the structure which enables the soul to govern the body on the basis of the principle of the infinity of space and eternity, through transforming the mass of consciousness into the mass of perception. At this stage of structuring consciousness the World is perceived in all its interconnections and it becomes possible to concentrate the signals of the external and the internal world, as well as energy, on certain functions. In this case the optics of consciousness work on the basis of the principle of gravitational interaction: the higher the concentration, the more precise will be the reaction of space to the impulse. Consciousness of this level is aware of everything that is happening and controls the entire situation, both with respect to events that are close and ones that are remote.

True consciousness – True consciousness has the ability to reflect all of reality in each of its segments, that is, in each segment, true consciousness of all of reality exists at the same time, and develops at the same time

453

with the entire World in all its manifestations. It reflects all of the reality of the world in any space, in any time. In this condition it is not possible to have an intersection of the initial information concerning an object with developing information about itself; that provides an opportunity for the resurrection of a person or restoring any object.

True consciousness is a space-time form which is reflected in the eternity and infinity of the constructive creation.

Let's try to summarize:

Soul plus spirit is a spiritual structure; the operating principle of control through consciousness. This dyad has enormous power and is capable of transforming one dimension of space into another. Manifestation of the soul in the dynamic of the spirit creates feelings.

Spirit is the will of the Creator, the impulse, which transforms the light of knowledge of the soul from the external to the internal, and from internal through the soul to the external, from the manifest into latent and back, when the Creator thumps his staff and says: "Let it be!". For any object there exists a reflection in the areas of information. That is why in the hierarchy of making decisions it is fixed: spirit controls consciousness. Spirit is an action of the soul; it exists outside time and space.

Consciousness is the generalized reaction of an object to its informational environment. Therefore, it appears only where information is available, external or internal. And as we already mentioned, the highest form of development of information is the soul. Therefore, in the general sense of the word consciousness is a structure that unites the spiritual and physical matter.

Ability to work with one's consciousness may result in a radical change to the structure of the world. And then it is not the world that will determine the structure of a person, but quite the opposite. This is what

454

happens when Igor and I are visited by people with cancer or AIDS, – we change the situation in the world of that specific person. Because all the space of the world is built on the basis of consciousness. And consciousness, when necessary, can re-create any element of reality – for example, the gall bladder that was removed from the body by a surgeon many years ago. It is the consciousness that can replace, using its technologies, the procedure of physical process, because all the phenomena of the world are reflected by the local factor of the person. For many serious scientists this literary description of a complex biophysical process is unlikely to seem interesting. So, this is especially for them: initiation of growth of internal organs and tissues is achieved trough an impulse directed onto the areas of chromosomes which are informationally responsible for the functioning of the lost organ. This way it's more clear, isn't it?

Consciousness is a form of the mind. And the mind is the idea of the manifestation of the person. If you divide the Russian word meaning "mind" into two, you will see two words meaning: "one" and "intelligence". Now find the beginning of that end with which the beginning ends. This exhortation is not playing in paradoxes, but comes from a desire to awaken your consciousness, you, reader.

And a few more definitions which will help you to properly perceive events in this book.

Reality is the connection of the body of information with the boundary of the perception thereof. It is important to know that the factual and the real are not necessarily identical.

Information is the point of connection of the worlds, manifested in consciousness. It can be static and it may be dynamic. In the material world information is manifested through form. The dynamics of information is a change in volume or shape.

455

Time: on the one hand, it sort of exists, but on the other it does not exist in the conventionally accepted way. Think what is located on which side. On the side where it exists, time can be looked at as some sort of a space transformer. It's like lines along which the dynamic of events is transmitted.

An element of time can be also considered with respect to the structure of information. In this case time depends on the consciousness of the person. Therefore, time can be also be defined as a coordinate point at which consciousness is tied to the causal events of the external world.

At the level of real events the consciousnesse perceives information specifically at those points at which the horizontal and vertical lines of the structure of time cross. The time vector is an instrument of control.

And the last concept we need in order to understand the philosophy of resurrection and immortal existence is space.

Space is a construct of consciousness in order to implement the actions of the soul, spirit and body. In the dynamics of development of the plan of the Creator it gradually flows into the structure of the soul. In religion it is called the junction of the divine Kingdom and the Earthly Kingdom. Many might feel confused: so what was there first: space, consciousness or body? Don't worry yourself. At the beginning of all there was God, who already had all this.

In the future we shall repeatedly refer to these constants of the universe. And not only to these ones; we shall gradually add to their definitions and gradually broaden your understanding of the design of the Universe and the Earth, life and person.

And now pay attention: I am revealing to you the technology of resurrection. People are receiving it for the first time since Christ awakened consciousness. This is the will of the Creator, and we are fulfilling it, continuing what Grigori Petrovich Grabovoi started. At this point someone may want to smile sarcastically, someone like Hera who saw the Oceanid Electra in her palace will twirl his finger at their temple to indicate those people are mad – they will do as they will. Because the decision is taken by the person himself and he is himself responsible for the consequences of the decisions he has made. Most likely you will not become able, having read the subsequent pages, to resurrect anyone immediately, or attain immortality, but you will have a true guide, and you will be able to strive towards the absolute truth because of it.

First you must see the image of the person you are resurrecting, and then his outline. The next action is the alignment of the image and the outline.

Outline is a living form. In itself it reflects the entire world and its all-encompassing connections. The border of the outline separates the external and the internal.

Create the information point inside – the nucleus of a cell. Imagine it to yourself as an ideal gold standard: no abnormalities, no damage. It is fully in line with the concept of NORM. In this case an element of perception appears; but for visualization you should not use knowledge from anatomy atlases and textbooks on human morphology. Your consciousness understands much better than any specialists how and in what way everything is set up within your body, and will build everything by itself. At this moment your soul is transferring to your consciousness the knowledge that was requested.

Then the cell will start to divide. From the central point something like a petal appears, and then the second, third, fourth one. And so now we see the flower bloom – the flower of the soul.

Have you ever heard about liquid crystals located within the cell

457

nucleus? No? That's not a problem. Just imagine to yourself, on the left of the flower of the soul, a crystal of consciousness; then superimpose the liquid crystal and the one that you have imagined – because it is not quite the same. But don't you doubt – there is knowledge within your soul, and it will help you.

Consciousness is already a form of access to reality; it gives the soul a capacity to control the body.

Therefore, we now have the form (outline), the inner filling (flower), the petal (internal content) and the crystal, which is something that is contained within as a control mechanism.

Now we need an impulse. It must be strong and fast. Remember, I talked about it when we discussed the work with archiving points. You send an impulse – and the division of cells initiates. It starts under the influence of the penetrating and the single one, the movement and life. Even though it is in a small, negligible volume, but it is the real life which will contain all the elements envisaged by the Creator, and the monsters cloned in a lab.

The cells divide. It is necessary to combine the multitude into a single entity. In the outline, in the area of the solar plexus, imagine the horizontal sign of infinity and make it move clockwise. Only through infinity can we obtain a multitude, and from the multitude a single entity.

The way of the soul leads to the crystal, or logos, where the soul follows the connections of the world. The connections of the world are infinite. They are manifest and can be perceived via clairvoyance; they are seen as silvery or golden threads around the crystal, flower, cell, area. If you look at it from above, you will see how the soul travels along those threads.

In this way the infinity of the internal world opens with the help of the soul and the way of the soul.

Soul comes out on the way to the crystal, flower, cell, area; it is guided by the Holy Spirit along the connections of the world. It reaches infinity, where it takes the knowledge, creates a cell and builds the multitude. After that it returns from the Divine Kingdom, again travels through the area, cell, flower and crystal, thus receiving life. It arrives via this pathway on Earth, where it receives bodily life.

Spirit enters the soul – it paves the way for the area of the consciousness. The latter comes into the cell of the soul.

After that the person starts breathing. His heart starts beating. He inhales from the external world – inhales into the internal world and exhales into the world external, in this way connecting the consciousness and the soul along the penetrating and the single [pathway].

Many readers will consider this technology either very strange or very difficult. I understand. But believe me – you are never alone. And in each good deed you will find that you have a lot of helpers. Many of them are invisible. And so what? Look how they help the lesser animals among us.

Looking at the patterns of the nests of African termites, it is hard to believe that they were not built by a highly advanced civilization. Balls, structures that look like pitchers and bell-shaped domes, the walls of which are formed by ascending spiral columns; a complex system of galleries that cross and flow into one another. And everything is flawlessly precise, as if carved out of stone. How is it possible that tiny blind bugs that do not have a drawing and are unable to look at what they have created could build enormous structures, all these pyramids and cathedrals? South African biologist Eugene Marais spent a lot of time observing the termites repairing the breaches in their structures. They rush to the hole from all sides and start work, precisely restoring the complex shape of their dwelling as if following a precise plan. Marais performed a simple but effective experiment. He destroyed the top of termite mound and placed in the hole a metal plate which precluded workers from different sides from communicating in any way. Despite that, the termites built up two halves – one on each side of the plate. When the plate was removed, the halves of the termite mound matched each other perfectly. The termite dwellings form entire villages. This is comparable with the size of Arkaim, the legendary settlement of the people of Bronze Age.

An even more fascinating example if collective organization is sometimes provided by the colonies of protozoa, which are so harmoniously joined in one entity, that sometimes it is difficult to distinguish them from an autonomous individual being. The highest achievement in this matter belongs to siphonophores, whose colonies form a whole number of "individuals" inhabiting the deep ocean and whose behavior is quite complex; besides, each individual within the colony is specialized and performs specific functions.

Let us take a look at one of the species of siphonophores as a sample of such an organization. At the top of the colony there is an organism that has turned into a bubble filled with gas. Below there are a number of organisms that have transformed into water jets, which issue streams of water to ensure movement for the entire colony. Through coordinated actions and in accordance with the size of the nozzle they change the direction of movement and thus enable the colony to move in any plane. Further down the column there are the "foragers" of the colony. They spread around thin stalks with which they catch prey, digest it and therefore provide nourishment for the rest of their colony mates. Small scale-like beings line the central stem tightly, protecting it from physical damage. And, finally, there are "sex" organisms, which produce the gametes that spawn new colonies.

Such specialized communities of individual organisms within the colony already act as organs within the organism, and some of them are even connected by a common nervous system. Those life forms may be treated both as a colony and as organisms, even though they are formed by individual beings. One could guess that similar forms are likely to occur, both in the Cosmos at large, and in the human community.

At this time science has accumulated a large number of observations which force one to admit that it is impossible to explain biological reality in such terms as "instinct", "behavior program" "information embedded at the genetic level", etc. A vast body of literature on ethology, which is the science of animal behavior, shows a large amount of material leading to the following conclusion: the lives of a whole number of "collective" beings demonstrate the presence of a phenomenon which the biologists have defined by the concept of "supraorganism intelligence".

That is something to think about, isn't it?

The path from the top down – is the path of initial creation, the Heavens descending down towards Earth.

Later on everything returns via the same path, bringing the Earth up to Heaven. Therefore, Earth and Heaven are connected and brought into equilibrium; at the first stage they come to the limit of contraction or concentration of consciousness; at the second one there is an expansion into the spirit and soul. After the second stage it is not the world which will define the structure of the person, but the person who defines the structure of the world. So LIBERATION comes.

The intersection of the initial information about a person and developing information about himself in the area of causal relations has occurred.

But this does not mean that you will see the resurrected person that

461

same moment. There is also the problem of connecting the incarnations. The past, present and future are structures independent of each other, or, to put it more correctly, areas of consciousness, even with respect to the impulse of consciousness of the one who is performing the resurrection, or from the standpoint of the one who is being resurrected.

Grigori Grabovoi expresses this last procedure with a well-coined formula: the past must be taken into account, the future must be formed, and the present – aimed at the technology. A few months will pass (this period may vary somewhat for each resurrected individual), and people who love each other will be able to meet again and become inseparable in full agreement with the will of the Father in Heaven as was at some point foretold by His Son Jesus Christ, so as to see and control the way of the soul from the infinite to the finite and from the divine to the earthly.

The dark veil of the Cosmos guards many a secret. Not too long ago the distance separating stars and planets from each other was called the vacuum. But a fascinating thing occurred: the astronomers observing the galaxies reached an astonishing conclusion: in order to explain the trajectories of the celestial bodies, there is not enough visible mass. There must be some "hidden" part which comprises over 90 percent of the total mass of the Universe. Which means – energy as well! It is being suggested that it makes sense to seek the "hidden" mass within the physical vacuum.

Seek – and you will find! But what will you find?

* * *

Unfortunately, many of the scientists, particularly the ones who work in the field of genetics, have no understanding whatsoever what dangerous games they are playing with the universe. And who is their partner in this crazy game – Life or Death? Quoting from the newspaper "Sovershenno Secretno" (No. 5, 2001), from an article "Phantom of the DNA": "There have always been enough volunteers to suffer for the sake of science here in Russia. Whether they were studying genetics, biology or biochemistry. They will not spare themselves. Particularly if the matter in question is the genetic apparatus of humans. One of those "kamikazes" was a colleague of Petr Garyaev. He was using a laser beam to study the DNA of his own sperm. Then he wrapped the beam into a laser resonator, broadened the beam of laser radiation and was within the area covered by the beam. The photons that turned into radio waves (this is a known scientific fact which was, according to the journalist, discovered by Garyaev's group quite recently – A.P.), read the information from the scientist's chromosomes in the dish and immediately attacked the experimenter. He immediately fell horribly ill and nearly died. Even Garyaev, who happened nearby at that time (perhaps he was just passing by? – A.P.), felt the pernicious influence of the radio waves. He also felt suddenly quite ill". I believe this is a very clear example of what the classic wrote about: woe from wit. And another thing comes to mind when you read things like that.

…When a group of scientists led by Petr Garyaev tried to find out what happens with physical fields of the cell nuclei at the time when they are destroyed, and in order to achieve this, heated DNA to 43 °C, the oscilloscope showed an "SOS" signal (perhaps the spectrum of the SOS signal – A.P.). DNA molecules felt "pain", and they were in a way "complaining" about that "pain". But the scariest part came during the subsequent temperature increase. The liquid crystals were melting, the ones where hereditary information is recorded within DNA; high-level genetic programs for development of the organism were being erased, and one could "hear" quite a chaos of "sounds"! The readings on the oscilloscope (I suppose they must mean a correlating device – A.P.) went just about off the scale. Liquid crystals of DNA molecules were dying... And this death was confirmed by the "cries".

By the way, "singing" of DNA or their "cries" can be heard as of recently. At the laboratory of one of the Moscow Institutes under the Russian Academy of Science Garyaev's team was able to record radio wave "voices" of DNA molecules. This is hard to believe, isn't it? However, this is now a scientific fact, one of those that is recognized by academicians of Krugliakov's sort.

...One time Petr Petrovich Garyaev was once again "melting DNA. There is no need to mention that it was painful even to look at the acoustic field it created on the oscilloscope because the DNA was "suffering" It was dying. After the necessary measurements were taken, the scientists placed in the sample compartment, which had already been cooled and cleaned, some normal DNA, which had not been subjected to heating. And, imagine that, it was behaving in exactly the same way as the previous one that had been melted! Same "screams", same peaks on the graph, even though no pain was inflicted on it. This led to suggestions that the phantom of a murdered person possesses a high level of biological activity and can influence the people near it in a number of various ways. It would have been useful also to take that further and suppose in what way our living space has been affected by all the phantoms of all the melted, tortured cells, ruined forests, lakes, rivers, oceans and life that had inhabited them. And also the air, soil, the underground world.

It practically begs the question – what game are you playing? Wave-derived immunity? Again vaccines for flue, for AIDS? I have to tell you the bitter news, you scientists, docents and PhD's: – no kind of wave,

464

chemical and genetic manipulations with genetic materials pass without a trace. Even if no one suffers in a specific laboratory, information about the event is recorded in the information field of the planet, and whether you want it or not, at any moment it can come into unpredictable interrelations with any positive or negative archiving point in space. Maybe you don't know that they exist? But it does not make it easier for the rest of the people. Because all these cancers, AIDS and new horrendous diseases besetting people are the result of those types of scientific activities. Space is psychophysical, and, whatever you do, it always reads and records the events that occur. What did you want – to torture or kill a living cell, which is a part of the universe? The pernicious orientation of your consciousness will be recorded by the planetary field, the consciousness of Earth to be precise. So why be surprised later at volcanic eruptions, hurricanes, technogenic catastrophes. Planet Earth also has feelings and power; it has a right to react. And sometimes it returns to humanity the fruit of the thinking efforts of the latter. Such as here, feel on your own hide what you are doing to me.

Please understand me correctly: I am not against people engaging in scientific research. I am against them doing it in such a manner.

In Garyaev's laboratory they were investigating what happens with physical fields of cell nuclei at the time when they are destroyed. For that purpose, they were placed in temperature conditions under which liquid crystals, in which hereditary DNA information is recorded, would start melting. And together with the crystals the genetic program for organism development was destroyed. When a live cell was placed in the cleaned sample compartment of the instrument where DNA had been melted, it behaved in that instrument in the same way as its predecessor, even though this time heating had not been activated.

I have repeated this fact on purpose – so that the reader will remember and think. What does it tell us? That information about any even, good or bad, never disappears without a trace; it always remains and keeps working.

That is, you should not eat an apple if you have not studied the technology which is used to create apples. I mean the system of direct prohibitions that should be in force in science, not the trivial physiological process.

The disease which is trying to reach the crystals in cell nuclei is fighting for every minuscule element of information structures, trying to defeat and damage them. This is a real war, in which viruses, bacteria, microbes are part of a powerful invisible army fighting against the person. Who would have thought that all these dark forces would find such a powerful ally as scientists who have forgotten the biblical story about the apple? Even though the meaning of that story is very simple. They were told: do not eat the apple – and they should have obeyed. Because one first has to be prepared to receive the knowledge, particularly if it's the Creator's knowledge. In other words – everything in its own time. And taking something by force that you don't yet know how to use is both dangerous and dishonorable. All the more so is to obtain knowledge by destroying life. Because a human cell has its own consciousness, intellect and purpose in life. By destroying it, researchers unknowingly activate large-scale programs of injury and destruction of people in informational space. The death of one living cell in a laboratory, outside of its natural aging mechanisms, may lead to the deaths of a large number of people who have nothing to do with the crazy experiments. It would be actually more correct to say that they are dying already, thus paying the price for the ambitious curiosity of their fellow humans. I would like to remind you again that the

466

complete destruction of one of the main elements of information leads to the destruction of the object of information. And the cell, its nucleus and DNA are specifically the main element. As the researcher, Petr Garyaev, also suspects, the information in the cell nucleus is something more than he had previously thought: "There is indirect confirmation that speech is recorded on DNA, among other things, and it is, so to speak, the speech of the Creator".

Therefore Garyaev admits that in the crystals – which he melts – the intellect of the Creator is recorded, Who placed there primary information in the form of codes, in accordance with which everything living on Earth develops. And if the program is disturbed, then various freaks are born, diseases proliferate in the world, humanity suffers from losing the meaning of its existence.

What I have stated above was not said in order to throw stones of condemnation at any of the researchers, but to call on them to exercise caution. Because they have come into the House of the Creator. Should one really behave in His House in such an inappropriate manner, as if one were part of a SWAT team on a mission?

Besides, it is unsafe to do so.

Perhaps to some of the knights of science with their motto "I want to know everything", my warnings would seem like copybook moralizing. "Enough of that, you are boring us." I remind them of an old Korean tale. A wise man came to one couple and asked them: "do you want to learn to fly?" – "Yes, we do!" – "Here, take those magic robes; once you put them on and button three buttons, you will fly up high! And in order to..." – "We know, we know!" – cried out the impatient spouses. – Give them to us now!" They put on the robes, buttoned the three buttons and took off. They flew around for a while, and it was time to go home. But they did not know how to descend, because they did not listen to the old man to the end. They fiddled with the buttons every which way, but nothing helped. You understand how it ended, don't you?

It's time for our empiricists and positivists to think not one move in advance, but ten or twenty, and see not only the queen (that is the person they love most – themselves), but all the figures on the chessboard of the universe. But the most important thing is to know the rules of the game which they continuously break, chasing ephemeral success.

Lately more and more employees of classified laboratories come to our Center asking for help. They have worked on developing some kind of ideas of their own, penetrating the secrets of the cellular nuclei, without delicacy, using violence, – and suddenly they noticed that next to them people were coming down with incurable diseases, the people closest to them: children, wives, parents. And the researchers themselves paid with their physical and spiritual health: someone gradually going blind because of irreversible calcification of the blood vessels of their vision system, some gradually turning into "vegetables" – that is, slowly losing knowledge and intellect as the information on their brain neurons was erased.

Why does this happen? It is easy to guess: if you are engaging in violence over any living object – whether it is a cell or a person, – a counteraction immediately forms in the information field of Earth and it strikes back. Sometimes the strike is quick and immediate, and sometimes it is prolonged and didactic, with the purpose of bringing you to an understanding of the absolute truth. This is like the last question, when you look eternity in the eye: "For the sake of what were you doing all this?"

And it is impossible to keep silence – it is necessary to answer. But what is the answer? I wanted power over others, or the wealthiest ones, and ran people over while fighting for my dream? Or – "They paid me and

I did it"? I can tell you in advance: none of those types of answers will count. When I see people who are sick and run down by life, I certainly want to help them. But there is the question: for what are they being punished in this way? This question should not only sound in my soul. The people who are thus afflicted in life must also think about the reasons for what happened. Because properly understanding one's misdoings and a fair sentence against oneself may frequently start in the organism a reverse process: the process of recovery. That is, the health of the body directly depends on your spiritual health, on whether you hear the voice of your soul. On sincere repentance. Whys is this not a technology? It is unusual? I agree. But still, it is a technology nonetheless. And the results are quite statistically meaningful.

So, employees of various classified laboratories are coming for help. They have experimented with nature a lot. Now nature experiments with them. One day a man like that came to us: very strongly built, even powerful, with a military haircut. A real colonel. His name was Sergey Aleksandrovich. The only problem was – his vision was deteriorating very quickly. At the Helmholtz Moscow Research Institute of Eye Diseases they tried a lot of things, but they were afraid to offer even a hope of recovery. And the dire prospects did not stop at blindness. The specter of a wheelchair was squeaking somewhere just around the corner.

The main problem was the cerebral cortex. Figuratively speaking, the grey matter of the brain is the computer, and the white matter is the receiver. The receiver refuses to convey to the computer the information that it is receiving. Even though both at the top, at the receiver level, and at the bottom, at the computer level – everything is working.

We looked at the eyes – the nerves were white. And they should be red, therefore, there had to be insufficient blood supply. The blockage started from the cervical area of the spine. There was flow towards the brain, but practically no outflow. Looking at this picture it was surprising not that the person was blind but that he was alive at all. Near the pituitary gland the picture was very strange: blood was practically not moving at all. Under the pituitary gland, in the Turkish saddle area, something was blocking the outflow.

The venous outflow showed insufficient blood pressure. While on the arterial blood side it was normal. We looked into the vessels. On the walls inside there was something whitish, like scale in a kettle. This was calcium. And further on, starting from the cervical area, there were blockages and blood clots everywhere. It was multiple sclerosis. And the medical specialists did not know what was causing it. That's why Sergey Aleksandrovich's hair growled as if on a corpse: sticking out in all directions in some sort of bunches. The electrolyte metabolism was out of balance. His blood became thicker. The Colonel said that lately he had stopped drinking water; he did not feel like eating meat. The organism was shutting down its desires one by one.

It was, of course, possible to run a battery of tests and establish the physical causes of the disease. But when looking at the course of events that brought Sergey Aleksandrovich to his current sorry state, first of all we were shown the laboratory, in which the walls were covered with tiles, and all the equipment was made of stainless steel. This was where our new patient used to work. There were mice, rats and hamsters. Incisions were made on their limbs. Some viruses were introduced in the wounds. Everything was clear: Sergey Aleksandrovich was involved in the development of bacteriological weapons. In this laboratory they were seeking new viruses which could instantly destroy cells. And in addition they were developing substances, stimulating psychotropic effects for influencing

470

people. And he came to us not only as a patient (even though this aspect of coming to the Center was quite real), but also as a person, studying our technology, trying to understand what lay behind it. The lies that were part of his objectives create obstacles for both himself and us. If he only knew how much it gets in the way...

We tried to help him, but insincerity or, rather, the halfway truthful attitude of the colonel again and again threw us – and himself – back from the positions we managed to fight off from the disease.

At this time the illness had surrendered many of its fortresses that seemed insurmountable earlier. Sergey Aleksandrovich felt considerably better than before. His relatives did not have to support him as he walked when he came to our Center; he could even write; he could also read large print, even though with difficulty. It was obvious that there was spiritual work going on inside of him. And despite the fact that from time to time he shared with us that he dreamt of returning to his laboratory, there were signs of doubt in him: should he really do that? It seemed that he had not yet made the final decision as to which shore he wanted to choose for coming out from the river of his troubles. Apparently we will also have to come back to this story in our future books. Because the choice has to be made. And not only the health of the individual person depends on this choice, but a lot more. Because every person by being connected to the world interacts with the entire universe.

Crystals of cell nuclei, with which laboratories of many counties are playing Gestapo, store the innermost information about man and humanity. Any damage to them immediately affects individual people and society at large.

There is a strange situation. On the one hand, the scientific and technological development of society is bringing humanity closer to truly demiurgic power, granting us the capacity to influence the processes of the material spheres and vacuum sphere space of the Universe. On the other hand, the conceptual positions with respect to the main areas of our perception of the world are not that different from views prevalent not only in the XIX, but even the XVIII century.

Naturally, the scientific library of the XX century contains many prophetic, heuristic statements and conclusions. Without thinking, off the top of one's head it is possible to name a dozen or more brilliant authors who warn about the relativity of modern knowledge and about global dangers: Poincare, Tsiolkovsky, Einstein, Saint Exupéry, Chesterton, Stanislaw Lem, Asimov, Mamardashvili, Sakharov and others. But for the overwhelming majority of our contemporaries they are just eccentrics sticking their tongues out at the world, like Einstein on the famous photograph.

Millions of ordinary intellectuals read their works for entertainment, like a sales girl from a vegetable shop reads a blood-chilling thriller before bedtime to compensate for her boring everyday wretched existence. Great ideas cannot break through the quarterly and five-year plans of scientific research institutes and laboratories, through the barriers of hospitals and clinics. Being determines consciousness – this ominous part of the formula of the universe has still not lost its applicability. But everything could be the other way around: the way consciousness is – and so it would be being as well. And no matter what is the attitude which heads of laboratories show towards various prophesies and warnings as they are having a smoke break, after returning to their working desks they will resume the job to which they are accustomed and which they find so convenient: we are just small people. They would not even think to consider themselves at a level equal to God, with His objectives, and feel responsibility towards Him.

Researchers still cannot decide on the veracity of concepts on the basis of which even the most outstanding results have been received. And that puts in doubt many of the fundamental positions of modern science, makes completely unacceptable dogmatization of any laws and theories, because in our changing world everything changes – including theories, laws and absolute truths. Therefore it is better to orient oneself not towards the vain conclusions of the human mind, but on the commandments of God. It is better to understand this today rather than tomorrow, when it will be too late.

Modern scientific views of outstanding theoretical scholars such as David Bohm with his holographic model of the Universe in which an image entirely identical to the original carrier can live its own separate independent life, and neurologist Karl Pribram who discovered that computer hardware roughly corresponds to the configuration of the human brain, make it possible to transform the reality to which we are accustomed into a new cosmogony, and touch the basis of life – the all-encompassing force that in the scientific circles is generally called Higher Reason.

Development and scientific study and application of the possibilities that this open could substantially decrease state expenditures in many areas of its activities, while at the same time significantly increasing the effectiveness of work in such crisis-prone and costly areas as education, medicine, astrophysics, environmental protection, nuclear power, prospecting for mineral resources, troubleshooting at nuclear power stations, oil and gas pipelines, banking and finance operations as well as many other areas.

And now, since you are so impatient, let's take a look at one of the crystals of the nuclear cell, peek into the inner sanctum, but gently and carefully, without violence. And bear in mind: this is on the informational level, not the physical one.

It is only possible to access the crystal through the dark plane. This is a major problem. It means that not everyone can enter but only those in whose soul there are no false goals, egotistical ambitions, who are ready to sacrifice themselves for others, not others for themselves. This is the first access code. If you dial it right – you are already inside. But for now let's look at the crystal from the outside.

It is very beautiful, similar to a cut diamond. It is elongated. One end is sharp, the other is a flat plane, like the Soviet logo of quality assurance. The Pentacle is the sign of life. If you count the planes of the crystal – on the top, at the side of the pentacle – there are 24 of them (there were twenty four Elders at the Altar). At the bottom, at the point of the crystal, there are 12 planes. But not all planes are visible, there are hidden planes as well.

Crystal is a very complex structure. Everything here is in symbols, everything is in code, and everything is encrypted. For example, the edge of the crystal. And what lies behind that? An edge is not necessarily where two planes cross; it is a point where a multitude of projections intersect. But one has to think not of geometry alone when dealing with the creation of the Creator.

There is an English word database, which means nothing else other than a database. But when you look at the House of the Father, you should think not only about the information you would like to have.

Each plane of the crystal contains information which is directly related to any of the planes that have common edges with it. It's intersecting information. Following the crossing points it is possible to find references to everything else. Convenient, isn't it? But is it with your personal convenience that you should be concerned while knocking at the door of the House of the Father?

474

If you look at any plane of the crystals, in it is possible to obtain from it the precise address coordinates of any of the edges. (In its structure this crystal is similar to "hypertexts" on which the Internet is based). But are you, coming into the House of the Father, going to wander around His universe on your own? I am warning you: you will see the address of everything, but not this plane.

Spirit shows the way, connects the coordinates. If you look where you need to, you will know precisely why you are sick. It's the same as using a reference file: if a kidney is affected, you look under "K" for kidney, and it tells you about everything with which kidneys interact.

Crystal is knowledge. The beam goes there and it arrives at the soul. The Sun has sent that beam. Having reached the ionosphere of Earth, the beam hits its resilient elastic surface; resonance occurs and is immediately transmitted via the intravacuum channels to each crystal for which it was intended.

I think, this is where we shall stop for now.

But I cannot refrain from a small epilogue.

In one children's film a magician made the right decision and gave up the occult. "Why?" – a guest asked him in surprise. The magician's servant clarified: "He understood that people should not be allowed near miracles. There are a lot of people in the world, but little honor. Not enough for everyone".

The experience of humanity is convincing: higher energies require a higher moral level. Unfortunately, people try to use any new knowledge not for spiritual purposes but for pragmatic and utilitarian ones. To benefit themselves and harm others. That leads to new trouble. Nuclear energy led to Hiroshima and Chernobyl. Powerful computers brought forth computer viruses and dishonest hackers. Therefore, when you touch your consciousness to the high and divine, do not forget the advice by Bulat Shalvovich Okudzhava: "The most important think is to have pure thoughts, and everything else will just follow".

Of course, we don't know and don't understand many of the laws of nature of both our world and other ones. We do use them, however, on the basis of intuition or by observing the pattern of events.

But here we are talking about a different thing. About the ratio of the strength of the feelings to the strength of the mind, as was Mikhail Prishvin's definition of morality. Because the troubles listed above occur precisely due to a lack thereof. "On our word of honor − it will not explode!" − the nuclear specialists stated when they commissioned the reactor of the Chernobyl nuclear power station. This word of honor is recorded in official documents. Then, computer viruses do not exist in nature by themselves; they are created and disseminated by specialists who are rather good at what they do. Either they are too determined, or certifiably crazy. And then pop music becomes more and more psychedelic − is it that magical formulas of satanic cults are used as part of it in order to turn the audience into zombies temporarily? There are statements that humanity on the whole is perfecting itself in terms of virtue; maybe that's why psychic terrorism has become so threatening in form. The war of the worlds, so to speak.

About ten years ago Anatoliy Kashpirovskiy was the idol of Soviet TV watchers. It is said that now he lives in New York and still conducts extrasensorics sessions. The audience is smaller, however, by several orders of magnitude: the congregation in Roman Catholic churches and synagogues. (The priests allow him to use temples for his unusual practices.) In the temples of other countries these methods of increasing attendance are not even considered extreme. However, the problem is not with the

476

personal failure of the healer, who all but considered himself a new messiah. The problem is in his methodology.

The users of occult psychic energies frequently underscore that their main purpose is therapy, healing patients using nontraditional methods of influence. So Kashpirovskiy at his sessions proclaimed: "I bring you only good; I set the objective for good!" It was left to one to guess what is the definition of good from the standpoint of the healer himself and what it is from the standpoint of the millions of his viewers.

Soul is not a part which is mass-produced, not a standard vessel made for receiving some kind of fluid. It is always individual – that's why we are all personalities. And everyone has their own understanding of good and evil. And to offer to everyone a common "goal" of a psychic who is not so well educated and who is far from saintly is a superstition at the very least.

The psychics who work with a large audience in huge halls are comparatively few these days. The majority prefer to attend to their patients individually. But again the same questions concerning order in the world rear their heads: what is the norm with respect to health, what is success in life, happiness after all? The influence on the patient is performed at the level of fine matter, subconsciousness, of the soul (each ESP school has its own terminology). And what happens to the soul during this intrusion?

Here is a small range of printed ads. "Mages of higher level sin-free magic" promise the return of the husband, "absolute elimination of the rival". "Absolute" – what do they mean by that? In all senses, that is, at the physical level as well? "You will feel the result immediately" – the mages promise. Apparently, it must mean that your rival will be killed in front of your eyes.

"Will return your loved ones. Real. Sin-free, reliable". "All types of magic! Fast acting sin-free love spells". "Breaking hex spells, evil eye spells, generational curse spells, curses of loneliness; weight loss without dieting". And so on in the same manner.

From hundreds of the advertisements that fill modern newspapers, it is easy to understand the circle of illnesses that puzzle extrasensorics specialists and parapsychologists. Everything that there is which is vain and selfish in the world, all possible material benefits are promised to come true practically in an instant. If you take a white mouse and place an electrode in its brain to excite the pleasure center – it will need nothing else, it will be happy to the point that it will not even feel like eating. And so it continues until it dies simply of hunger.

The saddest part is that those kind of healers do not feel any embarrassment exploiting the current attraction of entrepreneurs towards religions. It is as if they do not know that no magic can be "sin-free". Do not understand that "powerful talismans for business and successful trade" are the idols in the temple of the golden calf. Their understanding of good and evil is rather primitive and single-minded, as is their trusting clientele. They have a superficial understanding of illnesses, everyday and other problems as purely negative phenomena.

Both this book an the previous one are, in essence, research into the consciousness and internal world of a person. In the process of this research Igor Arepyev and I discovered that in principlee everything is available to the consciousness – from the first days of creation to events that have not occurred yet. Many people, once they get into the magic country of archetypes where virtual events transform into real ones, lose their orientation, start perceiving everything not as a path, but as the achievement of some magical status of existence. Therefore I perceive the self-classification by some people as magician, wizard, hierophant, etc. like a diagnosis.

I can believe that some of those psychics sincerely believe that the gift

478

of healing was sent to them from above, and not from "below". But they are still spreading evil, because they show indulgence to bourgeois cares and the feeling of comfort of "lesser ones" – that is, common citizens, who are far from spiritual needs. It says in the Bible: evil is inevitable in the world, but woe to someone through whom it comes into the world.

José Ortega y Gasset in "Revolt of the Masses" quotes the following joke. A gypsy came to confession. The priest asked him: "Son, do you know the ten commandments of the law of God?" To which the gypsy replied: "Well, Father, it's this way: I was going to learn them, but I heard talk that they were going to do away with them." It seems as though this is the situation in the world in which we live.

Someone would object that orthodox priests also engage in healing. This is true, but the principle there is fundamentally different.

People from all over the country come for healing to Prior German (Chesnokov) at the Holy Trinity Lavra of St. Sergius. (I spoke about him with deep reverence in my previous book.) He has been for many years healing people from diseases of the soul which are called, in the language of the Church, demoniac possession. The procedure of exorcism starts with the sermon "Prior to the rite of exorcism of demons from a person". Here are a few provisions of this sermon. I am quoting from the 1998 edition:

"Sinners and infidels, even as they lie sick, still refuse to, still do not want to understand that their flesh is full of sin ... No, they lie there and say: "Someone cast a hex spell on me, there are evil people, wizards, they cast an evil eye over me".

You should not have sinned, man!

Father German does not only heal, he also teaches. As it turns out, sickness and misfortunes are the consequence, the result of our unright-

479

eous life, or that of our ancestors. And then, after the person is healed, Prior German calls upon the person to lead a spiritual life, not try to attain the pleasures of the day.

In this context the promises of various mages to resolve the client's problems once and for all look so thoughtless. "Till the end of your life", as one quack promises. Oh well, those whose souls are lazy crave outside help – and they receive what they deserve because of their laziness.

But we are calling you to a different thing: you must understand that no disease comes without reason. Look for the source of trouble in yourself, in your thoughts. It happens sometimes though that someone has to pay for their kin: parents or ancestors. In any case there is a reason. The person must on his own, through the work of his soul, obtain and preserve his health and happiness. This position is well in line with all the world religions. We are just helping you to see the way. The way towards the absolute truth.

* * *

More new characters appear around us. A beautiful young woman, Katerina, came from the Ukraine. She has beautiful blonde hair and very expressive Polovets face. A strange combination of the fair-headed Slavs and Asian Steppe dwellers. Sometimes, when she forgets herself, her cheekbones show very sharply, and something ancient, powerful and dangerous appears in her face. But a second later the smile covers the internal substance with external gloss.

She says that she came from the Ukraine especially in order to guard Igor and me. She says that she had a dream, in which she saw holy divine hierarchs, who ordered her to abandon everything and find us. That was her mission. She left two children in Nikolayev – and so here she is, playing bodyguard.

All this looks like vaudeville to me. Igor treats her more seriously.

I am trying to explain to the volunteer that no one has requested such a sacrifice from her: to abandon her children and undertake a social project of some kind of guarding activity.

– But I did not do it by myself. I was forced, – Katya explains. – They practically made me abandon my home, my work, my children and come here to you.

– Who did that?

– Well, you are the clairvoyant ones, take a look at who is there behind my back.

So we take a look. Behind Katya's back several dozen saints and hierarchs of light appeared. So what is one to say? After that she started interfering in our work with the patients – in an active and demonstrative manner, as if for show. She has her own techniques, and they are quite effective. However, to say that this is the highest level possible would be a major exaggeration. For some reason I don't like her. And I try to interact with her as little as possible.

A few weeks later Katya became so active that she started literally filling everything with herself. Every morning she would come to work before Igor or myself, settle down in the office and see the patients as if someone actually asked her to do so.

Sometimes I try to object, send her out into the waiting area. But nothing helps: she waits till I leave, and gets into the office again. Igor does not send her away, on the contrary, he encourages her. And when I once pressured him about this situation, which I considered wrong, he suddenly confessed:

– Remember in the Divine Kingdom two angels helped me mount my horse? I was quite exhausted at the time.

– Yes, I remember.

– So, one of those angels was Katya.

– Are you sure?

– It seems to me so.

–You should make the sign of the cross over yourself when things seem to you, – I advised him.

– Well, you saw for yourself who was behind her. It was the light hierarchy.

A week later Igor started seeing patients together with Katya already in the open, even in a somewhat confrontational manner. Feeling this strong support, the light messenger started interfering in everything and bossing everyone. Our staff hated her. Because of her the Center started looking like a miniature psychiatric hospital of Andrei Bilzho*. But Igor does not see any of that or does not want to see. He openly supports the strange impostor.

Katya is continuously proclaiming something. She says that in her eye some kind of camera is embedded, through which all our actions are monitored. She tries to barge in to be seen by Grigori Petrovich, but not very successfully. She is always trying to find something out, and arrange something. But what is it?

One day she brought to the Center some kind of prayer. She walks around me with this sheet and mumbles something endlessly. I am not particularly given to church rites, even though I am not generally opposed to that. But when it is done in this pushy manner, and every day repetitive mumbling continues – it is bothersome. One day I could not stand it any more and asked her:

– Katerina, why don't you go to a church and read your prayers there.

* Modern Russian writer and cartoonist

482

– But listen, Arkady Naumovich, what words these are! – And immediately started reciting:

From the point of Light that is in the Mind of God,
May light flow into the minds of the people.
May the Light come down to Earth!
From the point of Love, that is in the Heart of God,
May the love flow into the hearts of the people.
May Christ return to Earth!
From the point of the Center, where the Will of God is known,
May the goal direct the small wills of people -
The goal which the Teachers are serving.
From the point of the Center, which we call the tribe of the people,
May the Plan of Love and Light come true,
And may the door be locked, behind which evil lurks.
May Light, Love and Power restore
The Plan on Earth. **

– Those are good words, – I confirmed, softening.
– So, say: "Amen!"
– Amen! – I gave in.
Katya's eyes suddenly widened and her lips began trembling.
– Light, – she cried out, – I see the light! – And ran out of the office. A few minutes later she returned together with Igor.
– Why, when Arkady Naumovich said: "Amen!", was there a beam of light from above? Who is he?
Igor smiled.

** This represents an original translation.

483

– Katya, maybe, we should call the men in white coats for you? – I suggest. – Igor and I set up this light especially during classes and diagnostic work. It is not difficult at all.

But for a very long time this unexpected light bothered Katya. Several times she tried to find out not only from me but from our staff about other instances when at my command this light appeared. It was almost like being in the middle of a "CSI" plot.

It is not clear what visions visited Katya that time. But after that incident with the prayer and light she began suffering. Her right arm started hurting a great deal. She explained to us that some man's fingers had been cut off with a circular saw and she had immediately rushed to help. Stopped the bleeding, closed the energy field around the stumps. In general, rendered some assistance, but since no one actually asked her to help and she acted sort of spontaneously – now her arm hurt. We tried to help her, and for a time she felt better, but then the pain would return.

During the time that Katya spent around us her hair grew out and black roots started showing. The blonde turned out to be not so blonde after all. The zone of instability around our voluntary bodyguard kept expanding. No one could tolerate her; the staff of the Center openly mocked and derided her; but, as the popular expression goes, she could not care less.

She openly said nasty things about Grigori Petrovich, called his secretary a demon because he did not let her through to see his boss. All this was so much at odds with the image of an angel she was trying to present and which Igor supported, strange as it may seem. If angels really are the way Katya is, it would be better to stay an atheist. Because of her I started quarrelling with Igor.

– Over the years we have been together through grave hardship; we split all the difficulties evenly, – I said to my friend. – Have I ever set any kind of conditions or stipulations that I would help you with something if you do this or that for me? I just did what needed to be done, without any conditions, not trying to make anyone owe me. But here comes a pretty face from the Ukraine, and now you and I see each other and work together a lot less than we used to. She is taking the first place for you in everything. You study our technologies with her several hours a day. But are you sure she is the kind of person she is trying to present herself as?

Igor was embarrassed, but stood his ground:

– But you have seen yourself that the hierarchy of the forces of Light is behind her?!

– And so what? Thoth-Hermes also hid behind the name of the God. The way she interprets all the events turns everything into a myth. Maybe that is what the ones who sent her are trying to achieve? And besides, you said that the angel who helped you mount had fair hair. And Katya's black roots are showing very clearly. She is not a blonde – quite the opposite. Remember, Kirill warned us that an angel of Darkness would come. Maybe that is the case here? Because things seem to become really chaotic around her.

– She has black hair? – Igor asked again.

– Yes, she does. And she has a Polovets face besides. Can't you see? I have a feeling that someone has put a glamour spell on you.

Igor is hesitating, but still objects:

– She was sent by the hierarchy of the forces of Light.

– Even if it was of Light, – I am almost screaming now. – Why so much pressure? And who altogether, even among the adepts of Light, would make such a strange decision – to part mother and children for many months? And again, everything is done from a position of force. Not how she talks: "Do as I say. Can't you see who is giving orders through me?!" And who is speaking through her? The Creator communicates with us directly, He does not need intermediaries. When the Father tells me "you do not depend on anyone; listen to your heart", – this is understandable. These are the words of One Who respects the freedom and will of the person. And I do not care on behalf of which hierarchy she presents herself. I have the Father, and I am not going to look for any other Fathers who would be better or stronger. Once a traitor – always a traitor. Even if all hierarchs, light and dark, unite against the Father, I will stand by the Father. He speaks with us, teaches us. And the things He teaches us are confirmed on a daily basis by our people's health. We have already lost many days because of this Katya. This is like the story with Kirill. The days are passing and how do we make up for what we have lost? Grigori Petrovich simply does not let people like that near him. Listen to what she says in the Center: "Why do you need to resurrect anyone – Christ will soon return and resurrect everyone". Is this what the Creator tells us? It does not match ...

The next day after our disagreement, however minor, our student Sergey stopped me in the hallway.

– Arkady Naumovich, I would like to talk to you.

– Sure, let's go to my office and have a one to one.

I sat down in an armchair. Sergey settled down nearby.

– I worked with Katya yesterday, – he said. – I clearly saw her core within her informational structure.

– And something bothered you in what you saw, – I encourage Sergey, seeing that he is feeling shy.

– There is a real demon there – complete with horns and hooves. He is hiding behind a dark veil. But it was possible to see it clearly a couple of times. I think she is being manipulated. Note the way she talks. It's like

486

a TV set when you turn it on. And if the power is cut – and that has happened several times already – her eyes just go completely empty and not a single bright thought in her head.

Naturally, I conveyed to Igor what Sergey had said. Katya also learnt about Sergey's observations. And she immediately raised a scandal and demanded arbitration judgment from Grigori Petrovich.

I did not want to bring this victim of schizophrenia to Grabovoi, but Igor firmly decided to put a decisive end to Katya's story and, as he said, ferret out the absolute truth. The three of us went. In the hallway about thirty people were waiting – as usual. Another ten or so were at the reception area. We told his secretary, Georgiy, that we were requesting a meeting of about twenty minutes. I was thinking to myself "This little piece of work is going to take more than twenty minutes to sort out".

But Grigori Petrovich, through the secretary, somehow separated our strange bodyguard from us and invited only Igor and myself into his office.

Every time I meet with Grigori Petrovich, one word comes to my consciousness, like a key describing the situation. This word is composure. It is amazing how well Grabovoi controls his emotions. No matter what is happening, what kind of wild situations and ranges of human passions are rushing into his office, he is always calm, unflappable, reasonable and, most important, knows what to do and how to help.

So in this case as well we did not even have to explain anything. He immediately, precisely and calmly explained the events.

– Guys, this is an elementary thing to do. One takes a snapshot. In this particular case it was taken at the time of Armageddon, when all the holy hierarchy was observing the battle. Then the negative was lit up with the sun a little – and the backdrop was ready. When your girl says "look at who is standing behind me, who sent me", – at that moment you are shown the backdrop: the negative lit by the sun.

He was not reproaching, just explaining. But there was puzzlement behind his words: how was it possible to lead you astray so? You were caught by such a simple trick.

Igor was embarrassed. His clairvoyance works better then mine. But it turned out that my intuition in this particular case led us better than his vision.

– Besides, you mentioned that her arm hurts, – Grigori Petrovich continued. – Don't you see what she has in her hand?

– A spear? – Igor finally regained his ability to see.

– Yes, it is a spear. And it is an unusual one. It's just that she has not decided yet which one of the three of us she is supposed to strike with this spear. The strike must be precise and reach its goal. The connections between the components of our structure are very fine. How do you hit them with such a large weapon? So she is looking for a place to hit the goal without missing.

– And we nearly brought her into your office, – I shared the belated comprehension of danger that we avoided by sheer luck

– No problem, – calmly responded Grigori Petrovich. – First of all, at this time she does not have the spear with her. And this means there is someone else whom you cannot see, and to whom she could entrust it. Because this kind of spear you can't just leave in the corner. It is only possible to transfer it from hand to hand, like a baton. Secondly, one has to peruse one's future events and place protection there or change the course of events if they are not to our liking. Because that is what we do – controlling clairvoyance. Control – you understand, what is in that word?

We discussed with Grigori Petrovich a few current issues, said our good-byes and left. In the hallway Katya rushed to us:

– So, did you find out about me?

– Yes, we did, and now we are going back – it was more of an order than a suggestion on my part.

Katya looked at Igor expectantly.

He confirms it.

– Katerina, it is late. Let us disperse and go to our homes. We will talk about everything in the office tomorrow.

She felt in his voice that everything had changed rather dramatically with respect to her, and she refused to put up with this outcome. She turned around, returned to the reception area, and, pushing away from the door Grabovoi's secretary, who is taller then our self-appointed "bodyguard" by a head, barged into the office. Georgiy rushed after her, but came out alone. Grigori Petrovich, after all, decided to sort things out with her.

About fifteen minutes later Katya came out to us. And she was a different person now. Not a word about why she came here, what it was that she had wanted to find out. We went to the car in silence, got in and drove to Pushkino. Katya looked out the window all the while. When she turned towards us, here eyes were clear and peaceful. It seemed as though she had forgotten all her obsessive paranoid ideas. Close to Pushkino she said in a calm normal voice:

– I miss my children so much.

The next day Katya simply disappeared. She left for her hometown of Nikolayev. But the spear that she had brought with her surfaced again some time later – in a most unexpected way, and in action, too.

The next day, while Igor was seeing the patients, Sergey and I sat down together to try to understand this whole strange situation around Katya. And right away we saw both the lit-up film and what was hiding behind it: that's what it means when your consciousness is oriented properly. It was a collage with skillfully inserted groups of the holy hierarchs in white and golden clothes. But why had we not seen before how obviously static they were? Everything was set and motionless, like a common photograph. Well, actually, this was a photograph. It was just a large one and glued into the backdrop. Apparently, Katya used something like hypnosis, so that we would not notice that the subjects were unusually still. However, ordinary hypnosis would not have affected Igor and me. So, there are some other technologies which we have not studied or understood yet.

Now we took a look at what was behind the film. And there were four medium-level demons sitting around in armchairs. Where had they come from? After our forays with Igor to the lower levels there was nobody left there. They must have hid somewhere and waited until it was over. Then they looked around. There was no one in charge – in fact, there was no one at all. What would they do? It is not possible to change the core of one's being just so. For millions of years the only things they had done were various nasty tricks and perfecting their skills in evil deeds. So they must have decided to change something.

Took a look to see who was available on Earth to work for their department. Brought in, you can say, a stray malefactor for this critical assignment. Likely they had not even explained how empty and quiet everything had become down there. They must have decided to play an all-or-nothing game: either they would win everything or lose everything. This is their nature: it draws them to extremes. In a word, they are gamblers. That's probably how they gambled away their souls at some point.

The demons in turn saw Sergey and myself and understood at once. It did not even occur to them to run and hide somewhere. And on the other hand – where was there to run to or where to hide? They were outlaws now. Running would only make it worse. You could get killed on the spot for that. Oh, what a time this is: not people are afraid of demons, but demons are afraid of people. They oink with their pig snouts, and make guilty expressions on their mugs. But they are not asking for anything. They understand that they are in it up to their ears.

We took them carefully by the scruffs of their necks, like guilty kittens, and dragged them to the Abyss, where under the sealed lid the great laundering of the dark part of the universe is going on. So we threw them in there for good measure. They plopped into the energy demon whirlwind, turning around, started screaming like a cat with pinched tail. We shut the lid again, and my double with a book under his arm neatly sealed it again.

Now that we were done with this, we started searching on the problem of: to whom had Katya given her sting? Who had it now, who was hiding nearby holding it?

We could see the arm that took the spear. It was slender and smooth. A young man or a woman would have skin like that.

And the spear is not so simple. The shaft is black. There is a flag on the end. This spear is left over from some old Armageddon. There is an informational mechanism inside it. If it hits the target accurately, the pike opens up and an energy torus appears on the end. It's just that there is a problem with accurate aiming. This is not the physical plane, but the informational one. It has its own tricks, protections, mirages and illusions. But it's only possible to hit once. It's unlikely that the offender would get another chance to use his weapon. And another important question – whom should you hit? If you miss, the last chance would be lost. That's why Katya was so tormented. At the end she became downright hysterical: time was running out and it was still not clear who should be hit with the spear and where to aim it. Any demon would just go crazy from all this.

We started looking through the levels to see if there were any stray inhabitants still there. Everything was empty. But in one of the rooms, at the lowest level, we saw an old regency style table. There was a book on it. And a chair next to it. To the side there was some kind of a folding screen behind which there were vaguely visible shadows. This seemed to be their office. We looked behind the screen – and saw transparent statues the height of a person. Like dolls. But this was what was there now. There used to be archons before, or, rather, their prototypes. This was like a jacket on the chair in the manager's office: if someone looked in, it would create the impression that the boss was somewhere nearby. As to whether it was really true – who knows? Only in their realm everything was based on so much fear that no one would dare look behind the screen. And so everything was running under the supervision of the puppets from dawn till dusk. Even though the latter are in short supply there, I mean dawns and dusks. There are just torches and lamps all around. Not much natural light though. What a life, nothing to write home about, frankly speaking.

Now we look at the informational traces – and found a familiar one right away. Lapshin worked here. And he was not even an archon, just a gofer for an archon. When time started approaching the end of times, it suddenly dawned on him that it was just the prototypes of archons sitting behind the screens, not the archons themselves. Actually, he had just enough brains to not look behind the screens. He understood that even though there were dolls sitting there, but the informational trace from his entry would remain and he would be noticed. Therefore he started to look, very carefully, into the book that was lying on the desk.

This was the book of Satan himself. And it was written with blood. It dealt with technologies of managing events. On the dark brown cover there was a large circle and within it a triangle, a pentagram, and a red eye above it, surrounded by twelve symbols. So he started reading this book on the sly: he was scared and nervous, his tail was shaking like that of a frightened cat, but still he kept reading. Must have been thinking about his career advancement.

At first he read everything very thoroughly. Then he started hurrying, skipping pages. Then he was just leafing through it. Then he decided to do another trick and smuggle the book through the levels onto the Earth.

It was a good idea: it does not matter who you are now; in the end everything is determined through its incarnation in the image of a human. Whatever you achieve as a person that is going to be your fixed level for eternity to come. And again it was a gambler's psychology: all or nothing at all. Because if it did not work, most likely they would have him answer for that from the bottom and blow him to smithereens at the top. But still the devil dared.

He started to drag the book through the levels. But on the fourth level he encountered sort of an invisible membrane: it would let him through, but not the book. It was possible, of course, to ask someone for help. But how does one ask – does that mean that one will have to share the power? Viacheslav always felt incredibly tense about that.

He came back and started reading again. He read about half when suddenly a possibility for incarnation presented itself in Feodosiya. A three-year-old boy, using his thoughts, by accident set up an interspace tunnel. So Viacheslav took advantage of that and performed a replacement.

So what shall we do with this book?

– Maybe we should burn it, – Sergey suggested.

– But would then happen to the people who came to receive their incarnations from the lower side? – I asked him.

– They would disappear as well.

– And what would happen to the harmony? Let's look at it from the analytical point of view.

Sergey understood the task. So he started analyzing.

– If the book were to burn, the individual information of demons who had received the incarnation would be destroyed as well. While previously that information had not been erased. When a demon came to reside within a child – and he can see all the subtle matter world. But the knowledge would still have the hidden, latent form. He would not understand why he sees things besides the physical world, the energy and informational worlds. He would think that everyone else sees things in the same way. Then all of a sudden at the age of 10-12 years his knowledge would be transformed from the static area to the dynamic. The demon should start working on accomplishing its mission, and, depending on the results it achieved, would then receive a new status in the Dark hierarchy.

– What if we set as our goal not to destroy the book, but to transform it, bring light into it? – I asked Sergey. For him this is not just an interesting adventure in life, but learning the technologies. – Because each page there is someone's life.

– Then the people would not die, but they would change. They would stop serving the Dark forces. There would be coming to Light.

– So, shall we try?

Sergey was happy about that.

We directed at the center of the book a beam of the Holy Spirit. The circle lit up, but it did not burn – rather, it looked like it was melting. Nine cells filled with fire. Space and time compressed. The book was not without its own system of protection, but it failed.

Then we started working with two beams – using a gold beam in this

494

process in addition to the silver one. On the cover all the magical signs were as if caught in an earthquake. Their vibration was distinctly visible. But the book did not burn; it was transformed.

The letters that had been written on it in blood turned into normal typographic print. Knowledge of destruction changed to that of creation. On the cover their previous sign peeled off; the red sphere separated completely, and instead of their magical signs silver zodiac signs appeared.

The pentagram and sphere which had separated rolled up as well. Underneath them appeared a light-blue film, and a cross clearly appeared on it. After that the book became transparent and sort of dissolved, disappeared. We saw points over Moscow, St. Petersburg, Astrakhan, Murmansk. There were not too many of them, a little more than forty. These were the archiving points, through them the book was connected to its users. Now all their knowledge would become static, and they would no longer have any advantages over other people. Moreover, they acquired a spark of light. And if they were to use it correctly, they could receive a chance for forgiveness. Even though at some point those people had voluntarily agreed to serve the Dark ones. Exactly in the same way as young recruits select the place of service: one wants to be a submariner, another wants to serve in the artillery or in the aerospace troops. In the same way these ones made their choice: "you give me a nice life on earth, and I give you my soul". Apparently, they managed to reach agreement. Who would have known that such a mishap would happen with Armageddon. Because everyone believes that things will turn out for the best – the Dark ones believe in the best of the dark, the Light ones – in the best of the light. And how will it work out? God knows.

That was it for Katya who had appeared out of nowhere and disappeared into nowhere. At the last moment Sergey suddenly saw her sitting by the window in a train. There were tears in her eyes. One would hope that these were tears of repentance and purification.

But again, again and again – why is it that what arises as personal sequences of events of our consciousness with Igor, would suddenly – sometimes smoothly, sometimes rather abruptly – expand beyond the individual boundaries of personal thinking and become some publicly meaningful process? Who are we? And why is this happening to us?

* * *

No one can live without having the feeling of being needed, being important. No one! But how do you live, if you do not even know who you really are? Our transient lives, as it turns out, are just fleeting scenes and acts of the endless run in the circle of incarnations. We spend enormous effort to achieve something, to become someone, but all this is not worth a thing: if the goal is false, the achievements are but illusions. You can become the most outrageous conman in the world and then all of a sudden discover that as a result of all your effort you will be doomed to start a new circle of life, where you will be the victim of those who you had deceived in your previous incarnation. This would be your reward for dishonesty and trickery. Murderers would turn into targets of other murderers and in full measure feel the evil they had spread around in their previous lives. But only a few know and understand this.

I want to know: who am I, where do I come from? I want to understand my previous incarnations – who was I, what did I do? Can I be proud of my past or should I lower my eyes in shame when others look me in the eye? And so I ask Natasha from Ivanteyevka village to go again to the library of the Valley of the Kings and look if there is any further information there about myself, Igor, or Grigori Petrovich?

We gathered in Pushkino, in our Center. Many of the students at the Center, who have already heard about fascinating stories of Natasha which she had told in a state of clairvoyance also wanted to take part in this. We allowed it for those who already had a well-working internal vision screen. So there was no lack of recorders.

Natasha is within the Egyptian library. I told her:

– Ask the keeper of the library if there is a book here about me, Igor and Grigori Petrovich.

Natasha picked up a very old book. She placed it on the stand and said:

– From one side it is possible to read this book, and from the other side – watch it.

– What is more convenient for you?

– To watch it like a film.

– Then watch.

The images started appearing. This is Olympus again. The familiar palace where in the hall with the large pool Hera was, giving orders to servants.

Hera was all dressed up and irritated. She settled on the throne (the stairs from the pool led right up to it). She was angry and sent everyone away. A girl came in looking somewhat similar to modern Natasha (she had long hair). She presented a scroll from Poseidon, that is, her father. Hera read it. Poseidon was suggesting that Hera should not "harm" some person. Hera became angry and threw the scroll in Natasha's face.

The Goddess told Natasha that the latter was not here, that not a single God would provide any advice to her. That's it, she had the girl thrown out of the palace. Now our scout was walking along an alley, among the trees.

Cupid was flying behind Natasha on the left. Natasha walked quickly and was irritated. Cupid attempted to calm her down.

– Cupid is Igor, – Natasha suddenly told us in great amazement from her distant past.

She resumed walking. She left the cypress alley, and now there were different palaces on all sides. Some were in Flora style, some in Fauna style. So those were their features or differences.

– After this it explains here how Thoth usurped power, – she stopped for a moment. – Should I read this?

– Yes, do take a look, – Igor agreed.

– Hermes came up to each God and persuaded them that they should not share knowledge with people that the gods were higher than the Creator. He formed a conspiracy, even though he failed to convince everybody. But still the majority were in favor, and the others had to give in. Hephaestus was also convinced by Hermes' eloquence. So they formed a "circle" – and Hera joined in at once.

Some just left Olympus. For example, Pan – the forest god. The argument Hermes put forth was the darkness that stood behind him. Hermes said that the Dark forces may come out on top should the gods fail to agree. The Darkness is one of the impersonations of the fourth son of Nature.

– That is clear, – I interjected in the viewing of the events. – But let's take a look at what happened to those three children whom you have already seen, one of which was consoling you just now?

– I am returning to the palace where I was the last time.

Demeter was talking to Aphrodite. Demeter was tending to stand between the two boys. The book had no light to shed on who those three brothers are. They seemed to be in a special position. And it seemed that the women taking care of them were not their mothers.

Demeter loves the child a lot and has become very attached to him; she does not want him to know that she is not his real mother. This boy was Arkady Naumovich. I could hear the continuation of a conversation between Demeter and Aphrodite, criticizing Hera, talking about their problems. Demeter knew that if the boy were to read some book, it would be necessary to work. And he was still small. She, like it had happened during the previous time, did not want him to assume such responsibility.

How strange that was: looking at those children one could not trace who their mother or father were. They were on Olympus only for upbringing. These Goddesses were just teaching them.

There was a wicker bed there. The boy whom Demeter was bringing up liked to lie in it. Actually, at that point he was rather too large for this little basket bed. Demeter was always next to him. She had a wreath made of ears of grain on her head and a light blue cloak over her shoulders.

As for the Goddess who was with Grigori Petrovich, – she wore a wreath of laurels. She went around with some books, and carried a terrestrial globe. She seemed like a strict math teacher. She knew architectural science really well too.

Next to Igor there was Aphrodite. There was some man there as well. No one could see him. His facial features were changing all the time. He could become a wall, or some insurmountable partition. He could divide everything apart by means of his own self. This man was saying little, but if he did say something that would be final! He said so and that was it.

Now I could see a different picture. Arkady Naumovich was the oldest among the children: he was about eight years old. He was lying down in his wicker basket bed. He liked to lie there playing that he was still a little baby.

Natasha was not speaking caustically, just stating the facts, but I felt somewhat uncomfortable. Because I knew that I really like that – even when I work, I prefer to either be lying down or half-sitting. I place books and drafts around myself. And I can spend many hours that way. And when someone from the family tries to scold me for lying down a lot, I deflect that with a joke "I work only lying in bed, that's the best way to work". This is a quote from a poem by Nikolay Antsiferov about mine workers. Note that as a hint.

So that's the origin of my predilection for setting myself up in comfort for work process. You could say that this rebuke came from the depths of time: you are lying around too much. Even though, on the other hand, it does not affect productivity in any way...

– Grigori Petrovich came over. He brought a book. It had a green cover. Demeter again was trying to prevent the connection between me and work that would lie ahead. Igor flew up somewhere watching from above as to what it was that Grigori Petrovich brought. He was curious. The person who came with Igor showed himself and made a sign with his hand to Demeter, telling her to step away.

She did obey, but sort of half-heartedly. And she was very unhappy.

Grigori Petrovich said: "By the will of the Father I brought you a book. And now it belongs to you."

And then he stuck the book under your arm. He turned around. Oh, and on the table over there were some sheets of paper. They were white. But once the book was placed under your arm, text started appearing on them, all by itself.

Grigori Petrovich went off towards the door. Igor was there, hovering just under the ceiling. Grigori Petrovich stopped again and said: "I have to leave now and do something that the Father directed me to do. Once I come back, I will always be with you".

That was it – the images finished appearing. The book closed.

* * *

After this trip to ancient Olympus the number of questions did not diminish. I had seen something like that before – in the form of excerpts. Now some pieces started fitting together somewhat better. But at the same time I still completely did not understand the mechanism of materialized virtuality which from day to day had shown its specific activity which could be also checked and observed using instruments.

These were not just the feelings of my consciousness isolated from reality. Particularly since not only my consciousness took part in everything that took place. Events could not be considered the internal play of the imagination of the brain because the effects that appeared as the result were not only internal, but external as well, which drew into their orbits hundreds of people.

At the same time I felt that Igor and I were in a way trying to penetrate layer after layer through sheets of consciousness, which stores in its bottomless repositories all the history of the universe – from the first days of creation to this day. But this breakthrough was, for some reason, not only our personal business but was related, and related directly, to the evolution of all mankind. In essence, it was a transformation of consciousness, which pulled after it, like a mountain avalanche, hundreds, thousands, hundreds of thousands of other consciousnesses, inevitably changing, therefore, the world in which we live.

In the evening of that same day we sat down with Igor in order to once again take a look at and give a thought to what Natasha told us.

At first Igor looked over the situation in general.

– Hermes had been building his structure for a very long time. We know whose help he used. Death has no structure. She is nobody. The name of death is Nobody. And Mugen Is Nobody as well. Following the advice of Hermes, he brought the female aspect into the male principal. In this couple one is crazy and the other one is too smart. That's why Hermes at Olympus was creating gates through a woman, who accepted an alien principality for herself.

When, based on the advice of his mother, who felt uneasy because of the ancestral mistake, Mugen had exhaled his force into the man, he had also exhaled into him his male principal and then he immediately became Death himself. The only principal remaining in him was the female one. Even though his appearance was male. But extremely disgusting. We saw him. After that – what was there for the gods to do? Hermes had caught them in a tight bind.

Then the Father divided the levels – to the right and to the left. Some decided to stand to the right, some – to the left. And some just went below altogether. Everything was democratic to the extreme. Some from then on belonged to the earthly world, and some to the celestial. To each one his own. Time came, and each left for his house. Those who belonged to earth went into the earth. They had no immortality, just reincarnation until the end of days. But why does the earth accept people into itself, why would it not change the situation? This would be something that still needs to be figured out. Something we still have not understood in the complex relationships within the universe. You are probably right since you are trying to investigate this. In order to know the future, one has to understand the past.

Igor gave praise – that was a rare thing for him. But I was more and

502

more interested about the situation with the boys. Perhaps that was true for Igor as well; but information concerning Hermes kept coming and coming from somewhere.

– Even in the dark side there was an even more terrible force which was uncontrollable. It was deep under the surface. Hermes descended down there to understand this mystery of mysteries. In his hand he carried a torch, and he was going from one cave to another, into the very bowels of the earth, where a still lake of black water was sitting.

He stood on a stone above that water and said: "Black mother, I came to enter into an alliance with you. Come with me. I will show you the path to destruction." – "I cannot, – moaned the black water, in which a female face was outlined and approached the surface. – Even the light of your torch is unbearable for me."

Hermes answered to her that he could not put it out, because then he would not be able to find his way back. He said: "I want to march against the Father in Heaven, for the sake of him and you".

This alerted me.

– "For the sake of him." Who was he implying by that?

– Wait; I may be losing the information, – Igor asked. – She said: "If you come out victorious, I will come out and blot out the light. If you lose, I will flow into many streams. If the light falls on me, I will dry out. For your sake I am tolerating the heat of the fire from your torch. But do not deplete me. Raise the torch higher, and I will wash you with my water".

Hermes brought the torch up, and a black wave washed over him. But the black water did not touch his chest, since the light of the torch was falling there.

She was talking again: "Go. Give him his fire and come back to me. Now my force is with you – no one will be able to overcome you".

– So that means that we were battling Hermes himself, – I could not help but comment again. – And that's why he had taken Death to the lower levels when the Father brought him to the edge of the absolute truth: his heart had not been touched by the black water.

– Yes, this is so, – Igor confirmed. – Now, about the boys.

Grigori Petrovich was going around carrying the book and wanted to give it to you. The book is a responsibility. And my brother was all the time hanging around the adopted mother, or the nurturer, whatever you want me to call her? He was loved and cherished. The book was not what was on his mind. Meanwhile the second brother …

– Are you talking about yourself? – I interrupted him.

Igor did not respond; he continued as if the question had never been asked:

– The other brother was there with bow and arrows. He was learning to shoot. He was playing naughty. Aphrodite showed how to nock the bow, how to aim properly. And no one could see that when the boy was shooting he was standing on a very thin edge, like a blade. He was learning to shoot standing on the edge of the absolute truth. And there was another teacher nearby, visible to no one.

– So that means everyone was busy, and I was cooling my heels in the wicker bed?

– No, not really; when Grigori Petrovich left, you came out of your little basket. You came to the table and started reading. And then you no more turned your head aside from that. Your task was to write a book and give it to the people. This is a special book – The Book of Life, the Book of times. It has not been written yet. The one that you are writing now is a different one.

– And what happened after that?

– We became independent. I was learning, as before, to shoot while standing on the edge by myself.

– And do I have an edge?

– You do. But it is different.

– Would you be able to stand on it? – I was interested.

– My edge is narrow for you and wide for me. Yours is the other way around: It is narrow for me and wide for you.

– And what did we do later?

– Later, you and Grigori Petrovich came up with a way to improve the reincarnation system – the Dragon system. The Dark ones, when it fell to them through Da'at (Hebrew for "The Abyss"), they, in their foolishness, took it apart and created their own system of reincarnation. Someone took a ruby eye, someone – a black claw. So since then they are still running around with those trinkets. Then you invented a bicycle, then built manufacturing plants. One should hurry regarding the plants. The Earth is coming to the Center of the Universe, like the point of homeostasis. Did you understand that?

– Yes, I did. As for reincarnation – is it associated with the dragon?

Igor looked at me quizzically.

– There is some kind of a strange relationship between you and this dragon. Grigori Petrovich made it. And you, like a fool, dragged it off to your sephiroth.

– And what about you?

– And another fool pushed with all his might when he saw that that you were at the end of your strength. The dragon fell into Da'at. You balked and did not want to let it go. You were dragged waist deep in there as well. What do you think as to why here in this incarnation you have problems with kidneys, liver, pancreas, appendix, gall bladder, osteochondrosis and other troubles at the navel line? It's all because of that.

– You shouldn't have pushed, – I retorted.

– You shouldn't have pulled, – Igor insisted.

Several days later Katya's pernicious spear reappeared. One of the students brought it with her as she came in to be seen by Igor; she had come to the Center long before the "bodyguard" from Nikolayev. She was talking about this and that and then suddenly in between the phrases struck Igor with that hellish sting. However, the protection worked. The spear, deflected by the protection, fell down into the empty levels of the Dark ones, and with loud clatter rolled down the stairs to the vacant thrones of the Dark Rulers.

The terrorist could not figure out whether the strike had found its target, and was watching Igor with curiosity. Meanwhile, he was at that moment also thinking – what to do with a student like that. He decided that best of all would be to keep the person for correction, and pricked her black heart with a thin ray of light. From this point her mysterious female soul would now start becoming lighter.

And down below there was no one to take up the spear: the Dark realm was deserted. Later we broke it and threw it into a pile of old armor and weaponry.

So such is life – when you are asleep or awake.

Chapter 8

Finally Igor and I started working on a long-time dream – figuring out lipid metabolism. This is a topic that is directly relevant to my health, of personal importance. As it happened, previously there was not enough time to research this topic. And now, as they say, need forced us. The thing is that we completely accidentally discovered that the lymph has its own autonomous program for counteracting cancer and AIDS. Under certain conditions it may take the viral cells out of the body. And the way the program is launched is through geometric codes.

Disruption of lipid metabolism, as a rule, depresses the level of activity of the person. Therefore we have to first see on what the tonus depends. First of all, the pituitary gland, adrenal glands, and the walls of the blood vessels themselves. There are also areas on the spine which control this process on the whole, and the thyroid gland. Its control system is hormones.

We observe how the white balls of lipids enter into the blood serum. They move along the arteries and do not enter the veins. That's why sweat is actively exuded from the armpits. And fatty growths on the body are also associated with lipid metabolism.

Lymph, in the way that we see it, is not an auxiliary system, but a primary one. And it is an autonomous system, too. It can make independent decisions. It can even interrupt control from the brain. But all this occurs at the informational plane. That's why Grigori Petrovich likes to work with geometry so much. Indeed, this is very convenient. There, in the blood cell nuclei, we can see manifestations of cylinders, triangles, ensembles of other geometric figures. If some of them were to be transformed into pentagonal shapes, the organism would gain significant support for its functioning. It is possible, for example, to transfer the information of a cancer cell into lymph, having first limited its interaction mechanisms, then split and break it down. Based on the connections which hold the organism together, this informational procedure of transformation will rather quickly have an effect on the pathological changes that appeared.

But with stones this is not the way to work. Their geometry is different. Stones have to be broken down into sand grains. How is this done? If you remove from sugar, for example, the crystal that holds its form – sugar will disintegrate. At the informational plane the archiving point is clearly visible: it holds together the entire crystalline system of the stone. We can influence it and transform it into pentacles.

Everything is interrelated – lipid metabolism and kidney stones. If there are stones in the kidneys, the blood flow slows down. And as a result there is an accumulation of waste, weight gain, obesity, fatigue. One thing affects another. But the process of healing can be activated in the same way, through the original cause. Among the hexagon informational structures which are harmful for the organism in a specific situation, it is necessary to find the one which is the leader. In other words, find the boss of all hexagons. And then manage to transform it into a pentagonal shape similar to the Soviet logo of quality assurance. At the deep level this situation is somehow related to the carbon-based and silicon-based forms of life.

Carbon is us, because it constitutes the basis of organic chemistry. And silicon is a different, deep form of life; it is possible to call it proto-life. Almost 90 percent of the Earth's mantle consists of silicon compounds. And it is all like a giant crystal. A crystal is a form of order, a form of life. Unfortunately, humanity, while trying very hard to understand what is far away, the outskirts of the Universe, has only minimally studied the closest planet in the universe – the planet on which humanity lives. It seems as though in the next book we will return to this topic; meanwhile we have located one very important lead hexagon in the chest area. Its area of competency includes the liver, kidneys and adrenal glands. We changed its geometry and immediately directed our attention to the processes inside the kidneys. As we looked, we could not believe our eyes: the stones in the kidneys started melting like sugar. We added a little water (once we started experimenting – why not go the whole hog!). The stones are melting, losing shape, breaking apart. They are washed away by the water into the urinary excretory system. Once the radical in the center was removed, everything disintegrated.

The blood flow process was accelerating even as we watched. There was no time for lipids to group into waste clusters. Everything dissipated quickly. It was obvious that the load on the heart was reduced. The patient felt better.

Was that clear, why it happened? The kidneys are a filter. In this case the filter clogged up. So it was cleaned and the waste was removed. As a result, the blood flow increased. Because all that waste had taken up some space, it was preventing access of the blood supply to the organs. If the blood were to reach the heart without sufficient pressure, we would see external signs of that as well: shortness of breath, a feeling of fatigue.

Lymph in this case takes the bulk of the load on itself and sort of provides to the person some additional time limit, sort of saying: Pay attention to your health, correct the situation, don't let it fester.

So in this way through geometry, through symbols it is possible to resolve the problem. Symbols need to be treated very seriously. Hitler, for example, once had a dream. He saw the sign of Christ – letter "X". It would be possible to work very effectively with this letter and achieve wonderful results. But the one who had shown him this letter, had a different objective. He suggested that it be divided into two halves and bent. You know what that looked like: "SS". And it is also well known as to what came out of that.

Many people will read this book and say: this is a myth. But what is a myth? I can explain that to you: it is something that happened THERE, but it is known about HERE. And if a myth is implemented in our world, then it is not a myth anymore – it is REALITY. For example, Igor and I would like to cure people from cancer; if we were not successful – that would be a myth: that there were two people in the world who could cure people without instruments or medication. However, if it had been successful, then the word "myth" would no longer be applicable.

Or I am telling you: THE ONE WHO RULES ETERNITY – LIVES FOREVER. Why do I have such thoughts? But have you never had them? But you would read this and forget. You would go to your office and sink in your problems.

However, Igor and I do it differently: we start thinking about it, doing some research: is existence without death possible? What about the resurrection of the dead? Because among those who passed away there were many people who were close and dear to us. And one day we wake up. This can happen anywhere, not necessarily in bed. We just suddenly start seeing not within the narrow range of electromagnetic waves, in which we used to see before, but in a much broader range. So much broader that we discover next to us entire worlds, complete with their inhabitants and the Father, Who created this diversity. And Who regularly visits His garden, with a pitcher in His hand, and waters every flower that asks Him for help.

He waters one flower, but the threads of connections are extended to all the others. And the flower says: "I am alive! I feel good!" And all the rest repeat those pleasant words after it: "We are alive! We feel good!" And not in just one space they say this, but in all that are accessible to us now.

Everything is interrelated, everything is connected with each other. The word that was at the beginning and the one that we are saying now.

Logos, the flower of the soul, the crystals of consciousness. Sharing unity in diversity – these are the eternal absolute truths. As many times as you look, every time you will see something new.

If the flower of life, the flower of the soul blooms in one person, soon it will bloom in everyone.

The Father was watering the flowers of the garden. The pitcher in His hand, or maybe the bowl, is the allegory of the soul. Flowers are [the allegory] of the soul as well, of the souls of people.

Father from His soul provides aid to the flower, a living organism. He grants it His attention, His care, His love.

Water is consciousness. It falls down and it carries with it information. It combines with the soil – and this is an area of consciousness as well. The area of consciousness, with the information contained in it, is absorbed by the plant and, rising upward, corrects the damage to the organism.

This is an image, but also this is the technology and the knowledge. We, using this technology in accordance with the will of the Creator, to activate the procedures of resurrection. And so now other people are saying to us: "We have seen those who are dear to us, we see another world, and now we understand how everything is arranged".

Let us listen once again to the observations and vision of those who were participating in the program of resurrection. Because they were the first to go down the road which many should follow soon. In their diaries every small thing, every detail is of enormous significance.

We are again reading the diary of Galina Borisovna Kuznetsova:

"July 22, 2001.

We came to the village with Islam Umarov, a friend of my daughter Olga. We decided to have dinner outside, by the fire. While my daughter was preparing dinner, Islam and I made the fire. I looked at him, and it seemed to me that he was alarmed by something. I asked him: "Islam, is something wrong?" He replied: "I have a feeling that I am constantly being watched by someone". I told him very briefly about Sasha and the activated process of resurrection.

As we ate by the fire, I was observing everybody. The conversation evolved by itself with respect to the new treatment methods, alternative approaches to knowledge and science.

Suddenly Islam said: "Guys, what is it with you, can you not see?"

My son-in-law asked: "See what?"

Islam responded: "She (Sasha) just touched Olga's hair and now she is touching Borisovna by the shoulders while standing behind her".

Visually Sasha could not be seen; I did not turn around so as not to scare her away) (though I had already been through that).

Olga became very still.

At that time my son-in-law Alexander started seeing something as well. He said: "Now she is walking into the house ".

I put the guest up in Sasha's room (we were using it as a guest room then). I had noticed that everyone sleeps very well in that room, noting in the morning that they had never slept so well and felt so refreshed, energetic and rejuvenated. It would be useful to note that before we always used to entertain, and friends liked to gather for holidays and other celebrations at our place. My girls enjoyed receiving guests.

In the morning I had another conversation with Islam. It turned out that in the morning he, Islam, communicated with Sasha.

In brief, he said the following:

– She loves you a great deal. Until August she still has time to think... She likes this house, but does not want to be in it alone. And what about the city? My mother, the girl said, has no home. She does not have her own place – she is staying with someone else. I will have to think...

When I saw her, she would be wearing the striped dress, like in that photograph, or a grey suit".

Not only Galina Borisovna's relatives or friends see some fragments of the resurrection in progress. I have already mentioned that both Igor and I activated the processes of bringing back our own relatives. Igor returned from his trip to Trosna and said the following:

– There were already four people who saw my grandfather. Twice he was seen by my wife, Lenara. She had not met him during his lifetime. He died eleven years ago. She was still a schoolgirl then. She came to visit a neighbor, and there was a man sitting in the room. Meanwhile the neighbor was behaving as if there was no man present in the room. But this would be impossible! If one woman were to see a person, and the other one did not! Then Lenara described him. She mentioned even his favorite cap, his checkered suit and plaid shirt. That was grandfather for sure. He was a very neat and strict person. He had spent seven years at war, had a lot of medals and awards, and never boasted about it. We did not even know where he had been fighting or for what he had received the awards. He had been a very reserved and proper man.

What was typical for those descriptions was the distinct indication that the process of resurrection occurs in stages. This is not accidental. The thing is that a person is the result of the processes of disintegration and synthesis. It is very similar to the processes of thermonuclear reactions.

First we are divided into the negative and the positive; this is followed by the procedure of division by incarnation; then at the lowest point of separation of a structure that used to be connected into a single entity, the connections of the world activate the reverse process of the synthesis. The energy that is produced both during the process of personality disintegration and in the process of its synthesis is the most valuable in the Universe, psychic energy. We ourselves need it. Because it is with this energy a person could, once he achieved a combination of all of his aspects and, therefore, integrity, perform global transformations of the Universe and Cosmos. This is how one of the laws of the universe is implemented: FROM THE SINGLE – A MULTITUDE, FROM A MULTITUDE – UNITY.

Everything needs to be collected thoroughly – all previous experience, all the things of the days of old, and even the future that never occurred here but has long ago occurred there. And besides, remember, I told you about that – during the initial period those who have been resurrected have a discrete perception of time. They perceive reality as a series of slides combined into a film. For example, they see a rose. And on the next slide they see a rose with a bee sitting on it. And one needs to figure out before the next slide comes along, how did the bee get there? Different speeds of time passage here and there requires a serious adaptation of perception. When the person remembers everything and thinks it through, he receives the right to shape the events of his future, and arrives at the regime of immortal existence directly in the physical body. Through synthesis, by balancing in himself the negative and positive energies, latent and manifested worlds. The person who has achieved integrity becomes the basis of the homeostasis of the universe. It is a very comfortable position. But at the same time it involves a lot of responsibility. He is capable of everything, but everything he is capable of he has to measure against the goal he has set and the necessity. And also it is important to remember about responsibility. Because Thoth at some point was the kind of person who was capable of everything. And he called himself God. And he even was, for some time, a God. Meanwhile this person is not someone who existed – he does exist. Do not call yourself a God, even if you become one in reality. Because you are attaining your divinity, unlike the One Who creates it.

Resurrection and immortality is a very high technology. It has a multilinear direction. It is more complex than the technology of Merkaba, about which Drunvalo Melchizedek told in his works on sacral geometry. Merkaba is very useful and wonderful. But one has to understand that at its beginning there is a static source of information. In light of the events that have so rapidly occurred on Earth over the last two or three years, this is already in the past. It is interesting as the history of the issue, but is unlikely to help with resolving the objectives which humanity is facing at this stage. There are unshakeable rules of the Cosmos, and the main one among them is: *if at least one person is capable of perceiving cosmic amounts of information at the level of new technologies, all previous knowledge becomes no more than applications to what he learns.*

And the most important things now are the technologies of the soul and of the spirit, which have never been described by anyone on earth, with the exception of some elements of the technology of resurrection. The entire history of humanity is a story about what never came true, or was never implemented, or never achieved. All this is because the spiritual aspect of our existence was not understood, studied, or needed to the necessary extent.

There is a science called psychology. This is exactly the science that should be studying the soul. But the specialists practicing this discipline

515

still cannot come to a definitive opinion as to what is the subject of their studies. It is both sad and funny, but actually more sad than funny.

* * *

Sergey, the son of Liudmila Mikhailovna Litovchenko, came from England. He lives in Gilford, being a graduate student at the University of London. His mother had told him a lot about Igor and myself. In addition, the story with Caroline had unfolded before his very own eyes, so to speak. And he had his own small unforeseen difficulties in life that he had been wanting to understand for a long time. For example, Sergey by the power of thought could at his will change traffic lights. Or become invisible from time to time. His relatives would be meeting him in the airport – his mother, father, and sister. He went by them one way and then the other way; but his relatives were looking straight through him, as if he were made of glass, and did not see him. It could be some kind of coincidence had it only happened once. But no, it was a commonplace occurrence.

Sergey was still rather young. He had a law degree. In England he was preparing to defend his doctoral thesis in law. At our meeting a large number of people gathered: Sergey's mother, our students and our staff. Everybody was interested.

When Sergey and I were being introduced to each other Igor was rubbing his hands in glee.

– I had wanted for a long time to arrange for you two to meet. And so now you have met.

Both Sergey and I looked at him in bewilderment: why was he so glad, at what was he hinting?

However, soon we saw a ray of light in the darkness of the unknown.

516

Sergey had barely associated with us for a day or two, when he suddenly acquired clairvoyance abilities. His gift started working at full blast, as if he had had it since birth. And the first thing that he saw was the world which had been bothering the public attention of the inhabitants of Earth for a long time by its open and hidden signs. The notorious UFOs which were seen lately in a lot of different countries, even though previously they had preferred to hide behind the screen of natural anomalies. The alarming fact of the presence on Earth of a different mind, another civilization, alien intelligence. They were called The Grays, and they were the ones about whom we were warned by the demon, Kirill, – or, rather, he attempted to intimidate us by them. He called their world a confederation. And when Sergey started talking about them in clairvoyance mode, he also used that word – confederation.

– I am present at the meeting of the intergalactic assembly of the confederation, – Sergey said suddenly, right in the middle of our conversation on an entirely different topic. – This is a different world, not ours. No one can see me. It is just that a tunnel was formed – something like a giant telescope. And for some reason from my location I can see and hear everything that is happening there.

Sergey was speaking evenly and calmly. But all the signs were there indicating that he was also surprised by his first experience of clairvoyance into a parallel world.

I wanted to ask Igor: from where did Sergey have such access through interspace tunnels? But I was afraid to interrupt the connection. Actually, everything became clear soon enough. Meanwhile we were listening to the narration about what was happening in one of the intermediate worlds. We were listening to it without leaving my office.

– I could see a huge oval room. In the middle there was a table. About

517

twelve individuals were sitting around it. They were tall – over 2 meters in height. They had very large, elliptical eyes. In the bleachers, as it would be in the circus or at a hockey game, there were thousands of other beings. They looked similar to people, only they had very large eyes and small mouths. But they were not people. They were screaming, yammering and raging. They were not people. They had a different organic chemical composition? – Sergey underscored once more.

– What are they screaming about? – I tried to direct the process.

– They were unhappy with the results of the latest events on Earth. Readjustment of information fields would lead to active development of our world while their world would decline. They were contracting a lot of diseases which they previously knew how to utilize in our space.

– So, they were prospering at our expense? – I clarified.

– Yes, – confirmed Sergey. – And now what they used to dump here on us has turned against them. Panic has broken out among them. They were demanding that the latest results be reconsidered. And they were threatening to start a war with mankind.

– Star wars?

– Yes, just like that, – Sergey confirmed. – They had powerful military equipment, nuclear weaponry and other military advantages. They had been working on Earth for a long time, they had representatives, residents, and bases here. They had studied people quite well and were ready to resolve the problems with the aid of weapons, contrary to the laws of the Cosmos.

– And the ones in the center, sitting around the table, – what were they talking about?

– Those would be justices of the peace. This is what they were called. They were in doubt, but it looked as though there would be no other option.

They would not like to live like people – with suffering and diseases.

– Leave now, – Igor suddenly ordered. – They have noticed you. They could see the energy lens above.

Sergey quickly came out of clairvoyance mode and looked at us, his eyes shining. It seemed as though he was very happy with his new capabilities.

– It would be time to figure out: who is who? – I suggested.

– Then the two of you would have to take a walk to the sephiroth, – Igor suggested.

It seemed as though he already knew about everything that would happen there. Confederation and the threat of star wars did not seem to worry him much. When I asked him why he was so calm, Igor replied laconically:

– All this was already in the past. They were going into the past, like the Olympic gods.

But practically a few days later we had to meet the Grays. And this was not an easy meeting. And while we were finding out with Sergey from where he had acquired those phenomenal capabilities for transgalactic travels.

Just as Igor suggested, we went off to the sephiroth. And Sergey immediately went to the left row in the sephira of Saturn immediately, without spending time to follow the way that Igor and I had to pass at one point, before we started to feel comfortable with the Space computer. There he looked around. He saw a cloud and sat down on it, as if it were a comfy sofa, folding his legs as they do in the East. That gave me a slight shock. The thing is that it was impossible to enter into a sephira in this way! There were guards there, there were codes and a very complicated entrance mechanism. One would have to know it. Sergey knew it.

In front of him, out of nowhere, a pyramid appeared and started rotating. Six sticks appeared around the cloud and settled around it like petals around the flower center. Information started flowing from the pyramid directly to Sergey.

– Others would need a lifetime for that, and you were able to do everything in an instant and expand consciousness, – I expressed my surprise aloud.

Suddenly Sergey started speaking, and it became clear why everything was happening so precipitously.

– In ancient India I was considered a god.

– And so what? – I hastened to cool off his possible enthusiasm in that regard. – So, God, whatever. As you could see, no one fell out of their chair because of that. At the End of times, as a rule, very high-level entities would come up for incarnation. Otherwise how would one get into the New time? Get to work, dude.

– From sephiroth it is possible to assemble a plane, and each plane will serve as a transition path to another sephira. What this creates is an atom. But not a small one. It is a large one. There is so much information there – a whole day would not be enough to cover it. Everything changes so quickly. I am afraid to become disoriented. What should be done?

– You can create whatever you want here, – I suggest to Sergey.

But he was not inclined to experiment.

– I would like to hide in the farthest corner of the Universe and think, – Sergey said.

– But you could think right here. No one would disturb you here. For a couple of millions of years you could be thinking, or even longer.

– Look around, – Igor suggested. – Do you see a temple nearby?

– Yes, it looks like an ancient one – it has columns and a pediment.

Behind it there is another temple, looking like a blue block of crystal.

– That's right, – Igor confirmed. – And in front of the temple there is a cloud as well.

– Yes, and someone is sitting on it.

– Take a look – who is it?

– Oh, but this is Arkady Naumovich.

Everyone around laughed. We shook hands. Now we met there as well.

* * *

The next day Sergey wrote down and brought his account of impressions as to what happened later, already at home, a day after our trip to the sephiroth. I would like to quote the document almost verbatim.

"July 26, 2001, 7:00 – 11:00 a.m.

Having regained my composure after the discovery I made at the Center, and having told myself that I was myself, that there could be no doubts about that, I went to the sephiroth. Having entered in my sphere, I sat down on the cloud again in the lotus position and started to read the book which was there. Some time later I realized that these were my own notes, which had been made thousands of years ago. And that the book was mostly dedicated to various methods of non-surgical, non-pharmaceutical treatment of diseases. Besides that, the book contained a description of the secrets of levitation, teleportation, materialization and de-materialization. In addition, various predictions were included in the book.

A lot of time would be needed In order to read this, much more than I would like to spare at that moment. Therefore I left the sphere, and began practicing entering and exiting the sephiroth using as little energy as

521

possible and as quickly and inconspicuously as possible. The result was achieved about an hour later: I could instantaneously appear in the center of the sphere, at my place, and as I left I would put there instead of myself a gold Buddha figurine, hiding (and protecting) him within a pyramid constructed in a very interesting manner.

Having achieved what I wanted, I decided to take a look as to what else was located outside of the boundaries of my sephiroth. I immediately arrived at the upper sphere, but, unlike my visits from the previous life, I was not rotating around it, but was sitting having turned my back towards it. I immediately found myself face to face with the Indian Saint Sai Baba. I had a feeling as if he had been waiting for me on purpose. I greeted him, but all of a sudden he was swept off along the orbit. Instead of him three grey entities appeared. I fell on my knees and bowed to them in greeting, and at the same time I called on the Creator with a prayer. The elders threw off their gray coverings and showed themselves before me in their true appearance. I was given to understand that it was allowed for me to pass through the fire which suddenly appeared behind them. That was then what I did.

Having arrived at the other side of the wall of fire, I saw the Creator. I greeted him. He returned the greeting. His face was extremely large. It was so enormous that besides His face and hands, in which He was holding a large shining sphere, nothing else could be seen. At first His gaze was focused only on the sphere which He was holding. It was clear that He was deeply concerned with something, some problem. He extended the sphere to me, but I did not dare accept it. Then the Creator smiled as if trying to say: take it, take the sphere, do not be afraid. I took the sphere and looked into it. Inside it there was a galaxy in the process of formation.

I watched its formation for a while and then I started on performing

522

my direct responsibilities. I found myself in some house, where at a round table about twelve beings were sitting. In the middle of the table on a stand there was a sphere identical to the one the Creator had. The subject on the agenda was, once again, the displeasure of the confederation with the outcome of the latest Armageddon. That was already clear the day before; I learnt nothing more to add to what I already knew.

I returned back to my sephira (about 9:00 a.m.); A.N. Petrov was already there, working on his book. I greeted him, but he was so involved in his work that he seemed to not notice me. Then I started to read my book, the first chapter concerning the structure of the cell. I read to the level of forming a plant cell. I was even able to materialize some vegetables. That was followed by the pages on the structure of the person: it was shown that a person consists of three energies. In addition, I was shown a very interesting molecule and a figure eight which could be tilted; then something moved along it.

After that there was a small introduction on teleportation and expanding space. Time was coming to take a break. I left the sephiroth. I saw Igor for an instant. Then the cross started appearing. It would appear and then disappear again. When it appeared once again, I said: "Good afternoon, Grigori Petrovich. I know that this is you. Please do not hide any more". It felt strange to have said that. I had never previously met this person and only heard his name from Arkady Naumovich and Igor. A moment later Grabovoi appeared and we greeted each other. Then we parted, and I decided that perhaps I should eat. I knew, however, that in the physical world I had nothing to eat: my refrigerator was empty. I started creating vegetables and teleporting them into my stomach. I would have to admit that the feeling of hunger really did start abating. That was how all this ended".

During the subsequent days Igor and I watched with interest how Sergey was sitting in his sephiroth and reading the book. It seemed he liked it. It was obvious that he was contemplating what he had read, and how his consciousness was expanding. We tried not to disturb him. That was his work, and he had his destination in life. He needed to do his work and accomplish his mission. It was extremely complex and related to the synthesis of the seven major religions.

And, by the way, speaking about religions.

We visited Kali again. As we already knew, she gave birth to a boy – Ganesha. He was very cute: he had the head of a baby elephant. Shiva was close to the stage, but still had not crossed the border between light and dark. We were trying to find out why.

Ira did not at all advance with the translation of the song. After the recent events with the second personification of Kali – Death – her creative capacities fell into a sort of stupor. Everything was in a chaos – she was feeling ill; at work her boss was pressuring her more and more. Ira had lost the lever of controlling events and the situation was going to the dogs. It was a very dangerous period. She was creating in her consciousness negative informationи, as if everything was really turning out badly for her that her life was becoming a failure. And the people around her were feeling the negative attitude and would also start to play with her to force her to lose.

She should have been aware that the situation with Kali was dangerous and could reflect on many people. She had an agreement with the Goddess, and no one other than herself would be in a position to cancel that agreement. Only by honoring the obligations she had taken on could correct the situation in which she ended up.

It really is not done: you ask for everything for yourself, you take eve-

524

rything for yourself, and when the time comes to pay – you don't know what to do. Of course health problems will begin. Ira already had tumor growths in the gallbladder. It was necessary to help her in some way, but what was one to do?

She was in the state of prostration: would not do anything, did not want to analyze the situation, was going with the flow of events, like a twig which had no free will nor its own goal. Where would one arrive in this manner? Ira needed to come back to her senses: clearly indicate her goals and tasks; create a work plan; to not let events control her, but rather learn to control events. That would not be easy, but there was no other way. At least not for her.

* * *

Andrey Igorevich Poletayev from the Institute of Molecular Biology lately was working very intensely on the problem of regeneration of teeth. The events that occurred with Galina Borisovna Kuznetsova served as a good stimulus. She regularly visited dentists for evaluation, and they conscientiously noted all the positive changes. The teeth were growing – at that point no one was doubting that any more. They were growing – repeating the entire natural biological cycle. Andrey Igorevich was certain that it would be possible to perform an accelerated regeneration process. But he was also certain that this technology was closely related to dematerialization. And for that reason he prepared a number of various experiments. The simplest of them was dematerialization of a paper clip. We would sit down in my office with a few experiment observers. A paper clip would be placed on a clean sheet of paper, where Poletayev would record the time of beginning of the experiment and sign it.

Our task would be to achieve the disappearance of the paper clip, at least for some time, in such a way that this event could be recorded by a video camera. We had already tried to do that a couple of times, but had not obtained a positive result.

The analysis that we usually performed after each unsuccessful experiment each time revealed to us some details of the technology of dematerialization that we had not known about earlier. It seemed that this gradual movement towards the result was part of the learning technology. If you fell down – you should get up. If you fell down once more – you should get up again and go on. If you became too tired to fall, get up and continue on – that would be your own problem. You did not have to strive anywhere and believe that at some point everything would somehow come to you by itself.

When we worked with dematerialization, we used the technology of two spheres. We were looking sort of from inside one of the spheres, where the paper clip was located on the outer side. At the point of connection of the two spheres there was some twist. The spheres did not just touch, forming a structure consisting of two balls, but they also turned at the point where they touched, or rather, connected with each other. In that point not only did a passage appear from the external side to the internal, but another sphere formed there. And it had a different color – not the same as the two original spheres. In our work color was generally one of the important conditions of the experiment. We had been working with it a lot, and as we knew that the same thing could appear in completely different colors from the standpoint of our perception. For example, the three main colors which were the constants for world creation, – black, white and silver – in reality would seem a manifestation of the same color, the original blindingly shining Absolute. If the flow of Absolute were directed towards you, you would see white; if it were directed away from you, you would see it as black. This could be compared to the white (emitting) hole and black (absorbing) hole. If you were to enter the flow of Absolute and move within it at the same rate of speed as it was itself moving, you would see the silver ray of the Holy Spirit. Therefore it was not enough to see the sphere and know the way of how to transform the paper clip from the external to the internal, from the manifested world into the latent one. Neither would it be sufficient that you possessed the power necessary for such manipulations. Another necessary component was knowledge of how to work with the color, what needed to be done at first and what later.

We knew how to move the paper clip through the plane, dividing the internal and the external – and using the shortest way while doing so. But this would not resolve the problem, even taking into account the points which I listed earlier. Access of consciousness clearances would be needed as well. It would have to sanction the transfer of the object from the external side to the internal and vice versa.

Theoretically everything was simple. Knowledge activated consciousness. The latter would immediately create the projection of disappearance or dematerialization of one object or another. The object would immediately be dematerialized or taken into the fourth dimension. If a chronometer were not to be used to record the events at that moment, the observers would not even figure it out as to whether the paper clip had really existed. Because in the fourth dimension time did not exist.

During the first attempt, when Igor did not record time, the paper clip started falling altogether somewhere into the plane of the desk, inside. And no one noticed that. That is what one would have to take into account in order to move forward. Because these would not be miracles at all, but technologies. It was possible to master them and use them. In essence, it

527

was very close to nanotechnology. Close not in the sense that they were identical, but in the sense of understanding the transition to manipulation of reality using consciousness, spirit, and soul.

During the next time we attempted to take into consideration many of the points that I had already told you as a matter of preface. We could take a look at what came out of it. Below is the protocol of observation prepared by A.I. Poletayev.

EXPERIMENT DESCRIPTION

This description was prepared based on the results of the experiment conducted on July 29, 2001 by the employees of the Center: Petrov Arkady Naumovich, Arepyev Igor Vitalyevich and Kuznetsova Galina Borisovna with participation of Poletayev Andrei Igorevich, an employee of the Institute of Molecular Biology named after V. A. Engelgardt, in the role of an observer.

Experiment objective *– an attempt to alter the space-time status of a small physical object.*

As an object for the purposes of the experiment a standard paper clip made from a soft iron-containing alloy was selected.

The object was placed on the desk in office No. 1 of the Center. The object was placed on a sheet of white paper with a handwritten text as follows: July 29, 2001/3:40 p.m./ Poletayev. In order to record the progress of the experiment it was planned to use a CCD FX410 video camera manufactured by SONY, working in NTSC format, and a PowerShot S100 digital photography camera manufactured by CANON, working in Macro Mode recording.

At the stage of equipment preparation for recording, I .V. Arepyev suddenly informed me that the video camera would not work.

Prior to the beginning of the experiment (at about 3:40 – 3:45 p.m.), it turned out that it was not possible to operate the video camera in record mode, even though it did work in replay mode. (Detailed examination of the camera that was performed later in the evening of the same day revealed that the failure had occurred due to two faulty contacts in the camera operation mode switching unit. Subsequently the failure did not recur. – A.P.). Due to the above reason the recording of the experiment was performed only with the help of the digital photography camera.

After the beginning of the experiment at 3:40 p.m., I noticed that I acquired a previously not observed ability to voluntarily change the brightness of the image of objects observed around me. The experiment was held in an office with a medium level of lighting: 500-1,000 lux. However, the light level perceived subjectively by the eyes could be changed from very bright (analogous to direct sunlight illumination) to quite dark (equivalent to thick evening dusk). During the first attempt of the experiment the camera recorded the image of the object.

Repeat experiment (3:50 – 4:00 p.m.) was accompanied for me by the same peculiar features of visual perception of the surrounding objects as the first one. After the second attempt a photograph was made. The camera recorded a partial disappearance of the object and complete disappearance of the control inscription with my personal signature certifying the experiment.

Both photographs were taken under the same conditions without changes to parameters and settings of the digital camera.

The participants of the experiment, who were concentrating their attention on the object, reported that at the time of concentration they perceived the object to be located within a light halo and hanging above the table.

Following the completion of the experiment, I prepared a comment, the summary meaning of which was as follows. The object of the experiment did not change its status completely as an observed physical object for the reason that its objectives and coordinates for its movement within the space-time continuum had not been stated. "

Even that partial success provided us with serious materials for moving forward with the regeneration methodology. Just a few days later one of our patients with surprise discovered at the time of the medical examination not only that the functions of her adrenal glands had been restored, but also that the platinum brackets which had been installed during a surgical procedure now had dematerialized. Since the patient herself was a medical professional and observed the process of dematerialization on the screen, she naturally exchanged comments regarding the brackets that had disappeared with the physician who was conducting the examination. The shock that she experienced when she observed the dematerialization of the said brackets could be compared to the feelings of a person who was suddenly transported from Moscow to, for example, Paris. He had just a moment earlier been living in one world, and all of a sudden he was in a different one.

But we were not the only ones thinking about new technology. In the press one could see with increasing frequency reports about new discoveries by scientists who penetrated deeper and deeper, through methods using violence, into the secrets of the cell, nuclei and DNA. We respected scientists and never were against science. Moreover, it is part of what we do. But there should be some ethics code in obtaining knowledge. It's one thing for the Higher Intelligence, taking into account your mental settings concerning ethics, to lead you from one secret of the universe to another. And it is something completely different when violence is inflicted on living biological material, using Gestapo-like treatment of cell nuclei, chromosomes, and DNA.

There was another alarming report – received from Australia. A new virus was created; a few grams of it could instantly kill millions of people. I already explained in this book that the evil on Earth receives its shape counterpart and energy counterpart at the material fine plane through men. That is, we ourselves create phantoms in the world, and they acquire their own independent existence in the latent space and then strive to manifest themselves in the world of man in the form of diseases – cancer, AIDS, etc. These diseases in the subtle matter world can be seen in the form of devils, demons, three-headed firedrakes, Koshchei the Deathless and other nasty things, depending on the national and cultural context. Or even global concepts – Fate, Death, Doom. That is, everything that torments us, interferes with our life, poisons our existence, ruins our dreams and aspirations – this is all the spawn of our envy, meanness, villainy, betrayal and selfishness. If you have pain somewhere, remember, how you treated other people, what you wished for them, how you helped them. And what your ancestors did. Evil has been accumulating for millennia. The concentration of evil created so called "entities" which afterwards bring disasters to our world. It depends on the person what kind of entities will congregate around him – good or evil, demons or angels. And it is time, high time to think about the meaning of the words: entity, being, Absolute.

So, here is one more of those new creations. I am going to quote it:

531

"Recently scientists from the Australian National University located in Canberra, working under the lead of Dr. Ronald Jackson, have reported the creation of a new mutant virus which destroys the immune system in humans.

The appearance of this virus is an unexpected event. The original goal of the Australian scientists was a peaceful one. They were attempting, using genetic engineering manipulations, to change the attributes of mousepox virus in such a way that it would prevent mice from procreating. In this manner the researchers wanted to create a new biological weapon against mice and rats. The scientists inserted into a mousepox virus a gene that was to stimulate antibodies to destroy eggs in female mice, thus making the rodents infertile... But instead of the planned result a mousepox virus emerged with a drastically increased ability to cause the disease. The gene that was inserted in the mousepox virus completely destroyed the immune system of the animals in the experiment,; as a result the virus started multiplying rampantly, killing the majority of the mice and crippling the survivors. Even the animals immune to the normal mousepox virus were wiped out.

Unfortunately the mousepox and the smallpox virus are related. If it is possible to insert this gene in the smallpox virus, a very dangerous situation would arise. If you take into account that smallpox is considered an eradicated infectious disease and vaccinations against it have not been conducted for a rather long time, the mutant virus would become a superweapon, capable of destroying the major part of humanity on Earth!

Moreover, it is quite likely that inserting some human genes into most innocent viruses, for example, that of the common cold, could transform them into a terrible biological weapon! That is precisely why Dr. Jackson and his colleagues who made this horrifying discovery immediately

532

reported about it to the Australian government and to the military. Subsequently the decision was made to publish the data in the open media so as to draw broad attention to the possibilities that are so dangerous.

Practically no leading scientists doubt the veracity of the phenomenon as described by the researchers at the university in Canberra. Nobel Prize Laureate in immunology, Peter Doherty, who worked in a research hospital in Memphis (USA), spoke highly about the data that was received, underscoring the unusual phenomenon of the dramatic increase of the virulence of the microorganism following a relatively simple genetic manipulation. In particular, he said: "Giving the microorganism the ability to drastically interfere with the immune system of the infected organism and thereby to cause a deadly disease is a laboratory phenomenon which is of great scientific interest and causes natural concerns associated with the potential manufacture and use of bacteriological weapons".

Congratulations: due to the effort of scientists – for which they are likely to demand substantial payment and public respect for themselves, another monster has been created in the fine plane material world. For some time it will continue to form unnoticed in latent space. In there growth and development cycles are present as well. Meanwhile, latent space is not located in the nebula of Andromeda (even though it is present there as well) – it is much closer, it is practically next to us. Then the new monster, according to the exhortations on the billboards in the streets of Moscow, sponsored by the tax police, will come out of the shadows. And when it does come out – please, do remember the tax revenues used to finance those types of projects. Maybe it is high time to tell those who distribute the money that has been forcibly taken away from us for what it may be spent, and for what it may not. And this should be stated not only in our country. It should be proclaimed in all the countries of the world. The trouble will be common for all. It will start in one country – and then all the rest will feel the full force of it.

* * *

Several days after I had written those pages, which seemed to conclude my book, events turned out in such a way that forced Igor and myself to directly confront one of the worlds which negatively affected events on Earth. Those were the Greys about whom we had already been warned twice; unfortunately, we had not paid due attention to this warning. They had finished their lengthy debates. And made the decision. They did not want disappear in the past, in their collapsing world. They decided to push through into our world.

These events started during the night. And I at first had thought that it was a dream. I saw myself in a chair that looked similar to a dental chair. But there the similarities ended. Because the chair was tilted back to the extent of being almost horizontal, and I was attached to its armrests with wide metal bands – special restraints. They did not interfere with the blood circulation, but when I tried to test their strength by moving my arm, they did not shift even by a millimeter. I was chained to the chair very firmly.

Next to the chair about fifteen beings were fussing. They were very tall – over two meters in height, with enormous dark eyes under a thick skin flap where people have eyebrows. On Earth these beings were known under the collective name of "Greys". The name very aptly conveyed the first impression at seeing those aliens. The color of their skin was grey, what would be sometimes called "muddy". Their clothes were also grey or brown.

They placed some kinds of instruments all around me. There was a small table near my head; on it they placed tools that looked like surgical ones. It seemed to me that they were preparing to perform surgery on me; naturally, my first thought was to protect myself.

I immediately created, using my consciousness, a flow of violet and started to erase with it all the aliens who were working around me. The procedure proved quite effective, and panic ensued. The Greys were just licked away by the violet sponge of darkness which I controlled with my consciousness. The reactions of the dying beings were quite similar to what people would probably do under similar circumstances. They put up their hands to protect themselves, hid behind the furniture, hunkered down.

When there were no more experimenters around me, I carefully applied the violet eraser to the restraints that held me in place and extricated myself.

A moment later I was in my own bed again, but I was not feeling sleepy anymore. Fortunately, it was already morning, and I decided to get up.

Two hours later Igor and I started to analyze the situation. The dream turned out to be real. These events had actually happened. Moreover, they were continuing to happen.

– Yes, I can see them, – Igor confirmed. – That's impressive how many steel implements they brought over! What, did they want to open up your chest or something?

– And where was all this happening?

– In the sephiroth below Da'at.

– How did they drag me in? And how did I escape from there? – I asked Igor to sort out the events.

– How did they get you in? – Igor asked back. – They took you and

535

pulled. They have an entire world, a civilization there. The amount of knowledge they have is truly impressive! And as for having escaped... this is not quite so.

– What are you talking about? – I was alarmed.

– One of the areas of your consciousness remained there. They took it as a hologram and once again extrapolated it to create the entire object. Do you understand? So, friend, it's not like you really escaped – you did not, in fact, that's the thing.

– But I erased them with the violet color.

– And so what? You just erased a couple dozen. And besides, whom did you erase? Just those who were nearby. And further away – did you see who were standing there?

– Who?

– They called them judges. They were the most important ones there. They stood to the side, watched and kept silence. By the way, they all had ESP. They couldn't care less how many would die there – a dozen, a hundred or a thousand. They wanted something completely different. And quite possibly they received what they wanted. They obtained that hologram in the chair and seemed to be very pleased with that outcome.

– So, pull me out of there, – I was pushing my friend to work faster.

– "Pull me out", but how? Theirs is a complete world. They had created an interspace tunnel by using gravitational transformation. They protruded it into our sephiroth, like a pipe. And they were look-ing through it. Where was their galaxy? I could see them there. Their sphere. If one were to enter there using consciousness, they would see you the same way as they were perceiving themselves. I pushed a green stick through, and it became blue. I carefully inserted my hand – and it became furry. I was perceiving their world with my consciousness in the same way at that time as they were seeing it themselves.

– Do be careful there.

– They are trying to understand our system of sephiroth. At this time, this very minute they can see me in front of their interspace pipe. And they see me as similar to them, the way they would like to see me. But this is not so. And they see you the way they see themselves. And this is wrong as well. Therefore, our essence stays the same, but the external appearance changes. Why? Because that's what their space, their reality, their consciousness thinks.

– What are they plotting? – I was alarmed.

– What they are plotting is more advanced than Star Wars. That's what it means when you calculate everything properly, – Igor praised the Greys. – They are thinking on a large scale. So that's what they decided. They needed to capture the first person they saw. They looked out and there you were in your sephira sitting on a cloud in front of the temple. So they took you to use as a shield. And acting from behind this living shield they would try to pull their world into our world. The idea is similar to how AIDS acts – to trick the protective systems. They would present your hologram, and the guards of the sephiroth asking "friend or foe" receive the appropriate answer – the picture of your plump self. This picture is familiar to the guards. So the Greys had calculated everything very precisely. They have gained access here and they are looking around. And I am not doing anything; the guards of the sephiroth can see it all, but do not know how to act. That's quite something!

– Let's look at some analogies to see what is going on? How do they want to attain their goals? To what is that most similar? They have gained access here, looked around. So what next?

– It is similar to what they did with the hologram: they took just one

537

area of the consciousness and expanded it to the full volume.

– Or just one cell and then one could create anything they want out of it?

– Yes, this is similar to regeneration.

– Is the technology similar? – I clarified. – Then let us analyze that.

– Regeneration which is concentrated on one area; so that in all areas of consciousness there appears an organ which is transferred and grows. Right?

– Right.

– And here, to create a consciousness which had been removed and is located in front of you? Is it necessary to concentrate in order to move closer or extract this area of consciousness? Because through this area of consciousness they can generate different types of events.

– What if we go into the past? – I suggested to Igor.

– And so what? The present already exists. This area of consciousness is like a TV: it will show one channel or another.

– Yesterday this was not here. And now it is.

– There are suspicious people slinking around the sephiroth. They should be caught, so that they would not slink in. But how could that be done? You have seen what they use to shield themselves.

– If we were in the sephiroth! There are guards there. But we are not in the sephiroth. This requires optical knowledge. If you are looking at ten mirrors what will you see? How to perform the blending over? Why does the photograph develop, and the image appears in the form of tones and shades, and then it is fixed?

– This is a chemical process: gelatin, silver, contact with the developing solution.

– A combination of one with the other results in the development which also exists in reality. You can take a photograph yesterday and develop it

538

today or ten days later. But how do you expand a consciousness, if a fragment is missing? They made a copy. Because of course it is not possible to take away the consciousness itself.

– By pushing your image here, they receive the focusing of two of our sephiroth. When two sephiroth are combined, what do we receive? – Igor asked again.

– A picture of reality.

– Exactly.

– Now what they have to do is the focus adjustment based on those two sephiroth, develop the resulting image and push their world through to ours, but with the fragment of ours already embedded into theirs.

– It sounds similar to genetic engineering.

– It could be that the problem is not with you or me, but with some gal or guy who is sitting in a laboratory, chopping up human DNA or crossing it with the DNA of some pig or worse, and as a result a parallel world appears. Under other circumstances that world would have no chance to gain footing here, but now it gains a wonderful opportunity to intrude into the organism of our universe, into our space, and that is immediately reflected in the health condition of specific people in all places – in Russia, and in Australia, and in the Galapagos Islands if people live there.

– The focusing of our two sephiroth provides the connection and interaction. One crystal is attracted to another, and we see the developing image. They are using the principle of image development in order to gain access.

– And what does it look like in fact? – I asked even though I knew the answer.

– You are standing on the left. And I am not standing on the right. I am standing in the middle. There are already two sephiroth guards at the

539

ready. If they close the passage now, the Greys will retain fragments of the consciousness of some of our comrades. And given their curiosity, this is not desirable. So that is the problem. We need to confiscate their movie and take it into our space, but not the entire thing – just the part that is of interest to us. They have already built backdrops to go with your image. They do work fast. So, if we send really bright light through their pipe, we will be able to spoil their film, but first we need to extract the fragment we need and bring it here.

– What backdrops were there?

– They are adding on parts of their world – mountains, deserts, grey stone, their cities. They have layered a number of frames there. And now they are waiting for us to provide the light. They have done their calculations precisely, those parasites. And behind the frames there are their ESP experts, the ones that are leading the break-in. And behind those – there are too many to count. The world is a whole entity. If they squeeze in here – a whirlwind will ensue. And it will start to pull our entire world out through the Abyss Da'at into their space; meanwhile they, in turn, will be pushed from their space into ours. We will transition from the macrolevel to the microlevel, and they will transition from the microlevel to the macrolevel. At this time we have the most favorable chance for development in the entire universe. So that's why they decided to swap.

– They want some light. And how much would they need? – I was interested.

– Yes, I thought about that as well, – Igor says contemplatively. And it is obvious that his contemplation will bring nothing good to our cunning brothers-in-intellect.

– You know how movies are created, right? Our eyes can perceive twenty-four frames per second. But what if we were seeing forty or fifty frames? Then another world would appear. Add twenty or thirty frames for perception – and another world comes about. Some funny people would start running around through life. They fall out of their space, run for a hundred paces – and return back to their own world again. Thirty frames would be, for example, the level of the Dark ones, fifty frames – the space of the Greys. There could be a million of those worlds. After the Greys' world there would be another one, covered with stripes. Thousands of screens of consciousness – and each is showing its own film.

How are cartoons created? That is exactly how: there is a film with a drawing on it. The drawings are arranged in a certain succession. A stack of those films, frame by frame – this is what a movie is. Everything comes alive, it becomes dynamic, the plot thickens, events happen. The wolf chases the hare and screams "I'll get you!" Or you can do it the other way round and have the hare chase the wolf. Twenty five frames per second. And if the frames are shown faster than that – you will not be able to see anything. But this does not mean that your brain does not record what is going on. It does, but is unable to convey it as a visual image (until the time comes). So that is the case when they talk about intuition. If the person trusts it, he sort of guesses what is happening in reality outside of the boundaries of his personal perception. And he knows what is happening in reality even though he cannot see the events. Specifically, the Greys live at a higher rate of speed. This is their advantage, but it is a drawback as well. Because they have intellect, but do not have souls. Therefore, their way of thinking is closer to computer intelligence.

Based on this speed of perception, it is possible to calculate what lighting would be required for sending into their interspace tunnel, so as not to develop, but on the contrary, to overexpose all the films they have prepared for interaction with the Holy Spirit.

We found the solution. But we had never previously done such a thing. It's just that we had no practical experience of doing it in practice and not in theory. We hesitated. And our uncertainty spread through the connections of the world. Suddenly the Creator Himself appeared next to us. His face betrayed irritation. Apparently, even the Father was annoyed with the temerity the Greys were exhibiting while acting in the world that did not belong to them, on someone else's territory. Something was going to happen now. And it did happen.

Igor figured it out – and instantly pulled from their backdrop the film that contained an area of my consciousness. After that the Father moved Igor to the side, and from His staff unbearably bright light shot into the interspace tunnel. He did not just overexpose the films they had prepared, He melted the frames and burnt down everything that was hidden behind those stage sets. The entire galaxy, which had been trying to squeeze through into our world and enslave it, was instantly destroyed.

Now the Father was pleased. He looked at us and said: "You must be capable of protecting your world. Act decisively". And disappeared.

Igor and I were left together once again.

– Let us analyze everything once more, – I suggested.

– Sure, – my friend, brother and savior agreed.

He scrolled in his consciousness through the events that just occurred which were so strange and so dangerous for our world.

– The first peculiarity is that their optical vision is reversed. From my side what was happening appeared close. And once I looked from their side – it looked far away. The actual distance did not change; but if one were to look from angle, it would seem far; from another it would seem near. If one were merely to approach he would start participating in their movie.

542

– If you provide light to them – that will start their movie, – I clarified.

– So it means that it is necessary to bring the fragment which contains your consciousness close to us, light it up and confiscate it immediately. Each square of the film – white, dark and the border. And when you overexpose it, the whole frame will be gone. But if you happen to land in the center, the frame will come alive. And what if there are a million frames? Will I be able to overexpose all of them? It feels like I should be able to! But on the other hand, it's like the Father says: "Are you sure you can handle that?" So then, I think, I will bring it close fast, and – quickly, instantaneously extract it and then zap it with light. Full blast.

– The light may overexpose the film, or it may burn it up completely, – I adjusted the focus of his attention again.

– It is possible. But one needs to know how to do it? As for the films – there are thousands of planes there. I selected them at once and started bringing them closer. It happened very quickly. The area of consciousness started approaching, came out and went into a far corner, into a remote area of consciousness, but this time here, on our side. And the closer area started lighting up the edges. And when they lit up, I saw that radiation was affecting these squares. They were overexposed.

– How did they make off with a piece of my consciousness? Tomorrow they might hack off another piece! How are they doing it? – I was newly concerned about my recent kidnapping.

– How? They steal, of course, don't you get it? They create a picture, which is presented as dangerous for you. Then you use the violet to erase them. When such powerful radiation is emitted, it is easy to figure out its coordinates. And what initially proceeded as a movie during the dream, becomes a reality. They capture a part of your consciousness and on the basis of this area expand the full hologram. Then this hologram was used

543

as a shield, and they were standing under its cover, moving into the sephiroth interspace tunnel, which is built like a photographic lens. Or rather, it is similar in function. When the light ray came in they simply overcame it with light. The distance there is small. You started burning them, but those judges, that is, the most advanced among them, which means the experts most advanced in ESP, – they were observing at that moment very carefully. They could not care less how many of them you were burning up. They were watching and calculating the coordinates. They had time to record only one film – just one film, that's all they had time for. When you started moving they could not do that any more. It was unbearable to watch, really horrible, when you started whirling them around.

– How did they drag me into the chair and restrain me in it?

– Well, that was not so difficult – they simply caught you, that's all.

– What are you saying? Caught, and that's all! Does not anyone catch you? – I felt really indignant at his calm reaction to my capture.

– No, not me. I feel that kind of thing at once, if someone is trying to capture me. Previously there were many times when I was caught from behind. But now I can feel it very acutely, – Igor explained.

– But what if they catch me again? When this is the kind of choice one has to make, of course, one has to save the world. You will feel pity for me, won't you? – I was building a hard dilemma.

– Of course. We will figure out a way how to prevent that kind of thing in the future.

– They did not have time to send the information?

– No. As it happens, if the violet color travels back, at that moment it produces an impulse. They intercepted it from consciousness. A weak reflection of one area of consciousness. That was what they captured. There was not enough time for more. You came to your senses. They

544

started fighting, then left. But the frame remained. They enlarged this area of consciousness, extrapolated the full image from it and presented it as a front. Their goal was to gain access to our world.

They plugged in this area of your consciousness at the front. After a hundred meters the plots would be different. They placed films and then more films and yet more films. They were waiting for the light and were certain that soon they would receive it. That it would arrive. The world would come out of its latent state and would start to develop. How would it be possible to stop them later? There was a huge number of galaxies. And they gained a foothold as just one galaxy. The leading one. They took a fragment, but in order to keep up the development a result was needed. And there was no result. They took your consciousness in order to develop their world through it. But there was no world on the film. Just you. They needed the light. Then the dynamics would kick in and everything would start developing.

And then this development could be pulled out and transferred to the galaxy, the universe. Or sold, rather. How much would the price for a piece of technology be? This much. And give them only a small piece. That is the worst evil for us. They would bury the entire world in armaments.

– Their technology is this pipe from space, like an appendix? – I clarified, remembering our conversation with Kirill a long time ago. – Are they copying the organism?

– That's true, – Igor figured it out. – Through the appendix the projection of the left hemisphere is transmitted to the right. At least it used to be that way. Now the entire galaxy was destroyed.

– The Dark ones were done in, so the Greys started rearing their heads.

– There is twenty percent left of their galaxy now. But now they are not in a position to care for much. There are no leaders, no equipment.

545

The rest of the worlds are backward.

– Now the rest are looking at this and thinking: what happened? Those judges were the ones who were creating the illusion for the entire population.

– Now I am looking at my arm, and is normal. That's true, the judges created illusions, – Igor agreed. – They are almost the same as people. But their world used to be very grey – stones, deserts. And now it became similar to ours. Nature appeared, and it is beautiful and varied. Besides, it all happened in a moment – the light rushed in, and everything came to life. Even water appeared. For them this is a miracle. In front of their eyes, in their consciousness there was brown glass, all because of their judges. So because they were wearing it they saw everything in that way. And now colors appeared. The world was being transformed, and it was showing colors. The images of our world developed in their space. So that means that we actually helped them?

– Whatever, if it brings positive results, – I agreed. – Maybe now they will stop being so aggressive?

* * *

People came to our Center not only for assistance in healing. I have already mentioned that for over a year we had been working with Irina Karysheva – one of the most interesting translators of ancient Indian texts. At that time she was translating the song of love of the famous poet Kalidasa, his "Kumarasambhava".

Igor Arepyev – in the recent past a police officer who had never exhibited any interest in esotericism nor in ancient Indian literature, – with the help of clairvoyance helped Irina to understand the deeper meaning of this work, concealed from the attention of the common people.

Below you will find the transcript of this work.

Irina: – Last time we stopped at the "Address of the gods to the Creator", right?

Arepyev: – I remember where we stopped.

Irina: – The Creator said: welcome, you who have great power. Who have great power because you at the same time have long arms. Your own power is supported by forces and energies.

Arepyev: – Where the thought goes – energy goes; and where there is energy, there is power. This happens because thought is surrounded by energy and information is pushed through space. And this pushing is what constitutes the power.

Irina: – Then it will sound as follows: your own power is supported by energies.

Arepyev: – And this is thought, which is translated as long arms. There are very many thoughts: you think at the same time about work, about home, etc. Therefore, the thought is supported by energies and is pushed through by force. This is what it looks like… and this is how it is shown precisely… From this point to that point – this is thought. It is supported by energies and pushed through by force, but at the same time it is an arm. In the center of this there is an arm. And that is exactly what it says there. And by bringing it closer or further, that is, changing the distance between the points, we get reality. Shall we continue?

Irina: – The Creator says: your faces are like stars, shining dimly in the winter. Why does this inherent shining not stay as bright as before?

Arepyev: – Everything is correct. The matter in question is mirror reflection, that is, reality. It is spoken about consciousness. This is a very direct description. They have lost the original light.

Irina: – The weapon of the gods which does not radiate light because it has faded is like the blunt end of the thunderbolt of Indra [1] which killed Vritra [2].

Arepyev: – The Creator is perfect; He always creates such texts, so that I am quite astonished.

The radiation of light is altogether absolute. This tells us, first and foremost, [the connection] I just drew: thought – energy – power. And secondly, light illuminates. But as to what kind of light that is – it is the light of knowledge. And the Creator addresses them: what you have is some kind of glimmers, not light; you must open your souls and come to Me, then you will receive that light which I give you; and with this light you will be able to create, resurrect, rebuild the worlds, etc. I am already giving this to you, why is it that you do not comprehend? The text is direct.

Irina: – Beside that insurmountable enemy, the rope in the hand of Vritra, which causes the despondency of the one who had lost his strength… because of binding with the rope they are wise against the poison of the snake who lost its strength…

Arepyev: – How to translate it into Russian? Talking about consciousness, He compares it with direct thought. Then He talks about the rope – your thought is winding, and not direct, because it is following the track of the snake. But the way of the soul and consciousness must be direct … The Father is right – it is necessary to comprehend … It will be hard to read. The rope in hand – thought in consciousness… the rope… power in consciousness, which must have light… that is the key word.

Irina: – My translation in the text: the hand that cast aside the staff,

[1] Indra is the King of the Demi-gods and Lord of Heaven in Hindu mythology. He is also the God of War, Storms, and Rainfall.

[2] In the early Vedic religion, Vritra is a demon (an Asura) and also a serpent or dragon, the personification of drought and enemy of Indra.

like a broken branch of the tree affected by the suffering of consciousness.

Arepyev: – Once again... Power is in consciousness, which has the light... A consciousness which has a distortion – is like a staff that the hand cannot hold...

Irina: – The hand (arm) like a broken branch of the tree. The first expression, and the second one – afflicted by the suffering of consciousness that already tell about defeat...

Arepyev: – There are four meanings in one word. Thought, energy, power and this distortion. Yes, if the person has this distortion, he is like a broken branch of a tree, and is defeated ... This is in the physical plane... Father provides the text for people... and the third text: here (shows in the drawing). Concerning the defeated consciousness – this is the broken branch of the tree.

Irina: – There is spirit, soul and consciousness, I took that word...

Arepyev: – There are three meanings. And the four meanings he gave to us. The fourth meaning conceptually. The distortion is presented as like a broken branch in consciousness. And this is already the concept.

Four reflections in one word: thought, energy and power... how would that translate into Russian? Thought, energy and power, like a broken branch, which is reflected in consciousness. Everything through a concept: once it is understood – you have passed! These are the key words of the last text. He provides four meanings at once. But they are delineated on the top as well. Again, the key word is wrongness, distortion... Why did they come? The Father asked them directly. If you came for the light of the soul – I will provide it; if for the distortion – you should not have come to Me. You should rather look for the distortion within yourselves: you are sick, not receiving resurrection, no creation, just wars. The text is direct. Yes, His attitude towards the gods is not particularly favorable. He pointed the gods towards consciousness. The wise men spoke about true consciousness. One has to understand that the line – the thought, it goes here, it passes through infinity, but it is finite. So, whatever the person places in there, – anything might happen. When the person falls sick – the information is pushed through, which is a pathology. At the cellular level there is, for example, reddening – thickening, swelling… In order to prevent this from happening, the Father says: draw on the consciousness which is going to control each cell. This will provide resurrection, eternal life, absence of disease. Tell this to people, tell this to everyone. But you have to understand that, or else you will have distortion. Understand what I gave to you originally. Otherwise you (broken branches of the tree) will again come here, to the same place. The Father back then had let the gods know that they would be coming in a circle and would come here once again if they did not use the knowledge and the light of the soul. A person who is writing must understand what he is writing about!

Irina: – I translated a piece of text, and my stomach aches started again. I have to take a break: it is stressful! I have little strength to cope with this.

Arepyev: – The text is direct, and it is perfect. With it one can heal oneself and other people. In this form there are four formulas by which it talks about everything. Little, big … For me this is very big! The essence of resurrection. This cannot be measured by suffering of one person, or a thousand persons. How can it be measured? By meanings for the gods in one word. That means there must be a fifth one – to consider. And a sixth – in order to understand and translate that. In the Bible there are about ten versions provided for each paragraph. When you read [once] they are the same. When you re-read – everything is different… Consciousness! The perception is different. For what is it provided? For the concept. If you combine ten concepts – you will see

550

the true picture. You will control the absolute truth. You have to have the proper light in the soul, the light of knowledge. You must read not in idleness, but in order to help. And you must sit down to work on the text with the proper attitude of the soul: knowing that you will translate it. And the word "concept" – is the key! You have to understand: what are you doing, for what purpose, how?

Irina: – They don't let me work and translate…

Arepyev: – That should not be. Either you can do it, or give it up. We feel for each person, too, you know.

One could walk in a circle, or it is possible to stand in place and make the right decisions. To understand how life is proceeding, what corrections should be introduced? I think it is not worth it running in a circle. Everything is right with the text, but one must also see real life, see what is happening, and perceive it realistically. In this there is both an interest in and understanding of everything. This is my opinion. We can sit down in the office, translate the text till chapter eight, and, then life will flow around us in a different way, events will go on somewhat differently… Maybe it is necessary to have both at the same time – to live and to understand what you are doing?! And during this a person is not isolated. He is being useful. It is even more interesting that way. He is in reality. The Creator says: I am giving you light, freedom. Build. Create. For everyone. Don't look at your feet, I am looking you straight in the face. But you are going down a winding path. You must start with concept of consciousness. But it is distorted – how do you guess where to go? The planes are distorted. The absolute truth is needed to correct them. There many options… There are deep processes here. We have reviewed five positions for one direction. Besides the knowledge, you also receive technology – this is both fast and a lot…

The light of the soul, the light of the spirit and the light of consciousness – these are the three components! The one who provides the light of the soul – provides the light of knowledge. Provides the light of consciousness. And it is provided – through concept. Thought provides a section, different sections and speaks about infinity. The final result. And there is the optical form – the light. And we have reached the light. We are making way differently. We take the light of knowledge, illuminate with it and this is what helps us move forward.

A week later Irina brought this text. Listen to the voice of time, to the voice of great mystery, try to understand what the gods are speaking about.

"1. In that time the gods, being overcome by Taraka [3] , came led by Indra to the shining abode of Brahma.

2. Brahma [4] was standing in front of their beautiful dimmed faces like the Sun shows itself at dawn to the lotus flowers sleeping in ponds.

3. Bowing to the four-faced Creator of everything, the gods addressed properly the Master of eloquence:

4. "Greetings to you, Trimurti [5] , the one till the creation of the world, who then singled out the three qualities and reached the goal.

5. Oh the unborn one, you have fertilized the waters with your seed and therefore you are named the source of the entire world.

6. You are the only one who has radiated energy by your three forms and became reason for creation–continuation–destruction.

7. Man and woman are two parts of yourself, have created due to the desire to create a separate form, given the ability to leave progeny, like you, as you called Father and mother.

[3] Taraka – In Hindu mythology, an evil demon of night.
[4] Brahma – God the Creator, Creator of the world.
[5] Trimurti – the embodiment of Trinity.

8. By the measure of your own time you have separated night from day, such as the creation and destruction of all beings, which is sleep and wakefulness.

9. You, who have no womb, are the womb of the world, you, the immortal – are the end of the world, you, who have no beginning, are the beginning of the world, you, who do not reign, are the ruler of the world.

10. You understand yourself through yourself, you create yourself through yourself, you act through yourself and hide within yourself.

11. You are liquid and solid because of the conjunction, you are little and big, you are light and heavy, you are manifested and hidden, and you are free to manifest your force.

12. You are the source of speech; first the sound "ohm" is pronounced in three ways – and through the ritual of sacrifice receive the divine fruit of this.

13. They say that you are the Matter activated for the sake of the Person; they know that you are the Person impartially observing everything.

14. You are also the Father of fathers, also the God of God, also the Highest of the high and also the Creator of gods.

15. You are the sacrifice and the one who will perform the sacrifice; you are the food and the one who will consume the food; the Infinite; you are the knowing and the one who will know, you are the object and the one who will observe, the All-highest".

16. Such was their speech coming from the heart and in line with the purpose; the Creator listened to it mercifully and replied to the gods.

17. The beginning of the fourfold speech uttered in response by the four mouths of the most ancient of Masters, was as follows:

18. "Welcome, you who have enormous power through possessing long arms, whose power is supported by their own energies.

553

19. Your faces are like stars shining dimly in the winter; why is your shining not as bright as before?

20. The weapon of the gods which does not radiate light is like the blunted thunderbolt of Indra which killed Vritra.

21. Now the rope, which is ruthless to the enemy in the hand of Vritra, causing anguish in the defeated, like a snake who lost its strength because of the mantra used against its poison.

22. The hand that is not holding the staff, like a broken branch of a tree; the consciousness of Kubera [6] distorted by suffering is already showing defeat.

23. And Yama touches matter with the wand devoid of light, which became useless because of it, like a firebrand that went out.

24. Why those Adityas [7] , petrified because of lack of light, became visible as if painted in a picture?

25. The same way as because of the backflow of water it is possible to conclude that there is an obstacle to its flow, because of the gusty wind it is possible to see the embarrassment of Maruta [8].

26. Even the heads of Rudras [9], decorated with hair layered around their heads with the dangling horns of crescent moons, recognizing the destructive sound "hum", humbly bent down.

27. Why do you, o glorified, turn the general rules into exceptions and run away from the strongest enemies?

28. O children, tell me why you came here all together; for I create the worlds, and you protect them."

---

[6] Kubera – God of Wealth.

[7] Adityas – Twin gods, associated with wind, thunder, and lightning.

[8] Marutas – Twin gods, associated with wind, thunder, and lightning.

[9] Rudras – a weapon of Shiva.

The translation prepared by Irina Karysheva is not perfect, she would have to work with it quite a bit. I have provided the text simply as an example of work done by two professionals: a clairvoyant and a translator.

Because the practice in which Igor and I engage is in principle close to the tasks of a translator. What exists in the latent world, sooner or later travels to the earthly level. Not all of it happens automatically though; the transition is aided by both the Light and Dark forces. Healers help this process by eliminating the negative and using the positive. We seek optimal ways and methods for transferring information from one level to another.

And so here as we transfer information, we become akin to translators. Images, symbols, concepts surrounding us in the latent world are adequate but not identical to the ones on earth. They have the same essence, but are expressed differently. The same things are stated "in different languages". The Lord and Teachers speak our native tongue, but do we understand them correctly? Another difficulty is added: there the problem is shown in general, but here - in a specific case.

We are different from translators only in that a writer may wrangle his head for two or three days over just one line, while we frequently do not have time: the patient is in a crisis, one needs to act quickly and decisively, while an error threatens be lethal.

And both translators and clairvoyants need to have as rich a vocabulary as possible. Moreover, it has not to be a "store of words", meaning that it is kept somewhere in a bunker, but more like ammunition, weapons that one has with him at all times, always ready for battle. The word – is an expression of concept, image, idea; the more words there are the more precisely it is possible to express the idea, the closer to the absolute truth will be the created image, the more correct will be your

555

understanding of the technology offered from "on high".

This is the problem that stumped everyone who has dealt with words, from the prophets of the Old Testament to our contemporaries. Andrey Bely* wrote in 1933 to Fedor Gladkov**: "Write the truth", – (...) it is seemingly easy to write the truth; but sometimes it takes hundreds of years for the word of truth to mature, and then it will be a word fit to crush stones. I frequently despair at my own inability of eloquence, stupidity, when I would like to think the truth..."

* * *

With that we reach the end of the second book of our trilogy.

All these observations, notes, words are like the bed of the brook of life, which is bubbling through the thick layers of time in order to flow into the huge river of human existence. Everything that is necessary for it is already there. There is just not quite enough water. And water is consciousness. This is the kind of water that is mentioned in the Bible. If you know what meaning lies behind every word, the meaning of the holy book reveals itself quite differently. It talks about resurrection in it, about immortal existence.

If there is a riverbed – there must be water. Otherwise the bed will become overgrown with plants. It is necessary to see the length and breadth of the river. And then you will understand how the rivers which flow into the ocean are created. Using your consciousness to widen the river and strengthen it. Everyone can do it. You can, too, but you get dis-

---

* Andrey Bely (pseudonym of Boris Nikolayevich Bugayev)
  – a leading theorist and poet of Russian symbolism.
** Fedor Gladkov – Russian writer known for his novels of
   industrialization and modernization in the Soviet era.

tracted – you look to the right, or to the left, or up, or down, at something unimportant.

Do not get distracted; fill the bed of your river with water. Clean the left bank, the right bank, and the bottom. And the water in the river will be clean.

You want to see the path of consciousness? But you have the path. And you have the riverbed. Look at it, look at the flow of life and be ahead of it. And then you will be able to control the river and your destiny.

How similar those words are to regeneration, to resurrection, to immortality. Understand their meaning and do not let the river of consciousness to overtake you. And then you will see where the river starts and where it ends. Even though it is infinite, but infinity contains the finite, if it does not become eternal.

So here is the truth. Many have sought it, many have read about it. But who has understood it? What is the riverbed, what is the water? When it pertains to the areas of consciousness, you see that it can be below you that you can control your organism, you can heal other people.

What is the wheel of fate? And what is an area of consciousness? Are those not the same thing? What is water? Is it not what is contained in that wheel, in that river, in the area of consciousness? And what is the power of the river? It is consciousness, which leads the thought. If you have come to the point that you control the area of consciousness, – you control the thought. Then you will see that no matter where you turn, no matter where you look – both thought, and the power of thought are directed there as well, and the river follows. You turn this river from one area to another, from one cell to another. And from one wheel to another as well. And you are independent. When you are not subordinate to the connections of the world, then you are the world.

557

The river is consciousness and the thought that slides on the surface of consciousness. And the river itself may also flow to become very wide and very long, because human consciousness can be very broad and very deep. And human consciousness can occupy all areas of the Universe in breadth, in length and in depth. But a person has the capability to rise above those parameters and control them – breadth, length and depth. To control the sequence of events, to control the past, present, and future. To change events, heal and resurrect people, regenerate organs. It is even possible to control time and be independent of time.

What has been listed above refers to the three spaces. And Thoth, Who created this, is in the fourth, fifth or tenth space. He does not depend on the three spaces. The depth in these areas is measured by the scale of the mind, the breath by intellect and the length – by penetrating thought. That is what needs to be studied and understood.

In order for one area to link to another – thinking is needed. And thinking connects one area with another, that another with a tenth one, the tenth one with a hundredth one, and that one with a millionth one. And so forth. And it is obvious how thinking operates. It can move as a spiral, as geometric figures, simply chaotically and in different directions. It is visible how consciousness interacts with the soul through the spirit, takes the knowledge – and healing occurs. The soul is waiting, when areas of consciousness and consciousness itself would enter the soul and take its knowledge in order to heal the physical body, the body which is part of the soul. The spirit always touches both the soul and the consciousness, and connects them. It connects them because a person appeals to God, to the Father in Heaven; the Spirit connects them in the same way as people stretching their hand out for help appeal to the Heavenly Father.

The physical body, like the Universe, has threads of connections going through it. Each cell is connected with the soul, spirit and consciousness, each cell is stretching towards the soul, spirit, consciousness for help, for specific help for growth, regeneration, for resurrection. They are requesting help, as well as everything living – like stone, like flowers, like soil, like sky. All these are manifestations of the Father in Heaven, all these are connections, all these are consciousness and soul, all these are spirit – and they are one.

Rise above the river, and you will always be with God. Rise above your consciousness, and you will be able to help others. You will always be Creators. Always in order to save and help, to be of use, like the Father. And to be the beekeeper tending his hives. To draw and be an artist like the Father, and give people joy, bring joy into the world. To be a gardener like the Father, and love everything that exists and that has been created by labor. And everything that has been created by the Father will love you. Create form like the Father. And bring elements of consciousness into it. And express yourself in this form, so that this form would give you love and express itself in your image, as you are expressed in the image of the Father. And all together would be expressed in the connections of the world.

Would you like me to show you the world? Treat it with love. Because if you love it, it will return to you tenfold. World – is a PERSON Who created it. Try to see what you are about to read.

The throne of the Father in Heaven. At the foot of it in the center there is a point. The point from which everything begins and at which everything may end. Father is wearing white today. Lately He has been appearing in white robes more and more frequently. And His face looks younger. There is less white in His hair. This is not an accident, and it is related to some global events in the Universe.

Father is holding a staff in His hand. The staff has no color. There are three rings on it – black, white and silver. On top of the staff there is the earth globe. Why Earth? Because nowhere else did the Father create in His own image. And because this is His throne. And because such is His will.

The throne is standing on four spheres. These spheres are – logos, paragon, sky, eternity. Logos is the word of the Father, paragon is He himself, the sky is the one that He created, eternity is what He achieved. And also there are to flows on the left and on the right of the Father – the white light and the black light.

There are two large crystals on the armrests of the throne. On the left is the crystal of life, and it transforms into a flower. This is day and morning.

The other crystal absorbs the flows of life, and the flower closes – evening, night. This is the way it always happens.

On the Father's finger, the index finger, there is His ring. The color of the stone in it is light blue. The end of the Staff rests on the Universe and it rotates. And on the top of the staff the Earth rotates as well. And all this rotation at the top and the bottom depends on each other and influences each other.

From the bottom of the staff fire shows. The fire is replaced by water which flows from the staff. Three rings disgorge lightning and thunder – in succession or all at once.

In front of the Father there is a large desk. There is a Book on it. His left hand is on the Book. There is a candle holder on the left of the Book. And from it seven lights light up half of the desk. One part of the desk is light, and the other one is dark.

On the right there are seven horses of different colors and a chariot. One wheel is the soul, the other is consciousness and what is between them is the Holy Spirit.

A what is above the Father – that is united and never changes.

What is ahead is divided by the Father. There is both day and night, good and evil. And it can be permeated by what is one, and from time to time that is what happens.

Behind the throne of the Father there is that which builds and creates. People call it the unseen. The Father controls all of this and states that this is controllable and will always remain so. It happens that He calls it eternity. It happens that this is called power or force. But no matter what it is called – for Him it is always controllable and He controls it.

Father goes into force for creation. And approaches people already with a creative path. He builds the way for us. The way of the children towards the Father.

The book was begun on April 8, 2001, and finished on August 8, 2001.

Contents

Chapter 1	31
Chapter 2	99
Chapter 3	140
Chapter 4	201
Chapter 5	252
Chapter 6	387
Chapter 7	433
Chapter 8	507

**Arcady
Petrov**

CREATION OF THE UNIVERSE

SAVE THE WORLD WITHIN YOU

Cover Design: A. Tomilin

For further information on the contents of this book contact:

SVET center, Hamburg, Germany, www.svet-centre.eu

Jelezky publishing, Hamburg 2011

ISBN: 978-3-943110-09-8

CPSIA information can be obtained
at www.ICGtesting.com
Printed in the USA
BVOW09s1000091117

499966BV00021B/1037/P